Ruptured Cerebral Aneurysms: Perioperative Management

VOLUME 6: CONCEPTS IN NEUROSURGERY

Ruptured Cerebral Aneurysms: Perioperative Management

VOLUME 6: CONCEPTS IN NEUROSURGERY

EDITORS

ROBERT A. RATCHESON, M.D.

The Harvey Huntington Brown, Jr.
Professor and Chairman
Department of Neurological Surgery
Case Western Reserve University
Director of Neurological Surgery
University Hospitals of Cleveland
Cleveland, Ohio

FREMONT P. WIRTH, M.D., F.A.C.S.

Neurological Institute of Savannah
Savannah, Georgia
Clinical Assistant Professor
Department of Surgery, Neurosurgery
Medical College of Georgia
Augusta, Georgia

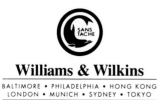

Williams & Wilkins

BALTIMORE • PHILADELPHIA • HONG KONG
LONDON • MUNICH • SYDNEY • TOKYO

A WAVERLY COMPANY

Accurate indications, adverse reactions, and dosage schedules for drugs are provided in this book, but it is possible that they may change. The reader is urged to review the package information data of the manufactures of the medications mentioned.

Printed in the United States of America

Library of Congress Cataloging-in-Publication Data

Ruptured cerebral aneurysms : perioperative management / editors, Robert A. Ratcheson, Fremont P. Wirth.
    p. cm.—(Concepts in neurosurgery ; v. 6)
  Includes bibliographical references and index.
  ISBN 0-683-09199-9
  1. Intracranial aneurysms—Rupture. 2. Intracranial aneurysms-Rupture—Surgery. 3. Subarachnoid hemorrhage—Treatment. 4. Cerebrovascular spasm—Treatment. I. Ratcheson, Robert A. II. Wirth, Fremont P. III. Series.
  [DNLM: Cerebral Aneurysm—physiopathology. 2. Cerebral Aneurysm—surgery. 3. Aneurysm, Ruptured—surgery. 4. Cerebral Ischemia, Transient—therapy. 5. Intraoperative Care. 6. Postoperative Care. 7. Preoperative Care. W1 CO459RK v.6 1994 / WL 355 R947 1994]
  RD594.2.R87 1994
  616.8'1—dc20
  DNLM/DLC
for Library of Congress   93-50107
                                                   CIP

94 95 96
1 2 3 4 5 6 7 8 9 10

Dedicated to

Peggy
Penny

Alexey　　　　　　　　　　　*Philip*
Rachael　　　　　　　　　　*Carolyn*
Abigail　　　　　　　　　　*Andrew*

Series Foreword

The Congress of Neurological Surgeons was founded in 1951 with the primary purposes of maintaining high standards of neurosurgery and promoting continuing education. Although the emphasis has been on the needs of the resident in training and the younger neurosurgeon, the programs of the Congress have benefited not only neurosurgery but also the neuroscience fields in general.

To help provide for the continuing education needs of its members, the Congress began publication in 1953 of an annual volume entitled *Clinical Neurosurgery*, which presents in detail the invited presentations made at the annual meeting of the organization. This volume has become an important reference source for neurosurgeons. Then in 1977, after several years of planning, the Congress began publication of a monthly journal entitled *Neurosurgery*, which proved to be an outstanding addition to the medical literature.

Now, under the direction of Doctors Fremont P. Wirth and Robert A. Ratcheson, the Congress is embarking on another publication series entitled *Concepts in Neurosurgery*. The goals of this publication, as proposed by Dr. Ratcheson during his term as President of the Congress, are to provide a monograph that will cover a specific area in depth with basic scientific knowledge and theory applied to practical neurosurgical issues. For the resident in training this publication can supplement the educational program or provide knowledge in an area that might not be covered in depth in a training program. For the trained neurosurgeon, each monograph will provide the opportunity to review recent knowledge about a practical subject and supply up-to-date information in an important area of neurosurgery.

The Congress has selected as editors Doctors Wirth and Ratcheson, two individuals who have been members of the Executive Committee for several years and have recently been officers. They have also had considerable experience with educational programs. They will be aided by associate editors, Doctors Robert L. Grubb, Julian T. Hoff, and Martin Weiss, who also have had broad experience with publications and continuing education endeavors.

The Congress is again providing a leadership role in an important area that will benefit all of neurosurgery.

Robert G. Ojemann, M.D.

FOREWORD

This is the sixth volume in the *Concepts in Neurosurgery* series sponsored by the Congress of Neurological Surgeons. The book represents the continuing commitment of the Congress to neurosurgical education. The editors, Dr. Robert A. Ratcheson and Dr. Fremont P. Wirth, have selected an outstanding group of authors to discuss issues concerning the perioperative management of ruptured cerebral aneurysms. The history of aneurysm surgery, the epidemiology of cerebral aneurysms, pathophysiological alterations following aneurysm rupture, and the timing of cerebral aneurysm surgery are covered in detail. Current concepts of the principles of management of subarachnoid hemorrhage and the management of cerebral vasospasm are presented. With this volume Dr. Ratcheson and Dr. Wirth are concluding their service as editors of the *Concepts in Neurosurgery* series. The neu-rosurgical community is indebted to these distinguished neurosurgeons for their efforts in starting this series of monographs and in making these volumes an important continuing educational resource for neurosurgery.

This volume fulfills the intent of the *Concepts in Neurosurgery* series by providing neurosurgeons and neurosurgical residents with current informational resources and their scientific basis. It will enable them to apply recent advances in knowledge to the care of patients with subarachnoid hemorrhage. The publication of this volume by the Congress of Neurological Surgeons will benefit neurosurgery and improve the care of neurosurgical patients.

Robert L. Grubb, Jr., M.D.
Julian T. Hoff, M.D.
Martin H. Weiss, M.D.

ix

PREFACE

This is the sixth volume in the *Concepts in Neurosurgery* series. It represents the ongoing commitment of the Congress of Neurological Surgeons to continuing education in neurosurgery. The management of the patient with a ruptured cerebral aneurysm remains a challenging undertaking for neurological surgeons. Despite major advances in operative technique and strategies, many patients succumb to the sequelae of subarachnoid hemorrhage. Advances, as measured by overall management survival rates, have occurred slowly and in small increments. These advances have been gained as increasing knowledge of the pathophysiology of subarachnoid hemorrhage has directed treatment. This book is intended to offer a foundation on which to base decision making for the management of patients who have suffered from a ruptured cerebral aneurysm. We have asked distinguished neurosurgeons and neuroradiologists to document the current status of pre- and postoperative management and describe accepted, new, and experimental therapies. They have offered information on the history, epidemiology, and pathophysiology of subarachnoid hemorrhage and described the principles of management of the sequelae of aneurysmal rupture with particular emphasis given to cerebral vasospasm. The book would not be complete without a description of modern neuroradiology's relationship to this disease. The editors hope that this book will represent the principles by which other volumes in this series have been guided—that of providing a scientific foundation which can be applied to practical management of patients. By the time this book is published, we hope that some of the information contained will be verified and other information rendered obsolete by advances in our knowledge. The management of subarachnoid hemorrhage and cerebral aneurysms remains a dynamic and vital part of neurological surgery that continues to stimulate our very best efforts.

The next volumes of *Concepts in Neurosurgery* will have new series editors, Drs. Stephen Haines and Paul Nelson. We wish them the joy of intellectual stimulation and of service which has accompanied this position. We would like to thank the Congress of Neurological Surgeons for the privilege and opportunity to have served as the editors of this series.

Robert A. Ratcheson, M.D.
Fremont P. Wirth, M.D.

ACKNOWLEDGMENTS

We would like to thank the authors for their contribution. Special thanks also goes to Lois Hengenius and Carolyn Thompson for their priceless assistance and to Carole Pippin and Trudy Rutherford of Williams & Wilkins for their time and effort in helping with the production of this book.

Robert A. Ratcheson, M.D.
Fremont P. Wirth, M.D.

Contributors

SERIES EDITORS

Fremont P. Wirth, M.D., F.A.C.S.
Neurological Institute of Savannah
  Savannah, Georgia
Clinical Assistant Professor
  Department of Surgery, Neurosurgery
  Medical College of Georgia
  Augusta, Georgia

Robert A. Ratcheson, M.D.
The Harvey Huntington Brown, Jr., Professor
  and Chairman
Department of Neurological Surgery
  Case Western Reserve University
Director of Neurological Surgery
  University Hospitals of Cleveland
  Cleveland, Ohio

SERIES ASSOCIATE EDITORS

Robert L. Grubb, Jr., M.D.
The Herbert Lourie
Professor of Neurological Surgery
Washington University School of Medicine
St. Louis, Missouri

Julian T. Hoff, M.D.
The Richard C. Schneider
Professor of Surgery
Head, Section of Neurosurgery
University of Michigan Hospital
Ann Arbor, Michigan

Martin H. Weiss, M.D.
Professor and Chairman
Department of Neurosurgery
LAC/USC Medical Center
Los Angeles, California

VOLUME EDITORS

Robert A. Ratcheson, M.D.
The Harvey Huntington Brown, Jr., Professor
  and Chairman
Department of Neurological Surgery
  Case Western Reserve University
Director of Neurological Surgery,
  University Hospitals of Cleveland
Cleveland, Ohio

Fremont P. Wirth, M.D., F.A.C.S.
Neurological Institute of Savannah
  Savannah, Georgia
Clinical Assistant Professor
  Department of Surgery, Neurosurgery
  Medical College of Georgia
  Augusta, Georgia

George Allen, M.D., Ph.D.
William F. Meacham Professor and Chairman
Vanderbilt University
T4224 MCN/Neurosurgery
Nashville, Tennessee

H. Hunt Batjer, M.D.
Professor of Neurological Surgery
Department of Neurological Surgery
University of Texas Southwestern Medical Center
Dallas, Texas

Michael Buchfelder, M.D., Ph.D.
Division of Neurosurgery
Department of Surgery
Faculty of Medicine & Health Services
UAE University
AL AIN UNITED ARAB EMIRATES (UAE)

Robert M. Crowell, M.D.
Massachusetts General Hospital
Chief, Cerebrovascular Section
Department of Surgery
Boston, Massachusetts

Steven L. Giannotta, M.D.
LAC/University of Southern California Medical
    Center
Los Angeles, California

Daryl R. Gress, M.D.
Department of Neurology
Bigelow 12
Massachusetts General Hospital
Boston, Massachusetts

Roberto C. Heros, M.D.
Lyle A. French Professor and Chairman
University of Minnesota
Department of Neurosurgery
Minneapolis, Minnesota

Craig Kemper, M.D.
Vanderbilt University
T4224 MCN
Nashville, Tennessee

J. Philip Kistler, M.D.
Department of Neurology
Massachusetts General Hospital
Kennedy 802
Boston, Massachusetts

Peter D. Le Roux, M.D.
Department of Neurological Surgery RI-20
University of Washington
Seattle, Washington

Sun Ho Lee, M.D.
Chongno-ku, Yunkeun-dong 28
Seoul National University Hospital
Seoul 110-744 Korea

Michael L. Levy, M.D.
University of Southern California School of Med-
    icine
Department of Neurosurgery
Los Angeles, California

James G. Lindley, M.D.
Neurological Institute of Savannah
Savannah, Georgia

Bengt Ljunggren, M.D., Ph.D.
Professor of Surgery
Division of Neurosurgery
Department of Surgery
Faculty of Medicine & Health Services
UAE University
AL AIN UNITED ARAB EMIRATES (UAE)

R. Loch Macdonald, M.D.
University of Chicago
Section of Neurosurgery
Chicago, Illinois

Patricia Mancuso, M.D.
Department of Neurological Surgery
University of California, San Francisco
The Editorial Office
1360 Ninth Avenue, Suite 210
San Francisco, California

Thomas J. Masaryk, M.D.
Cleveland Clinic
Cleveland, Ohio

Marc R. Mayberg, M.D.
Associate Professor of Neurosurgery
Department of Neurological Surgery RI-20
University of Washington
Seattle, Washington

Jimmy D. Miller, M.D.
University of Mississippi Medical Center
Department of Neurosurgery
Jackson, Mississippi

CONTRIBUTORS

Sean Mullan, M.D.
The University of Chicago
Neurosurgery Section-MC3026
Chicago, Illinois

Christopher S. Ogilvy, M.D.
232 Washington Street
Winchester, Massachusetts

John Perl, II, M.D.
Department of Radiology
University of Wisconsin Hospitals & Clinic
E3/311 Clinical Sciences Center
Madison, Wisconsin

Robert A. Ratcheson, M.D.
The Harvey Huntington Brown, Jr., Professor
    and Chairman
Department of Neurological Surgery
    Case Western Reserve University
Director of Neurological Surgery
    University Hospitals of Cleveland
Cleveland, Ohio

Warren R. Selman, M.D.
Associate Professor of Neurological Surgery
Department of Neurological Surgery
Case Western Reserve University
University Hospitals of Cleveland
Cleveland, Ohio

Santosh Sharma, M.D., F.R.C.S.
Division of Neurosurgery
Department of Surgery
Faculty of Medicine & Health Services
UAE University
AL AIN UNITED ARAB EMIRATES (UAE)

William Shucart, M.D., F.A.C.S.
Professor and Chairman
Department of Neurosurgery
New England Medical Center
Tufts University School of Medicine
Boston, Massachusetts

Robert R. Smith, M.D.
Professor and Chairman
Department of Neurosurgery
The University Hospitals and Clinics
The University of Mississippi Medical Center
Jackson, Mississippi

Robert W. Tarr, M.D.
Department of Radiology
Case Western Reserve University
    Hospitals of Cleveland
Cleveland, Ohio

Steven J. Tresser, M.D.
Department of Neurological Surgery
Case Western Reserve University
University Hospitals of Cleveland
Cleveland, Ohio

Bryce K. Weir, M.D.
Maurice Goldblatt Professor of Neurological Sur-
    gery
The University of Chicago
Department of Surgery
Section of Neurosurgery MC3026
Chicago, Illinois

Fremont P. Wirth, M.D., F.A.C.S.
Neurological Institute of Savannah
    Savannah, Georgia
Clinical Assistant Professor
    Department of Surgery, Neurosurgery
    Medical College of Georgia
    Augusta, Georgia

Julian Wu, M.D.
New England Medical Center
Tufts University School of Medicine
Boston, Massachusetts

Howard Yonas, M.D.
Chief of Neurosurgery and Associate Professor
University of Pittsburgh Medical Center
Montefiore University Hospital
Departments of Neurosurgery and Radiology
Pittsburgh, Pennsylvania

Contents

CHAPTER 1

History of Aneurysm Surgery

BENGT LJUNGGREN, M.D., Ph.D., SANTOSH SHARMA, M.D., F.R.C.S.,
MICHAEL BUCHFELDER, M.D., Ph.D.

The existence of intracranial aneurysms, their symptomatology, and the results of rupture were recognized with increasing frequency from the early 1800s by many far-seeing physicians in Central Europe (8, 11, 12, 41, 49, 55, 97, 116). Joseph Hodgson (48) from Birmingham, England, in his *Treatise on the diseases of arteries and veins* containing the pathology and treatment of aneurysm and wounded arteries of 1815, recorded the case of a ruptured basilar artery tip aneurysm in a young lady described by his countryman John Blackall 2 years earlier (7). Hodgson made the important distinction that the fatal aneurysm rupture had caused a major accumulation of extravasated blood at the base of the brain under the arachnoid. He also described a case in which an aneurysm of the anterior cerebral artery in an incurable lunatic had undergone a natural cure and a third case in which the cerebral aneurysm sac was as large as a cherry and had ruptured (48). A decade later, Étienn & Serres (105) at L'hopital de la Pitié in Paris reported on a physically fit middle-age coppersmith who had a sudden apoplectic death. Serres stated that "the sudden journey between the living reaction to death made one suspect an arterial rupture in the interior of the cranium" and that he had found the cause of the fatal apoplectic insult. At autopsy he traced a major meningeal and intraventricular hemorrhage to a ruptured aneurysm in the same location as in Blackall's case. He also described a female patient who had experienced apoplexy, which at autopsy was shown to originate from a ruptured anterior communicating artery (ACoA) aneurysm (105).

In 1836 in Berlin, Armin Stumpff (107)

defended the first academic thesis (in Latin) that was focused upon intracranial aneurysms and described 15 cases reported by previous authors and one case of his own of an aneurysm exerting pressure on the oculomotor nerve, with 'rupture, apoplexia, and mors.' Following Stumpff's dissertation one or more new cases were added to the literature and published in Central Europe almost every year. Hermann Lebert (61) in Breslau in 1866 published a comprehensive study on intracranial aneurysms in the form of seven letters. His review also included an historical update. Lebert, who had identified a total of 86 publications on the matter, stated that sudden paroxysmal headache is typical of rupture of intracranial aneurysms and that in many but not all cases the first ictus is associated with an immediately fatal apoplexy. He gave a detailed account of clinical manifestations observed in cases of cerebral aneurysm at different locations and emphasized that associated third nerve palsy points to the origin of the aneurysm at the take-off of the posterior communicating artery (PCoA) from the internal carotid artery (ICA), while mental and/or visual disturbances favor an origin in the anterior cerebral artery segment. Lebert stated that "in a number of cases a diagnosis of cerebral aneurysm is possible" and concluded that "the prognosis in general is very gloomy."

CAROTID LIGATION

Robert Bartholow (5), lecturer at the Medical College of Ohio, in 1872 presented a study on the symptomatology, diagnosis, and treatment of aneurysms of the arteries at the base of the brain. This study was based on one actual case of basilar artery aneurysm and included a review of Lebert's 86 cases and a number of other published case reports. He concluded that "the remedial management of intracranial aneurysms is not an entirely hopeless undertaking." Thus, Bartholow referred to a note in *Holmes's System of Surgery* (vol. 3, 2nd ed) stating that Mr. Coe was said to have "cured an aneurism of the internal carotid artery by ligation."

The Norwegian physician Edvard Bull in 1877 (13) reported the case of a teenage girl who was treated by him for meningeal apoplexy with oculomotor palsy. He attributed the condition to rupture of a right ICA-PCoA aneurysm. Despite clinical improvement, he warned of the possibility of a second hemorrhage. The girl rebled 1 month later and at postmortem examination an aneurysm was found at the predicted location. Bull postulated that ligation of the cervical carotid artery might have prevented further hemorrhage.

In 1885, Sir Victor Horsley, upon lifting up the frontal lobes of the brain, exposed what was believed to be an aneurysm at the skull base, compressing the optic chiasm. He ligated both carotid arteries in the neck (6). William Keen mentioned this case in one of his publications (59), and later Horsley supplied Cecil Beadles (see below) with the additional information: "At the operation a large cystic tumor in close proximity to the internal carotid artery was seen, a diagnosis of aneurysm was made and was believed to be confirmed by the fact that a loud systolic murmur was heard in the temporal region. The patient died some years afterwards and the supposed aneurysm was described as a large blood-cyst." In a middle-age female who had presented with symptoms pointing to a tumor in the middle fossa, Horsley was reported to have found a large pulsating tumor having the characteristic purplish colour of the arteries and measuring 1.75 inches in diameter. He ligated the right common carotid artery in the neck. Beadles (6) stated that Horsley had told him that "at that time, about 5 years since the operation, she was in extremely good health."

In 1907, Cecil Beadles (6), Hunterian Professor, presented a classic lecture before the Royal College of Surgeons entitled "Aneur-

isms of the Larger Cerebral Arteries," which was subsequently published in *Brain*. He based his paper on the notes of 555 cases with a confirming postmortem examination, of which 441 were cases from the literature and the remaining 114 cases "fresh material." Beadles found that 46% had presented with an apoplectic attack, in most of which "the patient had, to all appearances, been in good health up to the moment of the attack." He noted that 47% of patients with ICA-PCoA aneurysms had oculomotor nerve compression symptoms, but he expressed his opinion that it is quite impossible to diagnose an aneurysm during life except in quite rare circumstances.

In 1924, the pioneering Norwegian neurosurgeon Vilhelm Magnus, upon exploration of the middle fossa of an elderly gentleman suffering from trigeminal neuralgia, came upon a large intracavernous ICA aneurysm, which ruptured with a "great gush of blood, that could not be stopped by tamponade." Magnus was successful in arresting the bleeding following carotid ligation, and his patient made a smooth recovery (34, 73).

In 1928, Dr. Nattrass (80), an assistant physician at the Royal Victoria Infirmary in Newcastle-upon-Tyne, reported a 52-year-old lady whose illness had begun abruptly, 6 weeks before admission on August 23, 1926, with sudden vomiting and severe general headache. She had curious mental symptoms for 2–3 years preceding the illness and had caused much trouble in the village in which she lived by spreading unjustified scandal about her neighbors. She was described as euphoric and garrulous and had monotonous 'sing-song' speech. Her mental symptoms were considered suggestive of a frontal lobe lesion (Witzelsucht). The acute onset without further progression of' symptoms, normal eye fundi, and cessation of general headache were considered against the diagnosis of intracranial tumor. The diagnosis was made of an aneurysm of the ICA in the cavernous sinus. Ligature of the cervical ICA was performed by Professor Grey Turner on November 8, 1926, and at 1 year follow-up the patient appeared free of pain and was in good health except for diplopia. There was no trace of anosmia, and not the least striking feature was the alteration in the patient's mental state, which by all appearances had returned to being perfectly normal (80).

DAWN OF RECOGNITION OF SUBARACHNOID HEMORRHAGE AND INTRACRANIAL ANEURYSMS IN THE UNITED STATES

In 1920, Harvey Cushing's first foreign graduate assistant at the Peter Bent Brigham Hospital, Charles P. Symmonds from Edinburgh, suggested the diagnosis of an intracranial aneurysm in a patient upon whom Cushing was about to operate for a suspected pituitary tumor. The Chief scoffed at the suggestion. An uncontrollable hemorrhage terminated the operation and the patient died within 24 hours (20).

It happened that the only time Cushing could attend the autopsy was the following day, on which Symmonds and a resident, and, as it turned out later, Cushing himself, had tickets for an important World Series baseball game. Cushing decided that the autopsy should be held at that time anyway and that they all must be present, which they were. When the aneurysm was disclosed Cushing turned to Symmonds and commented: "Symmonds, you made the correct diagnosis; either it was a fluke, or there was a reason for it. If so, you will prove it. You will cease your ward duties as from now and spend all your time in the library." The resulting paper (109) with additional comments on the subject by Cushing (15) appeared in 1923. Symmonds presumed that, for patients who do not die immediately from rupture of an intracranial aneurysm, this is because in many cases the pressure is evenly distributed throughout the subarachnoid spaces and the fine meshes of the subarachnoid compartment promote coagulation. He warned against the development of a pressure cone, in which case "lumbar puncture may lead at once to a fatal issue."

Walter Dandy's first operation for a cerebral aneurysm was performed in 1928, when Fuller Albright persuaded him to ligate the carotid artery in a patient with an ICA-PCoA aneurysm causing a third nerve palsy (2). This patient did not survive. In the following year Albright reviewed 30 cases published to that date, in addition to two of his own, and commented: "It is to be hoped that, as the diagnosis becomes more exact, some surgical technique can be developed to save this unfortunate group of patients." Albright also postulated intracranial ligation of ICA-PCoA aneurysms.

PIONEERING DIRECT ATTACK

Among the forerunners in the diagnosis and surgical treatment of intracranial aneurysms, Norman McComish Dott from Edinburgh deserves the honor of being a most distinguished pioneer (24, 99). In 1923, at the age of 26, he had been awarded a Rockefeller Travelling Scholarship, which enabled him to work with Cushing and Symmonds from 1923 to 1924. Dott enthusiastically adopted the pioneering work of Moniz on cerebral angiography, and 5 years after his return to Edinburgh from Boston he was the first in the United Kingdom to demonstrate by this method a cerebral arteriovenous malformation.

In April 1931 a 53-year-old Edinburgh solicitor and governor of the Royal Hospital for Sick Children had suffered a subarachnoid hemorrhage (SAH) confirmed by lumbar puncture. The first ictus was followed 8 days later by a second bleed and 6 days later by a third coma-producing hemorrhage. Dott had lost several patients with recurrent fatal hemorrhages and decided upon "the apparently desperate measure of directly exposing the aneurysm." He expected to encounter extreme technical difficulties while trying to expose the aneurysm obscured in surrounding clot and he felt uncertain whether the application of muscle would control the bleeding if this complication occurred during operation. The patient had recovered consciousness after the third bleed, although he was dysphasic.

Dott was only 33 years old. He later described his patient as "an able, middle-aged, legal gentleman, who ruled the medical staff as with a rod of iron, sometimes with whips of scorpions." Fortunately, Dott had the "feeling of rebellion against letting these cases die." The young unestablished surgeon proposed to tell the able lawyer that he appeared to be heading for certain death and that his only chance of escape was an untried operation carried out by one of the younger members of his staff. So well did he impart this information to an analytical mind and so well did he impart confidence that the operation was arranged. His patient was of Hunt and Hess grade III (52) and was subjected to early operation on day 2 following a third SAH within 2 weeks.

Under ether anesthesia on April 22, 1931, through a left frontal bone flap the left carotid artery was approached subfrontally and the arachnoid was uncovered up to the bifurcation, where "a comparatively recent blackish clot ... was gently detached ... with a blunt spoon." The middle cerebral artery (MCA) was "literally dug out of blood clot. As this was being done some frank arterial bleeding occurred; this appeared to come from the posterior surface of the middle cerebral artery about 1 cm from its origin." Meanwhile, his assistant, Dr. Wallace, had obtained a muscle graft from the lower limb. Dott controlled the hemorrhage by applying muscle "steadily maintained for 12 minutes" and wrapped the aneurysm; "muscle was now carefully packed in such a way as to clothe the middle cerebral artery for its first 2 cm in quite a thick layer of muscle." He then performed a subtemporal decompression before closing the wound. The operation occupied 3 hours and 40 min.

This very first directed attack on a ruptured aneurysm turned out most successfully. When asked about his important patient by Dr. Wallace on the day following surgery Dott could reply: "Oh! he's fine. All he complains of is his leg where you took the muscle from!" Actually, the patient recovered so well that 2 years later he was fully able to indulge in his previous hobbies of shooting, mountaineering, and fishing.

ANEURYSM SURGERY IN THE 1930s AND 1940s

Dott made two more direct attacks with muscle wrapping in patients with "tumor type" aneurysms, in 1931 and 1932. Unfortunately, the first patient rebled fatally within 24 hours while the second patient died from pneumonia 5 days after surgery.

On October 27, 1932, Dott performed his first carotid ligation on a 26-year-old hospital nurse, who had suffered a coma-producing SAH confirmed by lumbar puncture and associated with third nerve palsy. He first made bilateral subtemporal decompressions and when these became tense on October 23 he suspected an additional leak from the aneurysm and felt reinforced "to take the comparatively small risk of tying the left internal carotid artery." The patient subsequently returned to her nursing duties. Between 1932 and 1936 Dott performed ICA ligation in a total of eight patients, with a good outcome in five. One patient, a young married woman of 23 years with two small children, showed the typical syndrome of an ICA-PCoA aneurysm, which was confirmed by thorotrast angiogram in March 1933. She recovered cervical carotid ligation and eventually died 24 years later from hepatic duct carcinoma. Dott later concluded: "We were by no means unaware of the radiation hazards of thorium dioxide in 1933. It was a risk that we then accepted on behalf of our patients, when we believed the balance of withholding its use to be the greater risk. I still consider this lady's 24 years of motherhood justified that decision in her case, and there were many others that followed" (23).

Also in 1932, Herbert Olivecrona in Stockholm successfully operated on a 50-year-old man who was believed to be suffering from a posterior fossa brain tumor. At surgery, a large thrombosed aneurysm, probably originating from the posterior inferior cerebellar artery, was found. The aneurysm was occluded by trapping ligatures proximal and distal to the origin and the patient was reported to have remained in a good condition for at least 17 years (83).

In 1934, Wilhelm Tönnis (111), who received his training from Professor Olivecrona, split the corpus callosum and explored an ACoA aneurysm, which he covered with muscle.

Two years later, Loman and Myerson (70) introduced direct puncture of the carotid artery for visualization of cerebral vessels by injection with thorium dioxide. As mentioned, the contrast medium of this time had toxic side effects and cerebral arteriography was not without significant risks. Hence, its use was only very slowly adopted.

Walter Dandy in 1936 trapped a carotid artery cavernous aneurysm (17), and in the following year he successfully clamped the neck of an ICA-PCoA aneurysm with a McKenzie silver clip (16, 75). This clip was a modification of the silver clip described for brain tumor surgery in 1910 by Cushing (14), "for the occlusion of vessels inaccessible to the ligature."

The same year Tönnis inadvertently opened a large globular aneurysm in the cerebello-pontine angle, explored on the assumption it was an infratentorial tumor. Tönnis controlled bleeding by packing the interior of the sac with muscle and his patient survived without deficit (112).

One year later German (36) reported the excision of an aneurysm of the posterior cerebral artery after occipital lobectomy. In 1939, Dandy (17) reported on two more favorable outcomes following surgery for aneurysms located in the intracavernous portion of the ICA or just as the carotid artery enters the cranial chamber. His approach had been a trapping procedure with ligation in the neck and intracranial occlusion by a silver clip (17).

Richardson and Hyland (95) in a classical study in 1941 provided a new stimulus to the recognition of intracranial aneurysms. They presented a correlation of clinical and pathological findings which pointed to the diverse nature of cerebral aneurysms and the consequences of their rupture. Their attitude, however, favored medical management.

In 1941, Dott again boldly operated upon a 36-year-old West Highland nurse who had suffered a major SAH. She subsequently recovered from the ill effects of the bleeding and Dott then at exploration found a large MCA aneurysmal sac, which he stuffed with a lump of muscle. According to Dott, she "then continued to tend her flock" (23). McConnell in Ireland 4 years earlier (1937) had reported on having opened a "subchiasmal" aneurysm with packing of the sac with muscle, resulting in improvement of symptoms to such an extent that the patient was considered to be cured (76).

In 1944, Dott received a 33-year-old Dutch mariner who had sustained a major SAH at sea, 1 week before, from a ruptured ACoA aneurysm; Dott "duly clipped the left anterior cerebral artery and the patient was still well in 1964" following the Hunterian ligation (23).

It should be noted that apart from his case in 1941, for several decades Dott abandoned direct intracranial exposure and repair using muscle graft and preferred carotid ligation or intracranial exposure with proximal Hunterian ligation. In the early series his mortality rate was 67% for intracranial operation (two of three patients), whereas it was only 25% for carotid ligation.

Much later, in 1969, he commented, "Forty years ago surgeons were sadly helpless in the face of cerebrovascular accidents. Now, surgical treatment is well developed for aneurysms . . ." and regarding ruptured ACoA aneurysms: "In my opinion, the best operation for this particular aneurysm is obliteration of the aneurysmal sac with preservation of the parent arteries, when this can be accomplished with safety, and not proximal ligation of the anterior cerebral artery" (23).

MEDICAL OR SURGICAL MANAGEMENT?

Egas Moniz and Almeida Lima visualized the first intracranial aneurysm by arterial contrast injection in July 1932 (77). With their introduction of cerebral arteriography the stage was set for visualizing intracranial aneurysms and for subsequent consideration of their surgical occlusion. However, at this time the attitude regarding surgical treatment of intracranial aneurysms was justifiably very pessimistic and remained so, with few exceptions, for another 20–30 years. In 1934 Warner Ayer (4) reflected: "Can surgery offer anything? The possibility of clipping off a small berry aneurysm on one of the communicating branches might be considered, but it would be a most formidable procedure and exceedingly dangerous."

In 1944 Dandy (18) published his classical monograph *Intracranial Arterial Aneurysms*, which was based on a study of 108 patients with 138 aneurysms verified by autopsy, operation, or both. Concerned by the toxic effects and the thrombo-embolic complications associated with the use of contrast media of that era, he never used angiography and in his series only four aneurysms had been visualized prior to operation by angiography performed by his referring colleagues. He had experienced rupture while trying to clip the neck in four instances of ICA aneurysms and had then gone on to perform trapping, usually with clips on the artery on either side of the torn aneurysm base. He was concerned about aneurysms originating from the ACoA, and he remarked that "since both of the anterior cerebral arteries lie very close together, the risk of operative treatment is very great." All four patients with aneurysms originating from the MCA had died following surgery and Dandy concluded that "such aneurysms are always so intimately connected with the main trunk of the artery that it may not be possible to cure them without sacrificing this artery, and such a result would be worse than death, and there is therefore probably less likelihood of curing an MCA aneurysm, at least in leaving a useful citizen." When considering posterior circulation aneurysms Dandy cautiously stated, "I know of no successful outcome from an operative attack upon such an aneurysm, but for those on the vertebral and posterior cerebellar arteries, which afford good exposure, cures will certainly come in time."

The Swedish radiologist Erik Lysholm in Stockholm made major contributions which improved cerebral angiography and was able to visualize intracranial aneurysms with increasing accuracy (64). As less hazardous and sufficiently effective intravascular opaque material became available, the use of thorotrast was discontinued and cerebral arteriography became more frequently used in some units, particularly for patients having a SAH.

RECOGNITION OF CEREBRAL VASOSPASM

In October 1947, Graeme Robertson presented an outstanding lecture before the Royal Australasian College of Physicians in Sydney, which was published 2 years later in *Brain* (96). He fully recognized the phenomenon of delayed SAH-induced cerebral ischemic deterioration and cerebral vasospasm often accompanying aneurysmal SAH, and he stated that "an understanding of the pathology of cerebral lesions due to intracranial aneurysms is essential in planning the surgical attack upon this pressing problem." He showed that "ischemic lesions may occur after aneurysm rupture and may be due to arterial spasm which can involve vessel segments remote from the aneurysm." For a long time this very important study was unnoticed by most clinicians.

In 1951, Arthur Ecker from Syracuse, New York, presented a study in collaboration with Paul Riemenschneider (29). Their publication dealt with arteriographic demonstration of spasm of the intracranial arteries, with special reference to saccular arterial aneurysms. As the talk began, Ecker noticed negative head-shaking by some of the senior members in the rear of the auditorium. However, another man in the front seemed to smile approval. Ecker addressed the rest of his remarks to him. In the subsequent discussion some of the older men denied the existence of cerebral arterial spasm. Some younger neurosurgeons responded that they had not only seen spasm at operation but also deliberately produced it by touching the vessel. When the session was over, Ecker went to the unknown smiling man in the front row to thank him for his encouragement and support. He answered, still smiling, "I don't speak English" (28). For a considerable period of time Ecker's remarks went as unnoticed as Robertson's remarks in Sydney 4 years previously.

TECHNICAL IMPROVEMENTS AND FURTHER ATTEMPTS AT DIRECT ANEURYSM OCCLUSION

The use of "electrosurgery" had been described by Pozzi in Paris in 1907 for destruction of deep-seated tumors, a procedure called fulguration. In 1927, Cushing (10) first used and described the Bovie electrocautery for brain tumor surgery. Greenwood's (39) subsequent introduction of bipolar diathermy represented a major technical improvement.

In the 1950s Olivecrona developed a special, long, removable clip for occlusion of aneurysms that represented a major improvement over Cushing's conventional silver clip, slightly modified in the mid-1920s by McKenzie. In the United States, F. Mayfield and co-workers introduced the spring clip (74) and Scoville (104) added his lightweight torsion-bar spring clips. The introduction of removable clips was a landmark, in that imperfectly placed clips could be reapplied and clips could be used for temporary parent vessel occlusion.

Murray Falconer (30), in 1950, documented his results from surgical treatment of aneurysms. He originally attempted the old technique of carotid ligation, trapping or wrapping the aneurysm with muscle, and avoided clipping in most cases because "the placing of a clip across the neck of an aneurysm is apt to tear it and cause bleeding." He emphasized the importance of making a distinction between carotid ligation for leaking (ruptured) aneurysms and ligation for nonleaking aneurysms. At this time he considered carotid ligation as the "sheet-anchor" for the operative treatment of intracranial aneurysms, although he fully recognized its dangers and limitations. With the evolution of improved vascular clips, Falconer subsequently attempted to clip aneurysms whenever possible.

In 1953, Olivecrona and his scholar Gösta Norlén (86) published the results of a series of 63 patients whom they had subjected to a direct surgical attack in the "free interval quiescent period." It had been possible to ligate the aneurysm neck in 76% of the patients. In 15 patients operated upon "in the acute stage," that is, in the period between a few hours and up to 3 weeks after hemorrhage, the mortality rate was 53% and the success rate 40%.

That same year Dinning and Falconer published a study of 250 forensic cases of sudden death due to ruptured intracranial aneurysms, in an attempt to learn the natural history of the disease and to prove the benefit of active surgical intervention (21). They found that in 66% of the cases "the fatal attack seemed to have come like a bolt from the blue." Dinning and Falconer concluded that percutaneous cerebral arteriography should be performed in all patients who have had but a single and mild attack

of SAH, since "rebleeds are frequent and carry a very high mortality." In the United States, Wallace Hamby (43) at the same time made significant contributions to the state of the art and showed that MCA and ACoA aneurysms were not prohibitive.

Drake has depicted the mist and the misery in which the pioneers, in anxious efforts to prevent the disasters of recurrent bleeding, were trying to perform direct attacks in the 1950s: "I remember a few successes and several disastrous operating room scenes ... The brain was swollen with a red and angry look ... to glimpse the circle of Willis meant tapping the ventricle and even then firm, even harsh, retraction of the frontal lobe. These aneurysms proved to be very fragile, often bursting with the least manipulation. Application of the small silver clip frequently tore the neck. The bleeding obscured the field ... and often the parent artery or an important branch was occluded, sometimes deliberately to prevent the patient from bleeding to death" (27).

By 1955, according to the Cooperative Study on Intracranial Aneurysms and subarachnoid hemorrhages, a total of 278 patients had been been operated upon for intracranial aneurysm, with an overall mortality rate of 28%. Within various small series, however, the mortality rate varied from 8% to 86% (100).

BLIND ALLEYS IN THE TREATMENT OF RUPTURED ANEURYSMS

To facilitate aneurysm surgery in the early 1950s various strategies were employed which, however, turned out to be unrewarding. Temporary cardiac arrest was tried (71), as was systemic hypotension, but when the phenomenon of delayed onset vasospasm became increasingly recognized it was understood that these were dangerous approaches and they were generally abandoned. Lougheed, who had experienced many catastrophes in the operating room associated with inadvertent rupture of fragile aneurysms, together with Botterell (9) began to use hypothermia combined with temporary occlusion of the cervical carotid arteries or both carotid and vertebral arteries in the neck for up to 15 min. When it became apparent that deep hypothermia was associated with bleeding problems in the brain, this approach also was abandoned. Gradually it became recognized that with the surgical armamentarium and available anesthesia of the day, operations had to be delayed for at least 12–14 days after the bleed to obtain acceptable surgical results.

In 1968, Mullan and Dawley (79) introduced a new concept, the use of an antifibrinolytic agent to preserve the clot and seal the rent in the aneurysm for the 1–2 weeks, it might take for a patient to become a good risk for surgical treatment. With this illusion of safety, aneurysm surgeons became even more inclined to delay operation for at least 1 week. It was not until 16 years later that results were presented (63) that demonstrated that, although rebleeds are reduced by the use of antifibrinolytic agents, this is at the cost of increased ischemic complications, with the result that there is no benefit to outcome (33).

It was not until 1987 that the overall outcome following a general policy of delayed aneurysm surgery and lack of any specific treatment to prevent ischemic deterioration was documented (98). This study revealed that, of all individuals who had been alive upon admission to a neurosurgical unit in Denmark through the years 1975–1983, only 28% had made a good outcome, whereas the morbidity rate was 27% and the mortality rate was 45%.

POSTERIOR CIRCULATION ANEURYSMS

Dandy (18) in 1937 "shelled out" a large aneurysm of the left vertebral artery with almost no bleeding, although he failed to relieve the extreme pressure in the posterior fossa. In his monograph of 1944 he concluded that, although he knew of no successful outcomes from operative attack upon an aneurysm in the posterior fossa, " . . . cures will certainly come in time, especially for those easily exposed on the vertebral and posterior-inferior cerebellar arteries." Dandy obviously did not know that in 1932 Olivecrona had successfully operated upon a 50-year-old man who was believed to be suffering from a brain tumor in the posterior fossa.

At surgery, Olivecrona had found a large thrombosed aneurysm, probably originating from the posterior inferior cerebellar artery. The aneurysm was occluded by trapping ligatures proximal and distal to the origin, and the patient was reported to have remained in a good condition for at least 17 years (82). Nor did Dandy apparently know that Wilhelm Tönnis in the same year (1937) had inadvertently opened a large globular aneurysm in the cerebello-pontine angle. This exploration had also been performed on the assumption of an infratentorial tumor. Tönnis had been able to control the bleeding by packing the interior of the sac with muscle and this patient also survived without deficit (112).

The first record of vertebral artery ligation for a presumed left vertebral artery aneurysm was of that performed by Dandy (18), who ligated the artery between the axis and the atlas. Dandy was also able to ligate the vertebral artery safely in a patient with an atherosclerotic basilar artery aneurysm discovered at trigeminal root section. Dandy performed the ligation "to lessen the strain on the aneurysm." He also described an attempt in 1927 to occlude both vertebral arteries for a huge S-shaped basilar artery aneurysm which proved immediately fatal.

Falconer (31) and Poppen (92) used lower cervical ligation of the vertebral artery and Logue (68) was the first to describe intracranial ligation of the vertebral artery just proximal to two large fusiform vertebral artery aneurysms. In 1948, Schwartz (103) described the first deliberate attack on an aneurysm in the posterior fossa. He found a saccular dilatation in the cerebellopontine angle which ruptured as it was being freed from its attachment to the pons and was trapped with clips and coagulated (103). The patient remained well after surgery. In the previous year Stig Radner in Lund, Sweden, had published the first successful cases of selective catheterization and injection of contrast medium in the vertebral artery (93), and in 1951 he defended a thesis entitled "Vertebral Angiography by Catheterization: a New Method Employed in 221 Cases" (94). The gate had been opened also for radiographic localization of ruptured aneurysms of the posterior circulation.

In his Hunterian lecture for the Royal College of Surgeons of England in 1957, John Gillingham (37) reported five patients upon whom he had operated for aneurysms in the posterior circulation; three had died and one had survived in a vegetative state. He concluded that such aneurysms pose extreme technical difficulties. A few years later Drake (25) described four basilar artery bifurcation aneurysms treated by a direct surgical attack. In a report by Jamieson (54) in 1964, he expressed discouragement about his results in 19 cases with posterior circulation aneurysms; 10 had died, and only four of the nine survivors were employable. Norlén and co-workers (51) and Logue (69) in the 1960s also reported poor results from surgery of basilar artery bifurcation aneurysms. By 1965 Drake (26) was optimistic with regard to aneurysms along the basilar artery trunk, for "four or five cases had done well," but the results of basilar artery bifurcation aneurysms remained gloomy; of the first seven patients, only two did well, whereas one remained in poor condition and four had died. Surgery of posterior circulation aneurysms was then successively improved thanks to many eminent vascular surgeons such as Drake in Canada, Yasargil in Switzerland, and Sugita in Japan.

MICROSURGERY AND EARLY TIMING OF ANEURYSM CLIPPING

While working on his medical dissertation, "A Clinical Study of the Labyrinthine Fistula Symptoms and Pseudo-fistula Symptoms in Otitis," the young Swedish otorhinolaryngologist Carl Olof Nylén, in 1921, in collaboration with an optician, constructed a monocular microscope for exploration of the inner ear in laboratory animals. Nylén (1892–1978), who was a student of the Nobel Prize winner Robert Bárány, first presented his new operating microscope at an International Congress in Paris in 1922 (87). His ideas were further developed by his chief, Gunnar Holmgren (1875–1954), Professor of Oto-rhinolaryngology at the Karolinska Institute. Holmgren was a pioneering surgeon for fenestration operations in otosclerosis who developed the binocular microscope for otological surgery (50). Unfor-

tunately, there was a delay of more than four decades until neurosurgeons realized its tremendous potential for a safer exploration of ruptured intracranial aneurysms.

In 1964, at the 17th Annual Meeting of the Neurological Society of America, Adams and Witt (1) first reported on the use of the microscope in intracranial aneurysm surgery, and in 1965 Lougheed and Marshall (72) introduced the diploscope, allowing magnification of the operative field for both the surgeon and an assistant. The next year (1966) Pool and Colton (91) emphasized the advantage of good illumination and magnification of anatomical details during surgery, based upon their experiences in 13 cases of intracranial aneurysms (91).

The birthplace of cerebrovascular microsurgery was the University of Vermont School of Medicine, where Gazi Yasargil in the laboratory of Donahy performed a series of experimental small-vessel anastomoses under the microscope, this was followed by use of the microscope in neurosurgery in Zürich (38). Subsequently, the use of balanced operating microscopes was quickly adopted by aneurysm surgeons, who gained improved knowledge of microsurgical anatomy and were also aided by an armament of new microsurgical instruments.

As early as in 1958, Pool (88–90) pleaded for early operation of patients in good condition to prevent disastrous rebleeds or relieve progressive ischemic deterioration or cerebral vasospasm. In 1960, Hunt et al. (53) expressed the same opinion, and 5 years later (1965) Norlén, at the Annual Meeting of the Japan Neurosurgical Society in Tokyo, declared that he had become convinced that patients in good condition should be operated upon in the first or second day after bleed (84). Norlén concluded that the very high mortality rate for recurrent bleeds favored a more active surgical attitude, in terms of early surgery. The results of a study of patients subjected to medical management, at that time, revealed that the second bleed occurs early and implies a much more serious prognosis than the first, i.e., 14% mortality rate from the first bleed, compared to a 60% mortality rate from a second bleed, with three fourths of the recurrences occurring within the first 8 weeks after the first bleed (113). More recent work has indicated that rebleeds are more detrimental because the presence of clot in the subarachnoid spaces is more likely to force the stream of blood into the brain parenchyma (114). In 1975, Norlén reported on the results of aneurysm surgery within 1 week after a first rupture. He reported upon 45 patients with a mortality rate of 4% in his hands (85). In the following year, Suzuki and Sano at the AANS meeting in San Francisco presented smaller series of patients subjected to early surgical obliteration, also with encouraging results. These authors later published larger series of early-operated aneurysms (101, 108).

Computed tomography (CT) and the operating microscope opened a new era. In 1976 the senior author and two colleagues took up early surgery. Within a few years early operation gained a few more enthusiasts. The results of this approach, analyzed and presented at the American Association of Neurological Surgeons Meeting in April 1981 (65) and published in the same month (66), were met with considerable scepticism. It was not considered proven that early surgery with microsurgical techniques was preferable to delayed surgery. However, the pendulum appears to have swung in favor of early surgery for anterior circulation aneurysms. The results of the Cooperative Study on the Timing of Aneurysm Surgery, performed between 1980 and 1983, were not published until 1990 (57, 58) and pointed to major intercenter variabilities in terms of surgical outcome. This study left many neurosurgeons feeling comfortable with a cautious attitude towards immediate aneurysm referrals and operation procedure and may have deterred the development of acute-stage surgery in some centers.

In 1980, Fisher *et al.* (32) demonstrated that there is a direct relationship between the amount and distribution of CT-visualized subarachnoid blood and later development of cerebral vasospasm and/or delayed ischemic dysfunction. This study confirmed the ideas expressed 23 years previously (56) that subarachnoid hemoglobin and its degradation products in the cerebrospinal fluid are responsible for induction of delayed ischemic deterioration.

Recently many experienced neurosurgeons have adopted early surgery also for posterior circulation aneurysms. Le Roux, Elliot, and Winn (62) in 1992 reviewed their 5-year experience with 53 posterior circulation aneurysms, including 21 basilar artery tip aneurysms operated upon within 48 hours after rupture, and concluded that early surgery for basilar artery bifurcation aneurysms may be safely performed, with the exception of those pointing posteriorly. Similar results have been reported by Drake and his group (81) and from Australia (22).

CONCLUDING REMARKS

The history of intracranial aneurysm recognition covers two centuries, whereas the history of aneurysm surgery is significantly shorter. The progress has occurred stepwise from medical management to carotid ligation, to intracranial exploration with trapping procedures or Hunterian ligation, and then to a direct attack with clipping or ligature of the aneurysm base. These procedures could, however, not be consistently performed in the acute stage without disastrous effects, and management with antifibrinolytic agents did not offer the safe umbrella that was hoped would protect patients awaiting delayed aneurysm occlusion. Thus, aneurysm surgery had little major impact on overall outcome until the microscope was introduced. This, in combination with improved neuroanesthetic techniques and the development of microsurgical instrumentation, allowed for acute surgical intervention, which has been increasingly adopted. Early surgery for anterior circulation aneurysms was subsequently combined with anti-ischemic treatment with calcium channel blockers to reduce secondary cerebral ischemic dysfunction. In the 1990s early surgery is being advocated with greater frequency for posterior circulation aneurysms. The limitations of early surgical intervention to prevent fatal aneurysm rebleeds were not conceptual (early advocates expressed their opinion in the 1960s) but technical. It was the introduction of the microscope and CT in the 1970s that represented the cornerstones for the breakthrough of early operative timing. Transluminal angioplasty, originally described by Zubkov, Nikiforov, and Shustin from Russia and recently further developed and described at a number of American centers, is for some patients an important adjunct in the treatment of symptomatic vasospasm refractory to conventional therapy (117).

Despite major improvements in the surgical management of ruptured aneurysms, less than 60% of all victims who are alive upon admission to well equipped neurosurgical centers with a policy of early operation may be expected to have a favorable outcome (102). In addition, a significant number of individuals who recover physically without neurological deficits show persistent problems relating to emotional adjustment and psychosocial abilities, which interfere with their social and occupational reintegration (67, 106). Further improvements may depend upon future developments in endovascular obliteration. A review (3) of the prominent work in this area (19, 35, 40, 42, 44–47, 60, 78, 110, 115) indicates that the technique remains experimental; for unruptured aneurysms the results are worse than those of surgery and for ruptured aneurysms the results have yet to approach the value of surgery. Yet even at the present time (1993) endovascular approaches have already established their niche in the management of selected cases.

As always, the future is boundless. Cardiovascular surgeons have already produced major advances by using long, thin, flexible endoscopes introduced into the coronary arteries. Possibly specifically designed endoscopes for intracranial use under television monitor guidance, in combination with flexible thin laser fibers may be developed also for cerebral arteries so that intracranial aneurysms may be closed by laser-weld in association with the acute diagnostic angiographic examination. One can envision endoscopic techniques being developed to evacuate extravasated blood and irrigate blood-contaminated cerebrospinal fluid from the basal cisterns and to instill thrombolytic agents such as tissue plasminogen activator. The scenario of immediate localization of ruptured aneurysms, combined use of guided endoscopes with directed laser beams to achieve aneurysm closure, may

become realistic and could be the ideal approach to this continually challenging problem.

REFERENCES

1. Adams, J. E., and Witt, J. A. The use of the otological microscope in the surgery of aneurysms. In: Proceedings of the 17th Annual Meeting of the Neurological Society of America. Litchfield Park, AZ, 1964.
2. Albright, F. The syndrome produced by aneurysm at or near the function of the internal carotid artery and the circle of Willis. Johns Hopkins Hosp. Bull. 44:215–245, 1929.
3. Ausman, J. I. Current controversies in the management of aneurysms, AVMS and cerebral ischemia. In: Proceedings of the 3rd International Workshop on Cerebrovascular Surgery. Tokyo, Japan, 1992.
4. Ayer, W. D. So-called spontaneous subarachnoid haemorrhage: a resumé with its medicolegal consideration. Am. J. Surg. 26:143–151, 1934.
5. Bartholow, R. Aneurisms of the arteries at the base of the brain: their symptomatology, diagnosis, and treatment. Am. J. Med. Sci. 64:373–386, 1872.
6. Beadles, C. F. Aneurisms of the larger cerebral arteries. Brain 80:285–336, 1907.
7. Blackall, J. Observations on the Nature and Cure of Dropsies, Ed. 5, pp. 132–135. Longman & Co., London, 1813.
8. Blane, G. History of some cases of disease in the brain, with an account of the appearance upon examination after death, and some general observations on complaints of the head. Trans. Soc. Improvement Med. Chir. Knowledge 2:192–198, 1800.
9. Botterell, E. H., Lougheed, W. M., Scott, J. W., et al. Hypothermia, and interruption of carotid, carotid and vertebral circulation in the surgical management of intracranial aneurysms. J. Neurosurg. 13:1–42, 1956.
10. Bovie, W. T. Electro-surgery as an aid to the removal of intra-cranial tumors: with a preliminary note on a new surgical-current generator. Surg. Gynecol. Obstet. 47:751–784, 1928. (Reprinted in J. Neurosurg. 23:86–116, 1965).
11. Bright, R. Reports of Medical Cases, Vol. 2, Part 1, pp. 226–267, 613–614. Longman, Rees, Orme, Brown & Green, London, 1831.
12. Brinton, W. Report on cases of cerebral aneurism. Trans. Pathol. Soc. Lond. 3:47–49, 1852.
13. Bull, E. Acute brain aneurisma, oculomotor palsy, meningeal apoplexia. Norw. Mag. Med. 7:890–895, 1877.
14. Cushing, H. The control of bleeding in operations for brain tumors: with the description of silver clips for the occlusion of vessels inaccessible to the ligature. Ann. Surg. 54:1–19, 1911.
15. Cushing, H. Contributions to the study of intracranial aneurysms. Guy's Hosp. Rep. 73:159–163, 1923.
16. Dandy, W. E. Intracranial aneurysm of internal

carotid artery, cured by operation. Ann. Surg. *107*:654–657, 1938.

17. Dandy, W. E. The treatment of internal carotid aneurysms within the cavernous sinus and cranial chamber: report of 3 cases. Ann. Surg. *109*:689–711, 1939.

18. Dandy, W. E. Intracranial Arterial Aneurysms, pp. 1–147. Comstock Publishing Co., Ithaca, NY, 1944.

19. Debrun, G., Fox, A., Drake, C., et al. Giant unclippable aneurysms: treatment with detachable balloons. AJNR *2*:167–173, 1981.

20. Denny-Brown, D. Harvey Cushing: the man. J. Neurosurg. *50*:17–19, 1979.

21. Dinning, T. A. R., and Falconer, M. A. Sudden or unexpected natural death due to ruptured intracranial aneurysm: survey of 250 forensic cases. Lancet *2*:799–801, 1953.

22. Dorsch, N. W. C., and Siu K. H. Early operation for ruptured posterior circulation aneurysms. In: Congress Proceedings of the 3rd International Workshop on Cerebrovascular Surgery. Tokyo, Japan, 1992.

23. Dott, N. M. Intracranial aneurysmal formations. Clin. Neurosurg. *16*:1–16, 1969.

24. Dott, N. M. Intracranial aneurysms: cerebral arterioradiography: surgical treatment. Trans. Med. Chir. Soc. Edinb. *40*:219–240, 1933. (see also Todd, N. V., Howie, J. E., and Miller, J. D. Norman Dott's contribution to aneurysm surgery. J. Neurol. Neurosurg. Psychiatry *53*:455–458, 1990).

25. Drake, C. G. Bleeding aneurysms of the basilar artery: direct surgical management in four cases. J. Neurosurg. *18*:230–238, 1961.

26. Drake, C. G. Surgical treatment of ruptured aneurysms of the basilar artery: experience with 14 cases. J. Neurosurg. *23*:457–473, 1965.

27. Drake, C. G. Evolution of intracranial aneurysm surgery. Can. J. Surg. *27*:549–555, 1984.

28. Ecker, A. The discovery of human cerebral arterial spasm in angiograms: an autobiographical notes. Neurosurgery. *10*:90, 1982.

29. Ecker, A. D., and Riemenschneider, P. A. Arteriographic demonstration of spasm of the intracranial arteries: with special reference to saccular aneurisms. J. Neurosurg. *8*:660–667, 1951.

30. Falconer, M. A. Surgical treatment of spontaneous subarachnoid haemorrhage: preliminary report. Br. Med. J. *1*:809–813, 1950.

31. Falconer, M. A. Surgical treatment of spontaneous subarachnoid haemorrhage. Br. Med. J. *1*:790–792, 1958.

32. Fisher, C. M., Kistler, J. P., and Davis, J. M. Relation of cerebral vasospasm to subarachnoid hemorrhage visualized by computerized tomographic scanning. Neurosurgery *6*:1–9, 1980.

33. Fodstad, H., and Ljunggren, B. Antifibrinolytic Drugs in Subarachnoid, Hemorrhage. In: Fibrinolysis and the Central Nervous System, edited by R. Sawaya, pp. 257–273. Hanley & Belfus Inc., Philadelphia, 1990.

34. Fodstad, H., Ljunggren, B., and Kristiansen, K. Vilhelm Magnus: pioneer neurosurgeon. J. Neurosurg. *73*:317–330, 1990.

35. Fox, A. J., Vinuela, F., Pelz, D. M., et al. Use of detachable balloons for unclippable cerebral aneurysms. J. Neurosurg. *66*:40–46, 1987.

36. German, W. J. Intracranial aneurysm: a surgical problem. Zentralbl. Neurochir. *3*:352–354, 1938.

37. Gillingham, F. J. The management of ruptured intracranial aneurysm: Hunterian Lecture for the Royal College of Surgeons of England 1957. Ann. R. Coll. Surg. Engl. *23*:89–117, 1958.

38. Goldring, S. The need to trace our roots in difficult times: the 1985 AANS Presidential Address. J. Neurosurg. *63*:485–491, 1985.

39. Greenwood, J., Jr. Two point coagulation: new principle and instrument for applying coagulation current in neurosurgery. Am. J. Surg. *50*:267–270, 1940.

40. Guglielmi, G., Vinuela, F., Dion, J., et al. Electrothrombosis of saccular aneurysms via endovascular approach. J. Neurosurg. *75*:8–14, 1991.

41. Gull, W. Cases of aneurism of the cerebral vessels. Guy's Hosp. Rep. *5*:281–304, 1859.

42. Halbach, V. V., Hieshima, G. B., and Higashida, R. T. Treatment of intracranial aneurysms by balloon embolization. Semin. Intervent. Radiol. *4*:261–268, 1987.

43. Hamby, W. B. Intracranial Aneurysms. Charles C. Thomas Publishing Co., Springfield, IL, 1952.

44. Heilman, C. B., Kwan, E. S. K., and Wu, J. K. Aneurysm recurrence following endovascular balloon occlusion. J. Neurosurg. *77*:260–264, 1992.

45. Higashida, R. T., Halbach, V. V., Barnwell, S. L., et al. Treatment of intracranial aneurysms with preservation of the parent vessel: results of percutaneous balloon embolization in 84 patients. AJNR *11*:633–640, 1990.

46. Higashida, R. T., Halbach, V. V., Dormandy, B., et al. Endovascular treatment of intracranial aneurysms with a new silicone micoballoon device: technical considerations and indications for therapy. Radiology *174*:687–691, 1990.

47. Higashida, R. T., Halbach, V. V., Dowd, C., et al. Endovascular detachable balloon embolization therapy of cavernous carotid artery aneurysms: results in 87 cases. J. Neurosurg. *72*:857–863, 1990.

48. Hodgson, J. A. A treatise on the diseases of arteries and veins, containing the pathology and treatment of aneurysms and wounded arteries. pp. 76–78. Underwood, London, 1815.

49. Holmes, T. Aneurysm of the internal carotid artery in the cavernous sinus: post mortem appearances. Trans. Pathol. Soc. Lond. *12*:61–63, 1860.

50. Holmgren, G. Some experiences in surgery of otosclerosis. Acta Otolaryngol. (Stockh.) *5*:460–466, 1923.

51. Höök, O, Norlén, G., and Guzman, J. Saccular aneurysms of the vertebral-basilar arterial system: a report of 28 cases. Acta Neurol. Scand. *39*:271–304, 1963.

52. Hunt, W. E., and Hess, R. M. Surgical risk as related to time of intervention in the repair of intracranial aneurysms. J. Neurosurg. *28*:14–19, 1968.

53. Hunt, W. E., Meagher, J. N., and Barnes, J. E. The management of intracranial aneurysm. J. Neurosurg. *19*:34–40, 1962.
54. Jamieson, K. G. Aneurysms of the vertebrobasilar system: surgical intervention in 19 cases. J. Neurosurg. *21*:781–797, 1964.
55. Jennings, J. A. Case of aneurism of the basilar artery, suddenly giving way, and occasioning death by pressure on the medulla oblongata. Trans. Provincial Med. Surg. Assoc. *1*:270–276, 1833.
56. Johnson, R. J., Potter, J. M., and Reid, R. G. Arterial spasm in subarachnoid haemorrhage: mechanical considerations. J. Neurol. Neurosurg. Psychiat. *21*:68, 1958.
57. Kassell, N. F., Torner, J. C., Haley, E. C., *et al.* The International Cooperative Study on the Timing of Aneurysm Surgery. I. Overall management results. J. Neurosurg. *73*:18–36, 1990.
58. Kassell, N. F., Torner, J. C., Jane, J. A., *et al.* The International Cooperative Study on the Timing of Aneurysm Surgery. J. Neurosurg. *73*:37–47, 1990.
59. Keen, W. W. Intracranial lesions. Med. News. NY *57*:443, 1890.
60. Knuckey, N. W., Haas, R., Jenkins, R., *et al.* Thrombosis of difficult intracranial aneurysms by the endovascular placement of platinum-Dacron microcoils. J. Neurosurg. *77*:43–50, 1992.
61. Lebert, H., Über die Aneurysmen der Hirnarterien: Eine Abhandlung in Briefen an Herrn Geheimrat Professor Dr Frerichs. Berl. Klin. Wochenschr. *20*:209–212, *22*:229–231, *24*:249–251, *28*:281–285, *34*:336–338, *35*:345–347, *40*:386–390, *42*:402–405, 1866.
62. Le Roux, P. D., Elliott, J. P., and Winn, H. R. Basilar bifurcation aneurysms: results of early surgery. In: Proceedings of the 61st Annual Meeting of the American Association of Neurological Surgeons. 1992.
63. Lindsay, K. W., Vermeulen, M., Murray, G., *et al.* Antifibrinolytic therapy in subarachnoid hemorrhage: reduction of rebleeding without benefit to outcome. In: Proceedings of the Annual Meeting of the American Association of Neurological Surgeons, 1984.
64. Ljunggren, B. Herbert Olivecrona: founder of Swedish neurosurgery. J. Neurosurg. *78*:142–149, 1993.
65. Ljunggren, B., Brandt, L., and Kågström, E. Results of early operations on ruptured aneurysms of the anterior part of the circle of Willis. In: Congress Proceedings of the 50th Anniversary Meeting of the American Association of Neurological Surgeons, pp. 99–100, 1981.
66. Ljunggren, B., Brandt, L., Kågström, E., *et al.* Results of early operation for ruptured aneurysms. J. Neurosurg. *54*:473–479, 1981.
67. Ljunggren, B., Sonesson, B., Säveland, H., *et al.* Cognitive impairment and adjustment in patients without neurological deficits after aneurysmal SAH and early operation. J. Neurosurg. *62*:673–679, 1985.
68. Logue, V. The surgical treatment of aneurysms in the posterior fossa. J. Neurol. Neurosurg. Psychiatry *21*:66–67, 1958.
69. Logue, V. Posterior fossa aneurysms. In: Clinical Neurosurgery, edited by J. Shillito, and W. H. Mosberg, Vol. 2, pp. 183–207. Williams & Wilkins, Baltimore, 1964.
70. Loman, J., and Myerson A. Visualization of cerebral vessels by direct intracarotid injection of thorium di-oxide. Arch. Neurol. Psychiatry *36*:912–915, 1936.
71. Lougheed, W. M., and Kahn, D. S. Circumvention of anoxia during arrest of cerebral circulation for intracranial surgery. J. Neurosurg. *12*:226–239, 1955.
72. Lougheed, W. M., and Marshall, B. M. The diploscope in intracranial aneurysms surgery: results in 40 patients. Can. J. Surg. *12*:75–82, 1969.
73. Magnus, V. Aneurysm of the internal carotid artery. JAMA 88:1712–1713, 1927.
74. Mayfield, F. H., and Kees, G., Jr. A brief history of the development of the Mayfield clip: technical note. J. Neurosurg. *35*:97–100, 1971.
75. McKenzie, K. G. Some minor modifications of Harvey Cushing's silver clip outfit. Surg. Gynecol. Obstet. *45*:549–550, 1927.
76. McConnell, A. A. Subchiasmal aneurysm treated by implantation of muscle. Zentralbl. Neurochir. *2*:269–274, 1937.
77. Moniz E. Anevrysme intra-cranien de la carotide inferne droite rendu visible par l'arteriographie cerebrale. Rev. Oto-Neuro-Ophthalmol. *11*:746–748, 1933.
78. Moret, J. Endovascular surgery of intracranial aneurysms: technique, results and long-term follow up. In: Proceedings of the 3rd International Workshop on Cerebrovascular Surgery, Tokyo, Japan, 1992.
79. Mullan, S., and Dawley, J. Antifibrinolytic therapy for intracranial aneurysms. J. Neurosurg. *28*:21–23, 1968.
80. Nattrass, F. J. Aneurysm of the carotid artery in the cavernous sinus: ligature of internal carotid: recovery. Edinb. Med. J. *35*:30–32, 1928.
81. Nemoto, S., Drake, C. G., Peerless, S. J., *et al.* Acute surgery for ruptured posterior circulation aneurysm. In: Advances in Surgery for Cerebral Stroke, edited by J. Suzuki, pp. 643–648. Springer Verlag, Tokyo, 1988.
82. Norlén, G. The pathology, diagnosis and treatment of intracranial saccular aneurysms. Proc. R. Soc. Med. *45*:291–302, 1952.
83. Norlén, G. The pathology, diagnosis and treatment of intracranial saccular aneurysms. Proc. S. R. Soc. Med. *45*:291–302, 1952.
84. Norlén, G. Some aspects of the surgical treatment of intracranial aneurysms. Neurol. Med. Chir. *7*:14–27, 1965.
85. Norlén, G. Experiences with intracranial aneurysm surgery: results in early operations. In: Conferencia Magistral: Apartado de Actas y Trabajos del XVI Congreso Latino-Americano de Neurocirugia, pp. 235–245, 1975.
86. Norlén, G., and Olivecrona, H. The treatment of aneurysms of the circle of Willis. J. Neurosurg. *10*:634–650, 1953.
87. Nylén, C. O. Quelques observations au moyen de

la loupe et du microscope, en particulier dans les fistules labyrinthiques et au niveau des fenêtres labyrinthiques pendant et après l'évidement pétro-mastoïdien. Rev. Laryngol. Otol. Rhinol. *43:*810–812, 1922.

88. Pool, J. L. Cerebral vasospasm. N. Engl. J. Med. *259:*1259–1264, 1958.

89. Pool, J. L. Early treatment of ruptured intracranial aneurysms of the circle of Willis with special clip techniques. Bull. NY Acad. Med. *35:*357–369, 1959.

90. Pool, J. L. Timing and techniques in the intracranial surgery of ruptured aneurysms of the anterior communicating artery. J. Neurosurg. *19:*378–388, 1962.

91. Pool, J. L., and Colton, H. P. The dissecting microscope for intracranial vascular surgery. J. Neurosurg. *25:*315–318, 1966.

92. Poppen, J. L. Vascular surgery of the posterior fossa. Proc. Congr. Neurol. Surg. *6:*198–202, 1969.

93. Radner, S. Intracranial angiography via the vertebral artery: preliminary report of a new technique. Acta Radiol. *28:*838–841, 1947.

94. Radner, S. Vertebral angiography by catheterization: a new method employed in 221 cases. Acta Radiol. *87*(suppl.)*:*1–134, 1951.

95. Richardson, J. C., and Hyland, H. H. Intracranial aneurysms: a clinical and pathological study of subarachnoid and intracerebral haemorrhage caused by berry aneurysms. Medicine (Baltimore) *20:*1–83, 1941.

96. Robertson, E. G. Cerebral lesions due to intracranial aneurysms. Brain *72:*150–185, 1949.

97. Roe, H. Aneurism of the anterior cerebral artery. Trans. Pathol. Soc. Lond. *3:*46, 1852.

98. Rosenörn, J., Eskesen, V., Schmidt, K., *et al.* Clinical features and outcome in 1076 patients with ruptured intracranial saccular aneurysms: a prospective consecutive study. Br. J. Neurosurg. *1:*33–46, 1987.

99. Rush, C., and Shaw, J. F. With Sharp Compassion: Norman Dott, Freeman Surgeon of Edinburgh, pp. 198–203. Aberdeen University Press, 1990.

100. Sahs, A. L., Perret, G. E., Locksley, H. B., and Nishioka H. Intracranial Aneurysms and Subarachnoid Hemorrhage: a Cooperative Study, 174. Lippincott, Philadelphia, 1969.

101. Sano, K. and Saito, I. Early operation and washout of blood clots for prevention of cerebral vasospasm. In: Cerebral Vasospasm: Proceedings from the Second International Workshop, edited by R. H. Wilkins, and A. J. M., van der Werf. Baltimore, Williams and Wilkins, pp. 510–513, 1980.

102. Säveland, H., Hillman, J., Brandt, L., *et al.* Over-
all outcome in aneurysmal subarachnoid hemorrhage: a prospective study from neurosurgical units in Sweden during a 1-year period. J. Neurosurg. *76:*729–734, 1992.

103. Schwartz, H. G. Arterial aneurysm of the posterior fossa. J. Neurosurg. *5:*312–316, 1948.

104. Scoville, W. B. Miniature torsion bar spring aneurysm clip. J. Neurosurg. *25:*97, 1966.

105. Serres, E. R. A. Observations sur la rupture des anéurysmes des artéres du cerveau. Arch. Gen. Med. J. Janvier, *10:*419–431, 1826.

106. Sonesson, B., Ljunggren, B., Säveland, H., *et al.* Cognition and adjustment following late and early surgery for ruptured aneurysm. Neurosurgery *21:*279–287, 1987.

107. Stumpff, A. A. A. De Aneurysmatibus Arteriarum Cerebri: Dissertatio Inauguralis Medico-Chirurgica, pp. 1–33. Formis Nietackianis, Berlin, 1836.

108. Suzuki, J., Onuma, T., and Yosahimoto, T. Results of early operations on cerebral aneurysms. Surg. Neurol. *11:*407–412, 1979.

109. Symmonds, C. P. Contributions to the clinical study of intracranial aneurysms. Guy's Hosp. Rep. *73:*139–158, 1923.

110. Taki, W., Nishi, S., Yamashita, K., *et al.* Selection and combination of various endovascular techniques in the treatment of giant aneurysms. J. Neurosurg. *77:*37–42, 1992.

111. Tönnis, W. Erfolgreiche Behandlung eines Aneurysma der Arteria Communicans Anterior Cerebri Zentralbl. Neurochir. *1:*39–42, 1936.

112. Tönnis, W. Zur Behandlung intrakranieller Aneurysmen. Arch. Klin. Chir. *189:*474–476, 1937.

113. Trumpy, J. H. Subarachnoid hemorrhage: time sequence of recurrences and their prognosis. Acta Neurol. Scand. *43:*48–60, 1967.

114. Vermeulen, M., van Gijn, J., Hijdra, A., *et al.* Causes of acute deterioration in patients with a ruptured intracranial aneurysm: a prospective study with serial CT scanning. J. Neurosurg. *60:*935–939, 1984.

115. Weil, S. M., van Loweren, H. R., Tomsick, T. A., *et al.* Management of inoperable cerebral aneurysms by the navigation balloon technique. Neurosurgery *21:*296–302, 1987.

116. Wilks, S. Sanguineous meningeal effusion (apoplexy): spontaneous and from injury. Guy's Hosp. Rep. *5:*46–49, 1852.

117. Winn, H. R., Eskridge, J. M., Newell, D. W., and Mayberg, M. R. Angioplasty for vasospasm following subarachnoid hemorrhage. In: Congress of Proceedings of the 3rd International Workshop on Cerebrovascular Surgery, Tokyo, Japan, 1992.

CHAPTER 2

Epidemiology of Cerebral Aneurysms

JAMES G. LINDLEY, M.D., FREMONT P. WIRTH, M.D.

INTRODUCTION

Intracranial saccular aneurysms represent the most common etiology of nontraumatic subarachnoid hemorrhage (43, 56). A significant health problem, they produce death or disability in approximately 18,000 persons/year in North America (63). A potential aneurysmal rupture may be averted with modern microsurgical and endovascular techniques. It is the difficulty of detecting an unruptured aneurysm in the asymptomatic patient that unfortunately precludes most prophylactic therapy.

The prevalence or frequency of intracranial aneurysms in a given population is an elusive figure. It has been estimated from autopsy data as well as arteriograms. The frequency of both ruptured and unruptured aneurysms discovered at autopsy is between <1% of cases and 9% in different series (4, 7, 14, 16, 28, 30, 34, 45, 46, 47, 56, 59, 68, 71, 80). This figure should not be mistaken for the prevalence which is estimated from only those patients harboring unruptured intracranial aneurysms. This range, cited in the autopsy literature, is from 0.3 to 5% (7, 14, 30, 46). Bannerman *et al.* (4) reviewed eight autopsy series, which included a total of 51,360 patients, and found a prevalence of only 0.34% unruptured aneurysms. Berry (7) demonstrated 1% in 6686 cases, Chason and Hindman (14) 2% in 2786 cases, and McCormick (46) 5% in 2276 cases. In a recent series, Inagawa and Hirano (30) determined a prevalence of 0.8% in 10,259 patients. In that study, aneurysms measuring 4 mm or less accounted for 54% of the cases and were therefore of questionable sig-

nificance. McCormick (46), however, demonstrated that measurements made of aneurysm size at autopsy were low. The size of aneurysms in the unfixed nonperfused state was compared to that of the same aneurysms perfused at 70 mm Hg pressure. Aneurysms were on average 40% larger in diameter when perfused (45). Therefore, even small aneurysms found at autopsy may be significant.

An important limitation of autopsy series is the predominance of elderly patients and individual hospital population distributions, which may not be representative of the whole population. Additionally, aneurysms may be missed if brains are not carefully scrutinized at the time of autopsy.

The incidence of unruptured intracranial aneurysms is low in the general population and is 1% or less in larger autopsy series. The incidence of unruptured intracranial aneurysms peaks in the seventh decade (30, 46). Inagawa found no intracranial aneurysms in 903 patients of age 0–29 years and a 1.24% incidence for age 60–69 years. Females predominated, with a ratio of about 5:3.

Estimates taken from retrospective angiographic studies are consistent with the low autopsy figures and range from 0.5 to 1.1% (3, 20, 59, 75, 79). The limitations of these studies include inadequate evaluation due to a deficiency of bilateral carotid and posterior circulation studies and special projections necessary to definitively rule out an aneurysm. As with autopsy groups, these are predominately older patient populations. The series of Atkinson *et al.* (3) represents an attempt to remedy these deficiencies. Selecting a population that was unbiased toward the presence of an aneurysm, they evaluated only the anterior circulation, because many patients did not undergo complete four-vessel studies (3). They found a 1% frequency of asymptomatic aneurysms.

The overall prevalence from the autopsy and arteriographic data is 1% or less. The lower estimates are more likely to be correct, considering that both types of series are biased toward older patients more likely to have an aneurysm. The likelihood of finding an aneurysm in a given individual is less than has been previously proposed (18).

Routine angiographic screening is not practical due to patient risk, variability in the age of onset of aneurysm formation, and cost (50). Magnetic resonance (MR) angiography has not yet demonstrated sensitivity level adequate to detect intracranial aneurysms in all areas of the brain. Early data, however, indicate great potential for this noninvasive test (29, 44).

Types of Aneurysms

A saccular aneurysm is an acquired degenerative lesion related to hemodynamic stress (52, 72). It consists of an arterial outpouching and occurs at the bifurcations of the proximal arteries at the base of the brain. The mean age for ruptured and unruptured aneurysms is in the mid-50-year range, and there is a slight female predominance (30, 56, 58, 71, 73). Multiple aneurysms are noted in 14–33.5% of cases (30, 42, 49, 52, 53, 60, 73, 74). Anterior circulation aneurysms occur in about 90% of cases (25). A saccular aneurysm is significant because it may rupture into the subarachnoid space.

An arteriosclerotic or fusiform aneurysm is associated with systemic atherosclerosis. It is a tortuous dilatation of a vessel and commonly occurs in the basilar artery. Rupture is unusual, and it is more often associated with brainstem compression or embolic events when it is symptomatic. These fusiform lesions were detected in only 0.1% of 10,259 autopsies (30).

Mycotic aneurysms usually occur in the distal aspect of the middle cerebral arteries and are related to bacterial emboli, most often from subacute bacterial endocarditis. High-dose antibiotics are the primary mode of therapy and may lead to thrombosis. These aneurysms may rupture and have been noted in only 0.05% of autopsies (30).

Traumatic aneurysms are rare and usually associated with delayed intracerebral hematoma with a poor prognosis. Neoplastic embolic aneurysms are also rare and usually result from an atrial myxoma of the left atrium. They may be fusiform or saccular or the vessel may be completely occluded.

Incidental Aneurysms

The rate of subarachnoid hemorrhage from unruptured intracranial aneurysms is an estimate upon which major treatment decisions are made. There have been few large series with long-term follow-up with which to determine the natural history of incidental aneurysms. In 1977, Jane et al. (33) estimated a bleed rate of 5%/year, based on several small series of unruptured aneurysms including the Cooperative Study (43). Several years later, this estimate was revised down to 1% by Jane et al. (32). Dell (18) used decremental life-table analysis to demonstrate a 16% lifetime risk for a 20-year-old and a 5% risk in a 60-year-old. The prevalence used to calculate these figures was assumed to be 5%. Data already reviewed in this chapter suggest that the prevalence is probably <1% and would indicate that Dell's percentage lifetime risk figures are low. Heiskanen (27) observed 61 patients with multiple aneurysms for 10 years and found a 1.1%/year incidence of bleeding. The mortality rate was 0.65%/year.

Wiebers et al. (77) felt that the size of incidental aneurysms was the most important factor. They evaluated 130 patients with a mean follow-up of 8.3 years and found that 15 aneurysms had ruptured and all were >10 mm in diameter. Fatalities were noted in 93% of hemorrhages. Those authors concluded that only aneurysms measuring 10 mm or greater had a significant risk of bleeding (77). Solomon and Correll (70) presented a case of a 6-mm asymptomatic aneurysm that had hemorrhaged, and they felt that any lesion of >3 mm in size should be considered for surgery (70). Schievink et al. (66) reported three cases of subarachnoid hemorrhage in patients known to have previously unruptured 4-mm aneurysms. Kassell and Torner (38) indicated that aneurysms of <10 mm were not benign and recommended that lesions of >5 mm be considered operative (38). Crompton (17) demonstrated that a 4-mm external diameter was the critical size for risk of rupture. de la Monte (52) did not determine the critical size at which an aneurysm would rupture but did report 2-mm aneurysms which had ruptured.

Incidental aneurysms approaching 10 mm or greater in size appear to have at least a 1%/year risk of hemorrhage. Aneurysms between 4 mm and 10 mm also are at risk for hemorrhage, although the risk is probably lower. The mortality rate associated with hemorrhage is high and is therefore a significant factor. Because aneurysm size may be a major factor in determining the appropriate mode of treatment, it is important to note that aneurysms may enlarge with time and the risk of hemorrhage subsequently increases (26, 37, 78).

Subarachnoid Hemorrhage

Subarachnoid hemorrhage from ruptured saccular aneurysms causes 6–8% of all strokes (51). Approximately 80% of cases of nontraumatic subarachnoid hemorrhage result from a ruptured aneurysm (63). The incidence of subarachnoid hemorrhage did not decrease over several decades, while other forms of cerebrovascular disease did (12, 58). In North America the incidence of subarachnoid hemorrhage is approximately 11–12/100,000, based on the most recent report by the Cooperative Study Group and others (58, 63). That incidence remained constant over 30 years in Rochester, Minnesota. There are approximately 25,000 new cases of ruptured aneurysm per year in the United States.

The prognosis for subarachnoid hemorrhage is undesirable. Drake (19) in his review summarized the mortality rate as 50% within the first hospitalization and, if not treated, another 30% during the next 10 years. It is estimated that 10% die immediately and without warning and another 25% are disabled or die as a result of the initial hemorrhage. This leaves only 65% available for intervention (10, 37, 56, 58). Hospitalized patients have an average 40% mortality rate over the next several days to 1 month (8, 10, 19, 37, 56, 58). Mortality rates at 1 month are reported to be as high as 60% (56, 58).

In addition to the initial hemorrhage, rebleeding is a major cause of mortality and morbidity (19, 32, 33, 37, 43, 56). The highest incidence of rebleeding occurred within the first 10 days and resulted in death for 20% of initial survivors in the series of Phillips et al. (58). The rate decreased to 1.5%/year for the first 10 years after the first 30 days (58). Others have reported that the risk is greatest within the first 24 hours after the bleed (32, 33, 36). Juvela (36), in his series of 236 patients, included patients seen in the emergency room and patients not usually referred from another hospital. The peak incidence of rebleeding was noted within the first 24 hours (4.1%) and at the end of the first week (16%). The rebleed mortality rate was high, at 74% (36). In selected aneurysms the incidence of rebleeding within 6 months was 50% on the first day after subarachnoid hemorrhage and decreased to 35% by day 10 and to <10% by day 50 (33). Jane et al. (33) reported on the 20-year follow-up for the 213 remaining patients in this series who did not undergo surgery and survived 6 months after hemorrhage. Rebleeding was reported at a rate of 3%/year after 6 months, with a 67% mortality rate.

Aneurysmal subarachnoid hemorrhage is associated with a high mortality rate. The major contributing factors are the original hemorrhage and early rebleeding. In one series a 30% mortality rate at 10 days was noted but rebleeding was felt to account for only 43% of this (58). Vasospasm and medical complications also play a role in the early mortality. In the untreated aneurysm, late rebleeding is also a significant factor and approximates 2–3%/year.

Predisposing Conditions

A 25-year autopsy study of 125 patients with ruptured or unruptured aneurysms at the Johns Hopkins Hospital outlined many significant factors relevant to the development and hemorrhage of saccular aneurysms (52). Hypertension, cerebral atherosclerosis, vascular asymmetry at the circle of Willis, persistent headache, pregnancy-induced hypertension, long-term analgesic use, and family history of stroke were all positively correlated with the formation of berry aneurysms. A correlation was not found with cigarette smoking, diabetes mellitus, or congenital abnormalities.

Aneurysmal rupture was correlated with previously documented severe acute hypertension (diastolic pressure of >110 mm Hg), increasing size, the presence of multiple aneurysms, long-term analgesic use, excessive alcohol intake, and fatty metamorphosis of the liver (52). The postulated mechanism of action for some of these factors was the decreased production of prostaglandin E and hence decreased cerebrovascular resistance with increased cerebral blood flow. Other studies presented variable findings for any association with hypertension (13, 48, 73). Smoking was a significant factor related to subarachnoid hemorrhage in another study (5). Broderick *et al.* (11) demonstrated that blacks had a 2.1 times greater risk of subarachnoid hemorrhage, compared to whites, after reviewing the medical records and autopsy reports for all patients in the Greater Cincinnati area during 1988.

Heavy physical activity is not necessary for aneurysmal rupture, because patients were reportedly at rest in 30–40% of cases (52, 64). Physical and emotional strain, defecation, coitus, head trauma, and other activities all contributed to varying degrees in the remaining 60–70% of cases. It is logical that increases in systemic arterial pressure may increase the risk of rupture.

Geographic Factors

The incidence of subarachnoid hemorrhage in Finland, Japan, and the United States has been reported as high. It is low in New Zealand and the Middle East. Pakarinen (56) demonstrated an incidence of 16.3/100,000 in 1967, and rates from 14.4 to 29.7/100,000 have been reported subsequently (21, 22). The highest incidence was reported in Finland by Sarti *et al.* (65), at 29.8/100,000. When adjusted to the reference population by Fogelholm (21, 22), however, the incidence was more consistent with previous reports, at 14.4 to 19.6/100,000.

The incidence of subarachnoid hemor-

rhage in Japan is also high, and rates of 17.5 and 18.3/100,000 in two different cities have been reported (31, 55). A similar analysis of a larger and more rural area including one of these cities demonstrated an incidence of only 11/100,000 (31). Inagawa *et al.* (31) hypothesized that many patients are missed in rural areas. A startling incidence of 96.1/100,000 was reported by Kiyohara *et al.* (39). Patients were observed for up to 22 years, and >80% underwent autopsy to determine the cause of death. This study attempted to minimize loss of those patients dying suddenly who would ordinarily not be included, and it thereby increased the likelihood of an accurate diagnosis. Eighty-two percent of the subarachnoid hemorrhage patients had intracranial aneurysms. The series is not comparable to other studies because only patients of age 40 years or older were included in the data collection and the results were not adjusted by sex and age to the same reference population.

In Auckland, the combined male and female incidence was reported as 14.3/100,000 (9, 10). The rates were age adjusted and indicate an increased incidence in this population. An Australian series reported an incidence of 26.4/100,000 population, but this was for patients over age 35 years and was not age adjusted to the reference population and it is therefore not comparable to other studies (15).

The age-specific incidence in the Netherlands was reported as 7.8/100,000, but this is felt to be an underestimate (23). Gudmundsson (24) reported an incidence of 8.0/100,000 in Iceland. This is also felt to be an underestimate because the incidence in the rural areas and villages was much less than in the city, indicating that many patients were not accounted for outside the city. In Greenland, Eskimos were found to have a 9.3/100,000 incidence, compared to the Caucasian Danes in Greenland, with an incidence of 3.1/100,000 (40). The disparity is possibly the result of genetic differences. The incidence in Caucasian Danes in Greenland is consistent with the incidence in all of Denmark of 3.4/100,000 (61). The isolated population of the Faroes, however, was found to have a 7.4/100,000/year incidence of subarachnoid hemorrhage (35). Since this population derived from the same ancestral stock as Denmark's population, a lower incidence would have been expected.

Subarachnoid hemorrhage in the Chinese was reported to be low, but adequate numbers are not available (69). The incidence in India was also reported to be very low (61). The crude incidence in Rhodesian Africans has been reported to be one half that of their European counterparts (41). This low incidence in India and Africa may be partially due to a decreased incidence of atherosclerosis in the respective populations.

Subarachnoid hemorrhage is also less common in the Middle East (2, 54). The incidence is probably underestimated due to inaccurate diagnosis, lack of routine autopsy, and failure to refer to a medical center (1). Nogueira (54) attempted to factor out these problems in the Middle East by using the State of Qatar, which is small and contains one health care system. He included a percentage of sudden deaths, intracerebral hematomas, and unproven source cases in which the computed tomography (CT) results were highly suggestive of aneurysmal rupture and added these to the known incidence. The estimate was still only 5.1/100,000/year. Arteriovenous malformations account for approximately 30% of subarachnoid hemorrhage (1).

Familial Influences

Familial aneurysms affect two or more first- to third-degree relatives. The patients are usually younger at the time of rupture, with an average age of 42 years (6). When familial intracranial aneurysms are the only abnormality the mode of inheritance is usually autosomal dominant, but only 18 families have been described (4, 6). Familial aneurysms may also be related to other disorders, such as Marfan's syndrome, Ehlers-Danlos syndrome, pseudoxanthoma elasticum, polycystic kidney disease, and coarctation of the aorta.

Chapman et al. (13) recently studied 92 adults with polycystic kidney disease. Approximately 4% were found to have intracranial aneurysms, whereas in the general population the rate is 1%. Multiple aneurysms were noted in three of four patients. High resolution CT was used for diagnosis in 60 patients, four-vessel angiography in 21, and both procedures in 11. Angiography resulted in a 25% complication rate in these patients. The recommendation from the study was that patients with polycystic kidney disease and a family history of aneurysm should undergo high-resolution CT screening every 5–10 years and should not undergo routine angiography, due to increased complications with this type of patient.

Schmid et al. (67) reported that a CT scan with 1.5-mm slices and rapid bolus intravenous contrast produced an angiography-like image of the basilar arteries. They were able to demonstrate 97% of 76 aneurysms down to a size of 3 mm. In addition, MR angiography has demonstrated an ability to detect intracranial aneurysms to a size of 3–4 mm (57, 62). MR angiography appears to work well for aneurysms located at the circle of Willis. It does not demonstrate more distally located aneurysms, such as middle cerebral aneurysms, as well.

Financial Considerations

The detection of an aneurysm prior to rupture not only profoundly affects the patient's health but also may result in saving health care dollars. Wiebers et al. (76) estimated the lifetime cost for patients with unruptured aneurysms who are hospitalized and treated as $522,500,000/year in the United States. This is compared to a $1,755,600,000/year lifetime cost for patients suffering from subarachnoid hemorrhage (76). There is a considerable potential savings with good surgical results. Routine screening tests performed at ages of increased risk would be cost effective, particularly as MR angiography becomes more widely available.

Conclusion

Incidental intracranial aneurysms occur in 1% or less of the general population, which is less than previously proposed in some cases. The rate of rupture is apparently 1% or greater for those aneurysms. The incidence of aneurysmal subarachnoid hemorrhage in North America is significant at 11–12/100,000/year and carries a high mortality rate. The risk of rupture may therefore be even higher, and thus a strong case is made for defining populations, age groups, and persons with specific risk factors for routine screening. With an effective and relatively noninvasive technique, a cost-effective approach to lowering the incidence of subarachnoid hemorrhage would be available.

REFERENCES

1. Al-Mefty, O., Al-Rodhan, N., and Fox, J. L. The low incidence of cerebral aneurysms in the Middle East: is it a myth? Neurosurgery 22:951–954, 1988.

2. Ammar, A., Al-Rajeh, S., Ibrahim, A. W. M., et al. Pattern of subarachnoid hemorrhage in Saudi Arabia. Acta Neurochir. (Wien) 114:16–19, 1992.

3. Atkinson, J. L. D., Sundt, T. M., Jr., Houser, O. W., and Whisnant, J. P. Angiographic frequency of anterior circulation intracranial aneurysms. J. Neurosurg. 70:551–555, 1989.

4. Bannerman, R. M., Ingall, G. B., and Graf, C. J. The familial occurrence of intracranial aneurysms. Neurology 20:283–292, 1970.

5. Bell, B. A., and Symon, L. Smoking and subarachnoid hemorrhage. Br. Med. J. 1:577–578, 1979.

6. ter Berg, H. W. M., Dippel, D. W. J., Limburg, M., et al. Familial intracranial aneurysms: a review. Stroke 23:1024–1030, 1992.

7. Berry, R. G., Alpers, B. J., and White, J. C. The site, structure and frequency of intracranial aneurysms, angiomas and arteriovenous abnormalities. Res. Publ. Assoc. Res. Nerv. Ment. Dis. 41:40–72, 1961.

8. Biller, J., Godersky, J. C., and Adams, H. P., Jr. Management of aneurysmal subarachnoid hemorrhage. Stroke 19:1300–1305, 1988.

9. Bonita, R., Beaglehole, R., and North, J. D. K. Subarachnoid hemorrhage in New Zealand: an epidemiological study. Stroke 14:342–347, 1983.

10. Bonita, R., and Thomson, S. Subarachnoid hemorrhage: epidemiology, diagnosis, management, and outcome. Stroke 16:591–594, 1985.

11. Broderick, J. P., Brott, T., Tomsick, T., et al. The risk of subarachnoid and intracerebral hemorrhage in blacks as compared to whites. N. Engl. J. Med. 326:733–736, 1992.

12. Broderick, J. P., Phillips, S. J., Whisnant, J. P., et al. Incidence rates of stroke in the eighties: the end of the decline of stroke? Stroke 20:577–582, 1989.

13. Chapman, A. B., Rubinstein, D., Hughes, R., et al. Intracranial aneurysms in autosomal dominant polycystic kidney disease. N. Engl. J. Med. 327:916–920, 1992.

14. Chason, J. L., and Hindman, W. M. Berry aneurysms of the circle of Willis: results of a planned autopsy study. Neurology 8:41–44, 1958.

15. Christie, D. Some aspects of the natural history of subarachnoid hemorrhage. Aust. N.Z. J. Med. 11:27–34, 1981.

16. Cohen, M. M. Cerebrovascular accidents: a study of two hundred cases. Arch. Pathol. 60:296–307, 1955.

17. Crompton, M. R. Mechanism of growth and rupture in cerebral berry aneurysms. Br. Med. J. 1:1138–1142, 1966.

18. Dell, S. Asymptomatic cerebral aneurysm: assessment of its risk of rupture. Neurosurgery 10:162–166, 1982.

19. Drake, C. G. Management of cerebral aneurysm. Stroke 12:273–283, 1981.

20. DuBoulay, G. H. Some observations on the natural history of intracranial aneurysms. Br. J. Radiol. 38:721–757, 1965.

21. Fogelholm, R. Subarachnoid hemorrhage in Finland. Stroke 23:437, 1991.

22. Fogelholm, R. Subarachnoid hemorrhage in Middle-Finland: incidence, early prognosis and indications for neurosurgical treatment. Stroke 12:296–301, 1981.

23. Giel, R. Notes on the epidemiology of the spontaneous subarachnoid hemorrhages. Psychiatr. Neurol. Neurochir. 68:265–271, 1965.

24. Gudmundsson, G. Primary subarachnoid hemorrhage in Iceland. Stroke 4:764–767, 1973.

25. Hacker, R. J., Krall, J. M., and Fox, J. L. The incidence of intracranial aneurysm. In: Intracranial Aneurysms, edited by J. L. Fox, pp. 15–62. Springer-Verlag, New York, 1983.

26. Hashimoto, N., and Honda, H. The fate of untreated symptomatic cerebral aneurysms: analysis of 26 patients with clinical course of more than 5 years. Surg. Neurol. 18:21–26, 1982.

27. Heiskanen, O. Risk of bleeding from unruptured aneurysms in cases with multiple intracranial aneurysms. J. Neurosurg. 55:524–526, 1981.

28. Housepian, E. M., and Pool, J. L. A systematic analysis of intracranial aneurysms from the autopsy file of the Presbyterian Hospital, 1914 to 1956. J. Neuropathol. Exp. Neurol. 17:409–423, 1958.

29. Huston, J., III, Rufenacht, D. A., Ehman, R. L., and Wiebers, D. O. Intracranial aneurysms and vascular malformations: comparison of time-of-flight and phase-contrast MR angiography. Radiology 181:721–730, 1991.

30. Inagawa, T., and Hirano, A. Autopsy study of unruptured incidental aneurysms. Surg. Neurol. 34:361–365, 1990.

31. Inagawa, T., Ishikawa, S., Aoki, H., et al. Aneurysmal subarachnoid hemorrhage in Izumo City and Shimane Prefecture of Japan. Stroke 19:170–175, 1988.

32. Jane, J. A., Kassell, N. A., Torner, J. C., and Winn, H. R. The natural history of aneurysms and arteriovenous malformations. J. Neurosurg. 62:321–323, 1985.

33. Jane, J. A., Winn, H. R., and Richardson, A. E. The natural history of intracranial aneurysms: rebleeding rates during the acute and long term period and implication for surgical management. Clin. Neurosurg. 24:176–184, 1977.

34. Jellinger, K. Pathology and aetiology of intracranial aneurysms. In: Cerebral Aneurysms: Advances in Diagnosis and Therapy, edited by H. W. Pia, C. Langmaid, and J. Zierski, pp. 5–19. Springer,

New York, 1979.

35. Joensen, P. Subarachnoid hemorrhage in an isolated population: incidence on the Faroes during the period 1962–1975. Stroke *15*:438–440, 1984.

36. Juvela, S. Rebleeding from ruptured intracranial aneurysms. Surg. Neurol. *32*:323–326, 1989.

37. Kassell, N. F., and Drake, C. G. Timing of aneurysm surgery. Neurosurgery *10*:514–519, 1982.

38. Kassell, N. F., and Torner, J. C. Size of intracranial aneurysms. Neurosurgery *12*:291–297, 1983.

39. Kiyohara, Y., Ueda, K., Hasuo, Y., et al. Incidence and prognosis of subarachnoid hemorrhage in a Japanese rural community. Stroke *20*:1150–1155, 1989.

40. Kristensen, M. O. Increased incidence of bleeding intracranial aneurysms in Greenlandic Eskimos. Acta Neurochir. (Wien) *67*:37–43, 1983.

41. Levy, L. F., Rachman, I., and Castle, W. M. Spontaneous primary subarachnoid hemorrhage in Rhodesian Africans. Afr. J. Med. Sci. *4*:77–86, 1973.

42. Locksley, H. B. Natural history of subarachnoid hemorrhage, intracranial aneurysm and arteriovenous malformations: based on 6838 cases in the Cooperative Study, parts I and II. In: *Intracranial Aneurysms and Subarachnoid Hemorrhage*, edited by A. L. Sahs, G. E. Perret, H. B. Locksley, and H. Nishioka, pp. 37–108. Lippincott, Philadelphia, 1969.

43. Locksley, H. B. Report on the Cooperative Study of Intracranial Aneurysms and Subarachnoid Hemorrhage. Section V, Part II. Natural history of subarachnoid hemorrhage, intracranial aneurysms and arteriovenous malformations: based on 6368 cases in the Cooperative Study. J. Neurosurg. *25*:321–368, 1966.

44. Masaryk, T. J., Modic, M. T., Ross, J. S., et al. Intracranial circulation: preliminary clinical results with three-dimensional (volume) MR angiography. Radiology *171*:793–799, 1989.

45. McCormick, W. F., and Acosta-Rua, G. The size of intracranial saccular aneurysms: an autopsy study. J. Neurosurg. *33*:422–427, 1970.

46. McCormick, W. F. Intracranial arterial aneurysm: a pathologist's view. Curr. Concepts Cerebrovasc. Dis. Stroke *8*:15–19, 1973.

47. McCormick, W. F., and Nofzinger, J. D. Saccular intracranial aneurysms: an autopsy study. J. Neurosurg. *22*:155–159, 1965.

48. McCormick, W. F., and Schmalstieg, E. J. The relationship of arterial hypertension to intracranial aneurysms. Arch. Neurol. *34*:285–287, 1977.

49. McKissock, W., Richardson, A., Walsh, L., and Owen, E. Multiple intracranial aneurysms. Lancet *1*:623–626, 1964.

50. Misra, B. K., Whittle, I. R., Steers, A. J. W., and Sellar, R. J. *De novo* saccular aneurysms. Neurosurgery *23*:10–15, 1988.

51. Mohr, J. P., Caplan, L. R., Melski, J. S., et al. The Harvard Cooperative Stroke Registry: a prospective registry. Neurology *28*:754–762, 1978.

52. de la Monte, S. M., Moore, G. W., Monk, M. A., and Hutchins, G. M. Risk factors for the development and rupture of intracranial berry aneurysms. JAMA *78*:957–964, 1985.

53. Nehls, D. G., Flom, R. A., Carter, L. P., and Spetzler, R. F. Multiple intracranial aneurysms: determining the site of rupture. J. Neurosurg. *63*:342–348, 1985.

54. Nogueira, G. J. Spontaneous subarachnoid hemorrhage and ruptured aneurysms in the Middle East: a myth revisited. Acta Neurochir. (Wien) *114*:20–25, 1992.

55. Ohno, K., Suzuki, R., Masaoka, H., Monma, S., Matsushima, Y., and Inaba, Y. A review of 102 consecutive patients with intracranial aneurysms in a community hospital in Japan. Acta Neurochir. (Wein) *94*:23–27, 1988.

56. Pakarinen, S. Incidence, aetiology, and prognosis of primary subarachnoid hemorrhage: a study based on 589 cases diagnosed in a defined urban population during a defined period. Acta Neurol. Scand. *29*(suppl.):1–128, 1967.

57. Pernicone, J. R., Siebert, J. E., Potchen, E. J., et al. Three dimensional phase-contrast MR angiography of the head and neck: preliminary report. AJNR *155*:167–176, 1990.

58. Phillips, L. H., II, Whisnant, J. P., O'Fallen, W. M., and Sundt, T. M., Jr. The unchanging pattern of subarachnoid hemorrhage in a community. Neurology *30*:1034–1040, 1980.

59. Pitt, G. N. Some cerebral lesions. Br. Med. J. *1*:827–832, 1890.

60. Poppen, J. L., and Fager, C. A. Multiple intracranial aneurysms. J. Neurosurg. *16*:581–589, 1959.

61. Rammamurtni, B. Incidence of intracranial aneurysms in India. J. Neurosurg. *30*:154–157, 1969.

62. Ross, J. S., Masaryk, T. J., Modic, M. T., et al. Intracranial aneurysms: evaluation by MR angiography. AJR *155*:159–165, 1990.

63. Sahs, A. L., Nibbelink, D. W., and Torner, J. C. (eds.). *Aneurysmal Subarachnoid Hemorrhage: Report of the Cooperative Study.* Urban and Schwarzenberg, Baltimore, 1981.

64. Sahs, A. L., Perret, G. E., Locksley, H. B., and Nishioka, H. (eds.). *Intracranial Aneurysms and Subarachnoid Hemorrhage: A Cooperative Study.* Lippincott, Philadelphia, 1969.

65. Sarti, C., Tuomilehto, J., Salomaa, V., et al. Epidemiology of subarachnoid hemorrhage in Finland from 1983 to 1985. Stroke *22*:848–853, 1991.

66. Schievink, W. I., Piepgras, D. G., and Wirth, F. P. Rupture of previously documented small asymptomatic saccular intracranial aneurysms. J. Neurosurg. *76*:1019–1024, 1992.

67. Schmid, U. D., Steiger, H. J., and Huber, P. Accuracy of high resolution computed tomography in direct diagnosis of cerebral aneurysms. Neuroradiology *29*:152–159, 1987.

68. Sekhar, L. N., and Heros, R. C. Origin, growth and rupture of saccular aneurysms: a review. Neurosurgery *8*:248–260, 1981.

69. So, S. C., Ngan, H., and Ong, G. B. Intracranial aneurysms causing subarachnoid hemorrhage in the Chinese. Surg. Neurol. *12*:319–321, 1979.

70. Solomon, R. A., and Correll, J. W. Rupture of a previously documented asymptomatic aneurysm enhances the argument for prophylactic surgical

intervention. Surg. Neurol. *30:*321–331, 1988.

71. Stehbens, W. E. Aneurysms and anatomical variation of cerebral arteries. Arch. Pathol. *75:*45–64, 1963.

72. Stehbens, W. E. Etiology of intracranial berry aneurysms. J. Neurosurg. *70:*823–831, 1989.

73. Stehbens, W. E. *Pathology of the Cerebral Blood Vessels,* pp. 351–470. C. V. Mosby, St. Louis, 1972.

74. Suzuki, J. Multiple aneurysms: treatment. In: *Cerebral Aneurysms: Advances in Diagnosis and Therapy,* edited by H. W. Pia, C. Langmaid, and J. Zierski, pp. 352–363. Springer, Berlin, 1979.

75. Wakai, S., Fukishima, T., Furihata, T., *et al.* Association of cerebral aneurysm with pituitary adenoma. Surg. Neurol. *12:*503–507, 1979.

76. Wiebers, D. O., Torner, J. C., and Meissner, I. Impact of unruptured intracranial aneurysms on public health in the United States. Stroke *23:*1416–1419, 1992.

77. Wiebers, D. O., Whisnant, J. P., Sundt, T. M., and O'Fallen, W. M. The significance of unruptured intracranial saccular aneurysms. J. Neurosurg. *66:*23–29, 1987.

78. Winn, H. R., Richardson, A. E., and Jane, J. A. The long term prognosis in untreated cerebral aneurysms. I. The incidence of later hemorrhage in cerebral aneurysms: a 10 year evaluation in 364 patients. Ann. Neurol. *1:*358–370, 1977.

79. Winn, H. R., Richardson, A. E., O'Brien, W., and Jane, J. A. The long term prognosis in untreated cerebral aneurysms. II. Late morbidity and mortality. Ann. Neurol. *4:*418–426, 1978.

80. Winn, H. R., Taylor, J., and Kaiser, D. L. Prevalence of asymptomatic incidental aneurysms. Stroke *14:*121, 1983.

CHAPTER 3

Pathophysiological Alterations Following Aneurysm Rupture

STEVEN J. TRESSER, M.D., WARREN R. SELMAN, M.D.,
ROBERT A. RATCHESON, M.D.

INTRODUCTION

Aneurysmal subarachnoid hemorrhage (SAH) strikes approximately 25,000 individuals each year in North America (132), resulting in a high rate of mortality and severe neurological impairment for many of the survivors. In addition to the central nervous system, other organ systems including cardiovascular, respiratory, and endocrine can be affected by rupture of a cerebral aneurysm.

The most feared complication for survivors of the initial hemorrhage has been recurrent bleeding, which occurs in approximately 20% of unoperated patients and is frequently fatal. In recent years, a trend toward early operation has reduced the risk of rebleeding for selected patients (82). Unfortunately this lower rate of rebleeding has not resulted in a decline in the overall mortality rate or a significant increase in the percentage of favorable outcomes (81).

The consequences of cerebral ischemia, now the leading cause of death and disability following aneurysmal SAH, have largely negated the gains achieved by lowering the rebleeding rate. According to the International Cooperative Study on the Timing of Aneurysm Surgery, 13.5% of patients who experience aneurysmal SAH suffer delayed cerebral ischemia and incur permanent disability or death (81). Of the 1494 patients in that study who died or became disabled, delayed ischemia due to cerebral vasospasm accounted for 32.0% of the total; in comparison, the direct effect of the aneurysmal rupture accounted for 25.0% and rebleeding for 17.6%.

This chapter focuses first on the immediate effects of aneurysmal rupture on the brain and other organ systems. Since an understanding of the pathophysiology of ischemia resulting from aneurysmal rupture is of importance for designing rational therapies to prevent and treat this leading cause of morbidity and mortality, this chapter also describes normal cerebrovascular control and discusses specific pathophysiological mechanisms which produce cerebral ischemia in the setting of SAH.

EFFECTS OF ANEURYSM RUPTURE

Intracerebral and Intraventricular Hemorrhage

Aneurysm rupture almost universally results in SAH, although hemorrhage is not always confined to the subarachnoid space. Several reports have described intracerebral hemorrhage (ICH), intraventricular hemorrhage (IVH), and subdural hemorrhage. As might be expected, the location of the hemorrhage can affect outcome, and patients with massive intraventricular or intracerebral hematomas tend to die earlier than those without blood in these locations (194).

ICH can occur either from direct rupture of an aneurysm into the brain or from secondary rupture of a subarachnoid hematoma into the brain parenchyma. Compton

(17), in an autopsy study of 103 fatal aneurysmal bleeds, found that direct rupture into the brain accounted for 42% of the ICHs and occurred most commonly with aneurysms of the internal carotid (53%), pericallosal (50%), and anterior cerebral (33%) arteries. Secondary rupture into the brain from a sylvian SAH occurs commonly with middle cerebral artery (MCA) aneurysms. Overall, the arteries from which the aneurysms that produced ICH arose were the anterior cerebral artery in 44%, MCA in 26%, internal carotid artery in 21%, and pericallosal artery in 10% (17). Several other reports have described similar results (146, 149). ICH due to aneurysmal rupture can appear identical to hypertensive hemorrhage on computerized tomographic scanning, implying that angiographic evaluation of a "typical" hypertensive hemorrhage may be needed to prevent overlooking an aneurysmal etiology.

IVH following aneurysmal rupture is associated with ICH in up to 57% of cases (96, 108). IVH is found in 13–28% of the clinical cases of ruptured aneurysm and in 37–54% of autopsied cases, implying that hemorrhage in this location has a deleterious influence on patient outcome (108). It thus appears to be a significant predictor of poor neurological status and outcome. Mohr *et al.* (108) studied 91 patients with IVH due to ruptured aneurysms and found a 64% overall mortality rate. The degree of ventricular dilatation was the key prognostic indicator. Aneurysms causing IVH were located on the anterior cerebral artery in 40%, internal carotid artery in 25%, MCA in 21%, and vertebrobasilar artery in 14% of the cases (108).

Subdural hemorrhage following aneurysmal SAH is encountered rarely. Several large clinical series have reported an incidence between 1.3% and 2.8% (4, 178, 203), although the incidence in various autopsy series has been reported as nearly 20% (159, 176). Several mechanisms might explain the formation of subdural hemorrhage in this setting: arachnoid adherent to the dome of an aneurysm may tear when the dome ruptures, permitting blood to flow into the subdural space; a powerful stream of blood emanating from the ruptured aneurysm may force itself through the arachnoid at a weak point; or the arachnoid may be disrupted by an ICH, which then decompresses secondarily into the subdural space.

The consequences of hemorrhage into the brain parenchyma, subdural space, or ventricular system include elevated intracranial pressure (ICP) due to mass effect and acute hydrocephalus. Both of these conditions may require immediate treatment, either separately or along with treatment of the aneurysm.

Hydrocephalus

Hydrocephalus due to SAH can be classified as either immediate or delayed. Acute hydrocephalus, that arising within 3 days of the SAH, has a reported incidence ranging from 9% (173) to 63% (6), depending on the method used to determine the presence of ventricular dilatation. Clinically significant hydrocephalus requiring immediate treatment occurred in 15–20% of patients in various series (47, 58, 59, 107). Milhorat (107) found that the incidence of acute hydrocephalus closely paralleled the clinical grade of the patient. In 93% of his patients the development of hydrocephalus was manifest by a decrease in the level of consciousness, often leading to a downgraded clinical status (107). The effect of acute hydrocephalus on clinical grade, though, can be difficult to distinguish from that of the precipitating hemorrhage.

Various researchers have hypothesized that subarachnoid blood causes acute hydrocephalus by interfering with cerebrospinal fluid (CSF) outflow through the aqueduct of Sylvius, the fourth ventricular outlet, the basal cisterns, and the subarachnoid space (7, 84, 91, 173). In a rabbit model of SAH, in which cisternal injections of blood were given, Black *et al.* (7) demonstrated that hydrocephalus was due to increased outflow resistance in CSF pathways and that CSF production and absorption rates were unaltered. Factors such as IVH and a diffuse spread of SAH, which acutely compromise the flow of CSF, contribute to the development of acute hydrocephalus (47, 59, 108, 193). The presence of intraventricular blood has been shown to be the strongest determinant for the development of acute hydrocephalus (59, 193). This effect of intraventricular blood is presumably due to either blockage of the CSF pathways by blood clot or diminished CSF outflow as a result of substantially elevated CSF viscosity (59). In the absence of ventricular blood, blood in both ambient cisterns has also been found to significantly increase the risk of developing acute hydrocephalus (59). Increased age (6, 47), vasospasm (6), and the use of antifibrinolytic drugs (47, 126) have also been found to correlate with the development of acute hydrocephalus after SAH. The correlation between vasospasm and hydrocephalus is not surprising, given that both are closely associated with large amounts of blood in the basal cisterns.

Chronic hydrocephalus, usually occurring after the 10th day after SAH, results when CSF circulation or its absorption at the arachnoid granulations is inhibited by adhesions in the pia-arachnoid. Extensive leptomeningeal fibrosis that occurs after a period of at least 10 days following SAH and interferes with the absorption of CSF has been demonstrated by pathological study (84, 105).

Cerebral Edema

Cerebral edema, defined as an increase in the water and sodium content of the brain, can be classified as cytotoxic, vasogenic, or interstitial (34). Either the intracellular or extracellular compartment of the brain, or both, may be affected. SAH can produce each of these types of edema from a variety of mechanisms. Vasogenic edema, due to an increased permeability of brain capillary endothelial cells, is the type of edema most frequently seen following SAH. The breakdown of the blood-brain barrier to macromolecules allows the leakage of protein-rich edema fluid into the extracellular space. The accumulation of fluid is primarily in the cerebral white matter, where cellular components are less densely packed. It is this type of edema which is present in the acute phase following SAH and which can cause hemispheric shifts and the various patterns of cerebral herniation. Vasogenic white matter edema may also be seen following surgery in areas of retractor use.

Cytotoxic edema occurs when the blood-brain barrier is intact and intracellular water is increased due to disturbed cell metabolism. It occurs as a result of systemic disturbances that include acute hypoxia, acute hypo-osmolality, acute episodes of apnea, or cardiac arrest following SAH. In this form of edema, the cellular elements of the brain swell and the extracellular fluid space is reduced in volume. Acute hypo-osmolality, which may be due to acute hyponatremia on a dilutional basis or secondary to the syndrome of inappropriate antidiuretic hormone (SIADH), leads to cerebral edema as the osmolality gradient between the serum and the brain drives water into the cells.

Interstitial edema is seen with movement of CSF across the ventricular walls into the periventricular white matter. The fluid lies in the extracellular space, which may be increased by as much as 30%. Because the ependymal surface offers very little resistance to the flow of water (186), transependymal flow of CSF occurs under normal physiological conditions, with the direction and velocity of flow determined by hydrostatic and osmotic pressure gradients (151). Interstitial edema is almost always associated with the onset of acute hydrocephalus and can be reversed rapidly by CSF shunting procedures.

Seizures and Seizure-like Activity

Acute loss of consciousness with abnormal tonic or clonic motor activity frequently occurs in the early hours following SAH. In an extensive literature review, Hart et al. (57) found a range of occurrence of 10–26% for seizures and seizure-like events following SAH. Because ictal activity often occurs during the first few minutes following SAH, many episodes are not witnessed by a physician. Descriptions of seizures following SAH are often insufficiently detailed in the literature, and many episodes may not be truly epileptic; therefore, there is some uncertainty surrounding the exact nature of these events. Hart et al. (57) found a seizure occurrence of 26% in a study of 100 consecutive cases of SAH; 19% of the patients had a seizure within a few minutes of hemorrhage. The incidence of seizures associated with acute rebleeding episodes was found to be nearly identical to the seizure incidence associated with initial hemorrhage. In almost all cases rebleeding directly preceded convulsive activity. Because of this intimate temporal association between rebleeding and delayed-onset seizure activity, seizure development in a patient who has been stable after an initial SAH suggests rehemorrhage.

Several pathogenetic mechanisms have been proposed to explain the association between bleeding and seizures. Direct irritation of the cerebral cortex by subarachnoid blood likely plays an important role in the pathogenesis of early seizures after SAH. Another possible mechanism is suggested by the temporal relationship between either initial hemorrhage or rebleeding and seizure activity. Acute marked elevations in ICP, known to occur within seconds of aneurysmal rupture, have been related to tonic seizure-like activity in humans and dogs (97, 208). The ictus is generally described as regular opisthotonic spasms and tonic extension of the extremities, although departure from this typical decerebrate posturing is commonly seen. Jackson (74) believed that there were epileptic discharges originating in the brainstem. In more modern times, it has been suggested that this represents a release of brainstem reflexes (45). Lundberg (97), in a study of patients with brain tumors, found similar seizure-like activity to be well correlated with spontaneous elevations in ICP and electroencephalographic flattening. The occurrence of these seizure-like events after SAH appears to be closely related to periods of acute ICP increase and thus may reflect release of brainstem reflexes as opposed to true epileptogenic activity.

Other pathogenetic mechanisms have been considered. Vasospasm was first proposed as a cause of seizures by Robertson (149) in 1949. Although experimentally induced vasospasm can be biphasic, with an early component occurring in the first few minutes after hemorrhage (10, 26), there is little convincing evidence to support a causative role for acute vasospasm in the development of seizures. Rose and Sarner (150) found no correlation between the presence of intracerebral hematoma and the development of early seizures. Sundaram and Chow (179) found equivalent incidences of intracerebral hematoma in seizure and non-seizure patients after SAH.

Epilepsy develops in approximately 15% of patients who suffer a SAH (150, 199), with onset during the first 18 months in >90% of these patients (150). Major risk factors for the development of late epilepsy are poor neurological grade on admission, rupture of a MCA aneurysm, cerebral infarction secondary to vasospasm, and shunt-dependent hydrocephalus (150). The use of prophylactic anticonvulsant agents in the acute stage is considered standard therapy, although Hart et al. (57) were not able to demonstrate an effect on the development of chronic seizures.

Alteration of Respiratory Function

Neurogenic pulmonary edema, considered to be a mixed pressure and permeability edema characterized by the rapid onset of respiratory failure with a protein concentration greater than 4.5 g/dl in the edema fluid, may develop in patients who suffer a SAH. The rapid onset and occurrence in patients with no evidence of cardiac disease or volume overload indicate that its pathogenesis is noncardiac in nature. Common to other recognized precursors of neurogenic pulmonary edema, including head injury, cerebral tumors, and strokes, is the presence of raised ICP. A possible sequence of events to explain the formation of neurogenic pulmonary edema was derived from animal experiments: an acute rise in ICP causes hypothalamic irritation, which leads to a massive sympathetic adrenergic discharge, systemic vasoconstriction, systemic hypertension, a shift of blood to the lower resistance pulmonary circuit, and an increase in pulmonary capillary hydrostatic pressure (24, 147). Presumably, the homeostatic aim of these drastic circulatory adjustments is to maintain cerebral perfusion pressure (CPP) after an acute rise in ICP. Theodore and Robin (187) in 1976 demonstrated the high protein content of the pulmonary edema fluid, indicating that alterations in capillary permeability are present as well. This increased capillary permeability may result from damage to the pulmonary endothelium caused by large transient increases in pulmonary capillary pressure (41, 93). Direct endothelial damage leads to extravasation of serum and blood into the interstitium and ultimately into the alveoli.

The predominant physiological abnormalities seen in patients with neurogenic pulmonary edema are a right to left cardiac shunt caused by markedly elevated pressure in the pulmonary circuit; decreased lung compliance; and fluid accumulation in alveoli leading to alveolar collapse, ventilation-perfusion mismatch, and hypoxemia (205). Treatment of this condition includes reduction of ICP, mechanical ventilation with positive end-expiratory pressure, and optimization of cardiovascular function along the Starling curve. Knudsen et al. (88) have reported effective treatment of severe neurogenic pulmonary edema with dobutamine, a drug which reduces total peripheral vascular resistance and increases cardiac contractility. The incidence of neurogenic pulmonary edema following SAH was reported by Weir (205) as 13%; he observed that the incidence declined as the interval from the hemorrhage lengthened.

A less severe respiratory complication of aneurysmal SAH is the development of pneumonia, reported to occur in approximately 8% of patients during their hospitalization (81). If severe, hypoxemia and hypoventilation from pneumonia may require mechanical ventilation.

Effect on the Heart

Alterations of the electrocardiogram (ECG), both morphological and rhythmic, are seen in at least 50% of patients with aneurysmal SAH (56, 100). In a review of 15 series, totaling 256 cases, by Marion et al. (100) the most common ECG abnormalities were T wave enlargement or inversion in 47%, prolongation of the QT interval in 37%, ST segment elevation or depression in 30%, prominent U waves in 25%, and various arrhythmias including supraventricular tachycardia, atrial fibrillation and flutter, and premature atrial or ventricular contractions in 35%. These abnormalities have generally been attributed to increased circulating levels of catecholamines and deranged autonomic control of the heart, resulting from SAH-induced hypothalamic stimulation.

Initially it was believed that the cardiac effects of SAH were primarily the result of disturbances of ventricular repolarization caused by excess catecholamine stimulation. However, Koskelo et al. (90) first proposed in 1964 that ECG abnormalities reflect actual subendocardial hemorrhage and necrosis. Evolving evidence indicates that this is likely the case. Patients with SAH often have characteristic microscopic subendocardial necrosis at autopsy (18, 23, 89). Ventricular wall motion defects have been demonstrated by echocardiography (133) in a disproportionately large number of patients with aneurysmal rupture. Szabo et al. (184) demonstrated abnormal myocardial perfusion by thallium scan in 32% of patients with abnormal ECGs in the acute period after SAH. The frequent elevation of myocardial isoenzyme levels after SAH further supports the notion that cardiac damage occurs, although the ratio of myocardial-specific creatine phosphokinase to total-body creatine phosphokinase only rarely indicates that transmural myocardial injury has occurred (28).

Fluid and Electrolyte Disturbances

Hyponatremia, a common finding in patients after aneurysmal SAH, is usually associated with SIADH, although in some patients a true natriuresis or "cerebral salt-wasting syndrome" may occur (114). SIADH develops in approximately 10% of patients following SAH (22, 36, 209) and is most commonly associated with aneurysms of the anterior communicating artery (22, 115). It is believed that SAH interferes with supraoptic hypothalamic neurons that secrete antidiuretic hormone. Due to abnormal regulation of its secretion by the hypothalamus, antidiuretic hormone is secreted in the face of low serum osmolality and increased extracellular fluid volume. Water is excessively retained by the kidneys to the point of hyponatremic expansion of the extracellular fluid volume. A secondary depletion of sodium occurs as volume expansion causes suppression of aldosterone, which leads to a decrease in tubular sodium reabsorption. In cerebral salt wasting, as originally described by Peters et al. (130), the primary defect is believed to be renal loss of sodium in the absence of renal or adrenal disease or diuretic use. It has been postulated that this natriuresis is due to an unidentified natriuretic factor elaborated in the brain (86, 114).

The laboratory criteria for diagnosing SIADH are a serum sodium level of <135 mEq/liter, urinary sodium level of >25 mEq/liter, serum osmolality of <280 mOsm/kg, and urine osmolality greater than serum osmolality. Patients with cerebral salt-wasting syndrome generally satisfy the laboratory criteria for SIADH as well. Thus, assessment of the intravascular volume status, red blood cell mass, and body weight is essential to differentiate these disorders and direct proper treatment. Patients with SIADH have an increased intravascular volume with normal or increased body weight, a normal or low hematocrit, and normal cardiovascular status. In contrast, patients with true natriuresis have evidence of decreased intravascular volume, decreased body weight, elevated hematocrit, and postural hypotension and tachycardia.

Symptoms of hyponatremia depend both on the absolute degree of hyponatremia and the rate at which it develops. Patients with sodium levels below 125 mEq/liter usually develop symptoms of anorexia, nausea, vomiting, irritability, and alteration of mental function. Seizures begin to occur with sodium levels below 120 mEq/liter. Below 115 mEq/liter, almost all patients develop neurological signs, including arreflexia, weakness, pseudobulbar palsy, Babinski's sign, and stupor or coma. In addition to symptoms of hyponatremia, patients with cerebral salt-wasting syndrome can have symptoms related to hypovolemia. Due to decreased intravascular volume, patients with cerebral salt wasting are at risk for the development of delayed ischemic deficits secondary to vasospasm.

The mainstay of treatment for SIADH is fluid restriction. With restriction to 800–1200 ml/day, serum sodium levels should increase within 2–3 days. It is rarely necessary to correct the serum sodium level more quickly than this. In patients who are markedly hyponatremic and symptomatic, hypertonic (3%) saline can be used to more rapidly elevate the serum sodium level. No more

than one quarter of the total body sodium deficit should be replaced during the first 8 hours, with another quarter being replaced over the next 16 hours. The remaining half of the sodium deficit can be replaced if necessary over the following 1–2 days. It should be remembered that too-rapid correction of serum sodium can lead to central pontine myelinolysis (117). Although the best therapy for SIADH is fluid restriction, this is often balanced by the need to maintain a high intravascular volume in an effort to prevent the development of delayed ischemic deficits secondary to vasospasm. Patients with cerebral salt wasting require both sodium and volume replacement to replace their deficits. Usually isotonic saline is satisfactory; in severe instances packed red blood cells and colloid may be necessary.

Diabetes insipidus (DI) resulting from the failure of antidiuretic hormone release from the hypothalamus has been reported after SAH and is associated with a poor prognosis (185). Anterior communicating artery aneurysms are most commonly implicated. A mass effect due to progressive enlargement of an aneurysm can damage the supraoptic nucleus of the hypothalamus or the infundibulum. SAH may likewise damage the hypothalamus or infundibulum either during the actual hemorrhage or in a delayed fashion as a result of ischemia secondary to vasospasm. Patients with DI have a urine output of ≥ 300 ml/hr (with a specific gravity of <1.005 g/ml), polydipsia (if able to drink), and elevated serum osmolality and serum sodium levels. Serum osmolality and sodium determinations are essential to exclude the possibility of water overload, which would also manifest as hypotonic polyuria, especially in the postoperative patient. Therapy for DI includes careful monitoring of body weight, fluid balance, and serum and urinary electrolytes. Replacement of fluid loss should be with hypotonic solutions. It is a mistake to give replacement solutions containing significant amounts of salt, because these provide continued solute load to the kidneys and aggravate the renal loss of water. Aqueous vasopressin or desmopressin (1-Deamine-8-D-arginine vasopressin, DDAVP) can be given if replacement volumes become impractical.

CEREBROVASCULAR CONTROL AND ISCHEMIC THRESHOLDS

Cerebral Blood Flow Regulation

Insights into the pathophysiology of ischemia secondary to SAH can be obtained only with a thorough understanding of normal cerebral hemodynamics and metabolism. Critical to that understanding is an appreciation of the regulatory systems governing cerebral blood flow (CBF). Five major interdependent mechanisms, listed below, are involved in this control. This division is likely somewhat artificial, because these control mechanisms may operate in concert. Recent work has provided evidence that at least some of these controls may be mediated by a final common pathway regulated by endothelial cells.

Metabolism-Blood Flow Coupling

Normally there is exquisite coupling between the regional cerebral metabolic demand for oxygen and glucose, generated by local neuronal activity, and the volume of blood flowing through that tissue (48, 95). Several chemical species related to neuronal and glial activity, including H^+, K^+, CO_2, ATP, adenosine, and lactate, are able to alter local vascular tone and have been hypothesized as being responsible for the tight coupling between flow and metabolism.

Neurogenic Control

Traditionally, investigation of neurogenic control of the cerebral vasculature has focused on the role of efferent nerves which follow large arteries to innervate the cerebral vessels. Three types of extrinsic nerve systems, with their respective origins and neurotransmitters, have been identified.

1. Sympathetic neurons that arise principally from the superior cervical ganglion and contain norepinephrine and neuropeptide Y, both vasoconstrictors (192).
2. Parasympathetic neurons in the sphenopalatine and otic ganglia that contain acetylcholine and often coexpress vasoactive intestinal peptide (11, 161).
3. Sensory fibers that originate in the trigeminal ganglion and contain sub-

stance P and calcitonin gene-related peptide, both of which are vasodilators.

It is generally considered that, despite the abundance of these nerve fibers, CBF is regulated primarily by local metabolism, with only minor modulation by extrinsic nerves. The manner in which these peripheral neurons might contribute to governance of the cerebral circulation on a moment to moment basis during normal activity remains to be established.

The possibility that the brain could regulate its own flow was recognized by several early researchers in the field, although for many years it was not considered by most to be a potentially important regulatory mechanism (158, 174, 197). With the advent of autoradiographic methods for determination of regional CBF and positron emission tomography (PET) studies of cerebral circulation and metabolism in humans, as well as an explosion of techniques and knowledge regarding biochemical neuroanatomy, there is a growing body of evidence to support the concept that the brain, through intrinsic neural networks, can regulate its own blood flow (143, 145, 161). Cerebrovascular autoregulation and response to hypoxia may be regulated, in part, by intrinsic neural systems within the medulla oblongata and may not be, as traditionally believed, entirely dependent upon responses of vessel walls and/or endothelium (144).

CO_2

One of the earliest observations regarding cerebral vasoreactivity was that a decrease in $PaCO_2$ results in marked vasoconstriction. A linear relationship between $PaCO_2$ and CBF exists within a $PaCO_2$ range of 25–60 mm Hg, with a CBF change of approximately 4%/mm Hg (120). This highly regional regulatory mechanism is presumed to be a function of the local perivascular pH (198). Because a change in $PaCO_2$ is also detected by carotid artery chemoreceptors, this regulatory mechanism might also be mediated by a reflex pathway.

Autoregulation

According to the general equation of blood flow, CBF can be described by the relationship between CPP and cerebrovascular resistance (CVR)

$$CBF = \frac{CPP}{CVR}$$

where CPP is equal to mean arterial blood pressure (MABP) minus intracranial pressure (ICP).

$$CPP = MABP - ICP$$

Under normal conditions, ICP is negligible and CPP is roughly equivalent to MABP. In the presence of ICH, cerebral edema, or hydrocephalus, however, ICP cannot be ignored. Changes of MAPB over a wide range, approximately 60–150 mm Hg, produce little fluctuation in CBF (55, 94, 177). This cerebral "autoregulation," then, is mediated by changes in CVR, as described by the equation:

$$CVR = \frac{L\eta}{\pi r^4}$$

where L is the vessel length, η is viscosity, and r is the vessel radius as derived from the Hagen-Poiseuille equation, which describes the flow of Newtonian fluids in rigid tubes (210).

As seen from this equation, changes in the radius of cerebral blood vessels result in marked alterations of CVR. A decrease in CPP produces dilatation of the precapillary resistance vessels, whereas an increase in CPP produces constriction. Largely by variation in the degree of constriction of the cerebral resistance vessels, CBF is maintained at a fairly constant level, near 50 ml/100 g/min in the adult human brain at rest. Although myogenic, neurogenic, and metabolic mechanisms have been postulated, the exact nature of the autoregulatory response remains unknown.

Endothelial Factors

A growing body of evidence suggests that endothelium-dependent mechanisms function to determine the tone of cerebral blood vessels. Endothelium-derived relaxing factor (EDRF) is a potent vasodilator (39) that has the chemical and physical properties of nitric oxide (NO) (109) and is produced by activated neurons (12, 43, 44, 87), astrocytes

(112), and perivascular nerves (190). The presence of an endothelium-derived contractile factor has also been postulated. Synthesis of EDRF/NO or a closely related molecule derived from the amino acid L-arginine appears to affect vascular tone, both under basal conditions and in response to the application of specific agonists (29, 30, 152). The proposed mechanism for this effect is that EDRF/NO stimulation of soluble guanylate cyclase raises levels of cGMP in vascular smooth muscle and results in vascular relaxation (109). This L-arginine/NO/cGMP pathway appears critical for the control of vascular tone and is gaining favor as the dominant mediator of the autoregulatory response and the vasodilatory response to hypoxia (42, 92, 102, 138).

Compensatory Responses to Ischemia

PET has greatly enhanced our understanding of the pathophysiological alterations that occur in focal cerebral ischemia in humans. The simultaneous measurement of regional CBF, cerebral metabolic rate of oxygen (CMRO₂), oxygen extraction fraction (OEF), and cerebral blood volume (CBV) has permitted the identification of three successive stages of severity of ischemia (Fig. 3.1) (46, 134, 136, 137, 180). As CPP ini-

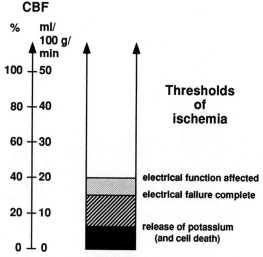

Figure 3.1. Ischemic thresholds for electric and pump failure. (Adapted from Astrup, J., Symon, L., Branston, N. M., *et al.* Cortical evoked potential and extracellular K⁺ and H⁺ at critical levels of brain ischemia. Stroke *8:* 51–57, 1977.)

tially falls, autoregulation causes vasodilatation of precapillary resistance vessels, resulting in an increase in CBV and maintenance of both CBF and $CMRO_2$. At the lower limit of autoregulation, maximal compensatory dilatation of cerebral resistance vessels occurs. Further reductions in CPP lead to a fall in CBF. The OEF then increases to maintain $CMRO_2$. If CBF reduction is modest, the increased extraction of oxygen and glucose from the remaining blood flow can maintain normal brain metabolism and function. A leftward shift of the oxygen-hemoglobin affinity curve as an effect of decreased local pH results in an increased transfer of oxygen from blood to tissue and is largely responsible for the increased OEF. When the OEF reaches its maximum (approximately 90%), no further compensation can occur. As CBF falls further, the metabolic demands of the brain can no longer be satisfied, $CMRO_2$ decreases, and "metabolic depression" ensues. The alterations of cerebral function that occur as these compensatory systems become overwhelmed in the setting of increasingly severe ischemia may be best understood in the context of ischemic thresholds and the ischemic cascade.

Flow Thresholds

Modern electrophysiological techniques and methods of blood flow determination have further defined the relationship between neuronal function, viability, and critical levels of regional CBF. Experimental studies of MCA occlusion in various species have demonstrated a gradient of blood flow, from normal in areas outside the affected territory, to moderately decreased in adjacent perifocal regions, to profoundly reduced in the ischemic core (110, 111, 183). The slope of this gradient is determined by the extent and functional capacity of collateral blood supply.

Different cellular functions, which require specific minimum levels of blood flow, are affected in these regions depending on the degree of blood flow reduction. Critical values for loss of synaptic transmission, corresponding to loss of neuronal function, are between 15 and 18 ml/100 g/min (9, 61). The threshold for membrane pump failure,

and thus cellular integrity, is approximately 10 ml/100 g/min (3, 8). The presence of these two distinct thresholds implies that some regions in the perifocal area contain cells that are electrophysiologically quiescent but nonetheless viable. These regions constitute the ischemic penumbra, defined by Astrup *et al.* (2) as areas with electrocortical quiescence and low extracellular K^+ levels.

The threshold for infarction in monkeys has been observed to be approximately 12 ml/100 g/min (76). The previous study also demonstrated that the duration, as well as the degree, of blood flow reduction is important in any consideration of ischemic thresholds. Infarction developed only if blood flow was reduced to below 12 ml/100 g/min for periods lasting 2 hours or longer. Since the time course for irreversible damage in complete global ischemia models is much shorter, *i.e.*, approximately 10 min (73, 85, 139, 140), it is reasonable to suspect that areas with more profound blood flow reduction in focal ischemia have a shorter tolerance than areas with higher levels of blood flow.

The Ischemic Cascade

While a comprehensive review of the pathophysiology of cerebral ischemia is beyond the scope of this discussion, an understanding of delayed ischemic deterioration in the setting of SAH requires at least a basic overview of the cellular events triggered by an ischemic insult. More detailed information can be found in several excellent reviews (142, 167, 168).

The mechanisms that cause irreversible injury in ischemia are probably multifactorial and interrelated. Several pathological mechanisms occur with the onset of ischemia and include alterations in energy metabolism, lipid metabolism, neurotransmitter release and reuptake, and ion homeostasis. The resulting energy failure, tissue acidosis, ion and water fluxes, altered calcium homeostasis, excitotoxicity, altered phospholipid metabolism, and free radical formation, as detailed in the sections that follow, may all contribute to processes resulting in cell death.

Energy Failure and Acidosis

The initial consequence of ischemia is energy failure, which leads to a cascade of events culminating in irreversible cell injury. Oxidative phosphorylation ceases with the onset of ischemia, resulting in a rapid depletion of high energy phosphate stores (phosphocreatine and ATP). Energy failure secondary to ischemia is an early event, and the cell is still viable at this stage. Cell death can be prevented if blood flow is restored. Continued lack of oxygen, however, stimulates anaerobic metabolism of glucose, which is less efficient than oxidative metabolism and supplies only 2 ATP molecules/glucosyl unit consumed, compared to 36 molecules/glucosyl unit from oxidative metabolism. Anaerobic metabolism is also the primary cause of tissue acidosis during ischemia (165). Acidosis in turn affects blood flow, blood-brain barrier permeability, edema formation, and mitochondrial function (13, 64, 77, 113, 119, 141).

In complete ischemia, tissue acidosis may be limited because glycolysis is restricted by the preischemic endogenous stores of glucose and glycogen. In incomplete ischemia, such as might be expected with ischemia from vasospasm, glycolysis may delay the onset of energy failure but the continued delivery of glucose may actually worsen the lactic acidosis. This lactate production increases tissue osmolality and contributes to the formation of cytotoxic edema. The acidosis inhibits mitochondrial phosphorylation, compromises the microcirculation, contributes to the denaturation of proteins and nucleic acids (78), enhances free radical reactions (164), and decreases cytosolic calcium binding (166). The aggregate of these actions results in an increase in ischemic damage with worsening acidosis.

Ion and Water Fluxes

Approximately 40–50% of neuronal ATP is used by the Na^+/K^+-ATPase for the maintenance of ionic gradients (2, 206). Movements of ions occur either in response to their electrochemical gradients or in response to receptor-mediated opening of specific ion channels. Active energy-requiring processes, or "pumps," are needed to restore the various anions and cations to their proper intracellular and extracellular concentrations for normal cell function. Some of these pumps are dependent on the hydrolysis of ATP for their energy source, whereas other transporters use the sodium gradient as an energy source. Since the sodium gradient is maintained by the Na^+/K^+-ATPase, these homeostatic processes are directly or indirectly dependent on an adequate supply of ATP.

An ischemia-induced reduction of available energy in the cell results in dissipation of ionic gradients, as evidenced by a rise in extracellular K^+ concentration (1, 52, 67). The extracellular concentrations of Na^+, Ca^{2+}, and Cl^- fall, together with a reduction in extracellular fluid volume (53). These rapid ionic fluxes are due to increased membrane permeability to these ions and are associated with depolarization of the cell. This depolarization not only results in the loss of the signal transmission capability of the neuron but also necessitates the consumption of precious high-energy phosphates in a futile cycling of ions.

The influx of sodium ions, with the obligatory movement of water, contributes to cellular edema formation. Cytotoxic edema is an early feature of ischemic injury and is a result of the movement of protein-poor fluid from the extracellular space into the cells. As the ischemic insult continues, the blood-brain barrier may become incompetent due to damage to the tight junctions between endothelial cells. This causes an extravasation of serum proteins and other molecules into the extracellular compartment, resulting in vasogenic edema. Vasogenic edema develops hours to days after the ischemic insult. Both cytotoxic and vasogenic edema may further worsen the primary ischemic insult, either by increasing the diffusion distance of substrates or by causing an increase in local pressure, thereby resulting in a further lowering of regional blood flow (163).

Calcium Homeostasis

Maintenance of a low intracellular Ca^{2+} concentration (10^{-7} mol/liter) is necessary for this molecule to function as a metabolic regulator and messenger. Loss of calcium homeostasis, leading to an elevated level of intracellular calcium, has been implicated in the etiology of irreversible cell damage in ischemia (19, 169). The normally high calcium gradient between the intracellular and extracellular spaces is maintained by export of Ca^{2+}. Intracellular Ca^{2+} is bound or sequestered in the endoplasmic reticulum and mitochondria. Both the maintenance of the calcium gradient and the intracellular sequestration of calcium are energy-dependent processes and may be impaired during ischemia.

There is substantial evidence that a massive influx of calcium occurs during ischemia. Cellular depolarization from energy failure leads to calcium entry through voltage-dependent calcium channels. Neurons also possess receptor-mediated calcium channels, which may contribute to the calcium influx when excitatory neurotransmitters are released during ischemia (166). Although both voltage-sensitive and agonist-operated calcium channels control the movement of calcium into the cell, the latter are predominantly involved in the initiation of the pathological processes associated with ischemia. The acidosis produced during ischemia decreases the capacity of the cell to buffer a calcium load (166). In addition, the breakdown of phospholipids during ischemia generates inositol triphosphate, which stimulates release of calcium from the endoplasmic reticulum (71).

Failure of the homeostatic mechanisms described above results in an increased intracellular calcium concentration. This intracellular calcium activates phospholipases A and C (212), leading to an alteration of phospholipid metabolism. It also activates proteases, which lead to the breakdown of both enzymatic and structural proteins, and acts as a second messenger in numerous intracellular reactions which, if not well regulated, can contribute to cell injury (170).

Excitotoxicity

Neuronal signal transduction is mediated by a calcium-dependent controlled release of neurotransmitters. Cellular depolarization and an influx of Ca^{2+} lead to a release of neurotransmitters. Normal neuronal function is dependent on mechanisms which control neurotransmitter synthesis, degra-

dation, release, reuptake, and inactivation. The energy for reuptake or sequestration of these neurotransmitters may be lacking during ischemia, and this can lead to pathological events.

There is now considerable evidence that excitatory neurotransmitters such as glutamate play a role in ischemic injury (16, 122, 123, 160). The exact mechanisms of injury from excitotoxicity are unclear but may be related to a continued increased metabolic demand which cannot be met in the face of reduced blood flow, the expenditure of energy in a futile cycling of ions due to neurotransmitter-induced alterations in membrane permeability, or the augmentation of calcium influx through receptor-mediated channels.

Phospholipid Metabolism

Four major alterations in phospholipid metabolism following ischemia occur which may have pathological consequences; these include overactivation of the cyclo-oxygenase and lipo-oxygenase pathways, the production of platelet-activating factor, and the activation of various protein kinases (168). The activation of phospholipases A and C by elevated intracellular Ca^{2+} promotes deacylation of membrane phospholipids, generating free fatty acids (FFAs), including arachidonic acid and lysophospholipids. Energy failure causes an arrest of phospholipid synthesis from FFAs by reacylation of lysophospholipids or by synthesis of inositol glyceride. Together, these processes lead to a rise in intracellular FFAs (207). Ischemia-induced phospholipid breakdown changes the membrane protein-to-phospholipid ratio. This may alter membrane characteristics, including permeability to various ion species and the function of membrane-bound enzymes, which may lead to cell death.

Free Radicals

Free radicals, such as the superoxide anion, hydrogen peroxide, and the hydroxyl radical, are highly reactive compounds. They are characterized by the presence of an unpaired electron in an outer orbit. These molecules are normally generated during the sequential univalent reduction of oxygen to water by the electron transport chain in the mitochondria. Free radicals can cause cell damage by initiating toxic reactions such as the chain reaction of lipid peroxidation. There are many naturally occurring free radical scavengers present in a cell, which together with the cytochrome oxidase reaction remove free radicals. The products of antioxidant neutralization undergo enzymatic detoxification by glutathione peroxidase and superoxide dismutase (200).

Although free radicals may be produced due to a lack of an electron acceptor (oxygen) at the cytochrome oxidase step (35), they are probably more prevalent during incomplete ischemia, such as occurs with SAH-induced vasospasm or during reflow. Active oxygen species may be formed during reoxidation of members of the respiratory chain, at the prostaglandin hydroperoxidase step in the metabolism of arachidonic acid to prostaglandins, and when xanthine and hypoxanthine are metabolized by xanthine oxidase (163). The free radical species have been postulated to cause cell death by damaging membrane structure (200). They may also play a role in the formation of ischemic edema (14, 162).

HEMODYNAMIC AND METABOLIC CONSEQUENCES OF SAH

Cerebral ischemia and infarction after aneurysmal SAH were first described by Richardson and Hyland (148) in 1941. With the advent of functional brain-scanning techniques, such as PET, a number of subsequent studies have confirmed that SAH can lead to a significant decrease in CBF and metabolism (50, 72, 135, 196, 202). These changes occur even in patients in good clinical condition (grades I and II by the Hunt and Hess scale) (70), although they are more profound in patients in worse clinical condition (grades III and IV). Several mechanisms can explain the hemodynamic and metabolic alterations following SAH.

The most straightforward effect of SAH on CBF can occur through an increase in ICP. Thus, acute hydrocephalus or an intracerebral hematoma may reduce blood flow by directly lowering CPP below the autoregulatory limits.

Another mechanism is an immediate and generalized effect of the hemorrhage on cerebral metabolism. Several investigators have provided evidence that, even in the absence of angiographically demonstrated vasospasm, SAH can lead to global reductions in both $CMRO_2$ and CBF (50, 65, 103, 196). This is presumed to be due to direct toxic effects of subarachnoid blood on brain metabolism, with a primary reduction in $CMRO_2$ and a secondary reduction in CBF governed by lowered tissue oxygen requirements, in accordance with the principle of metabolism-CBF coupling. Unfortunately, none of the cited studies conclusively demonstrated that cellular metabolism was reduced in response to diminished metabolic requirements. Measurements of OEF in one study varied tremendously (65), and no study documented normal lactate levels. Another possible explanation for the previous findings is that CBF was reduced primarily due to increased resistance in the microcirculation, which would not be evident radiographically, and that the altered metabolism was in fact a pathological response to an inadequate blood supply.

Undoubtedly, the most widely appreciated mechanism responsible for ischemia following SAH is that of vasospasm. In patients with radiographically evident cerebral vasospasm, an increase in CVR leads to a primary reduction of CBF, which then affects $CMRO_2$. Robertson (149) in 1949 first proposed this hypothesis, and Ecker and Reimenschneider (25) in 1951 were the first to demonstrate arteriographic evidence of vasospasm after SAH.

Despite intensive research spanning >20 years, the pathogenesis of vasospasm remains uncertain. Some relationship to the presence of a ruptured aneurysm appears to exist, because vasospasm in the setting of SAH due to nonaneurysmal causes is rare. A correlation between the amount of blood within the subarachnoid basal cisterns and the development of vasospasm also exists.

The most widely held theory explaining the pathogenesis of arterial constriction proposes that some substance released at the time of the initial hemorrhage acts on smooth muscle in the walls of small arteries and arterioles to cause vasoconstriction.

Eichlin (27) demonstrated in 1965 that marked vasospasm in exposed basilar artery could be caused by the application of fresh blood. More than 30 putative vasoactive substances, including numerous neurotransmitters, blood constituents or breakdown products, and autocoids, have been investigated as the source of smooth muscle contraction in vasospasm; none so far has been definitively established as the offending agent. Evidence implicating a breakdown product of red blood cells, most probably oxyhemoglobin, is compelling but by no means incontrovertible (38, 98, 99). Suzuki (181) noted that the development of vasospasm follows the same time course as the liberation of oxyhemoglobin from lysed erythrocytes. Fujita *et al.* (38) found oxyhemoglobin to be a much more potent vasoconstrictive agent than methemoglobin. They hypothesized that oxyhemoglobin acts indirectly through superoxide anion radicals derived from its oxidation to methemoglobin (38). Other investigators have likewise postulated that the auto-oxidation of oxyhemoglobin to methemoglobin produces oxygen free radicals, which in turn form lipid hydroperoxide (153, 155, 156). Steele *et al.* (175) have demonstrated that the effect of oxyhemoglobin on cerebrovascular smooth muscle cells is mediated by free radicals. Partial reduction of experimental vasospasm with administration of antioxidants (156) and iron-chelating agents (54) has been achieved. Okamoto (118) was able to substantially block vasoconstriction by administration of either prostaglandin synthesis inhibitor or antagonist. He concluded that vasoconstrictor prostaglandins intrinsic to the vessel wall mediate the effect of free radicals. The efficacy of antioxidant therapy in the treatment of cerebral vasospasm in humans is currently being evaluated. Findlay and Weir and co-workers (32, 201) have demonstrated that removal of clot from the subarachnoid space using intracisternal tissue plasminogen activator can reduce the occurrence of vasospasm.

Neurogenic constriction due to release of neurotransmitters from nerve fibers on cerebral vessels has also been postulated. The innervation of the cerebral vasculature utilizes a variety of classical amine neurotransmitters and neuropeptides. Despite several decades of research, the mechanisms capable of causing vasodilatation and vasoconstriction remain poorly understood. Fraser *et al.* (37) and Peerless and Yasargil (129) showed that experimental SAH resulted in depletion of catecholamines from perivascular nerves, leaving receptors empty and hypersensitive to catecholamines, found in high concentrations in extravasated subarachnoid blood. The acute vasoconstriction thus produced could be completely reversed by the administration of a long-acting α-receptor antagonist.

Another mechanistic theory holds that morphological changes of the arterial wall consistent with vasonecrosis or vasculopathy lead to a reduced vessel diameter. Vasospastic arteries subjected to pathological examination have revealed increased vessel wall thickness in addition to decreased vessel diameter (33). Degenerative changes in the tunica intima and media (33, 68), subendothelial proliferation, smooth muscle proliferation, collagen deposition (172), and ultrastructural changes in endothelial and smooth muscle cells (33) have been identified. In addition, platelet aggregation along the endothelial surface, especially near the site of aneurysmal rupture, has been seen (51). Although there is evidence that arterial wall mass is increased due to marked structural changes, this does not appear to be as important as smooth muscle contraction in the development of vascular constriction. One view proposed by Hughes and Schianchi (68) is that cerebral vasospasm actually gives rise to mural damage, probably through mechanical stress from sustained contraction of the smooth muscle or by accumulation of the pharmacological action of toxic metabolites in the vessel wall.

Constriction of vessels may also result from mechanical compression. In large vessels, this is primarily the result of brain displacement or herniation with entrapment of the vessel. In the microcirculation, increased local tissue pressure due to ICH or edema may cause the collapse of vessels due to markedly diminished transmural pressure (171).

Vasospasm can be diffuse, involving many of the major arteries at the base of the brain, or limited to arteries in the vicinity of the ruptured aneurysm. The arterial constriction can range from a very mild stenosis which is clinically inapparent to a severe, hemodynamically significant narrowing with attendant neurological dysfunction (204). Whereas radiographic vasospasm has been documented in 60–70% of patients in the second week after SAH, only 20–30% develop delayed ischemia (80).

Several factors must be considered to understand why vasospasm does not lead to clinically evident ischemia more frequently. First, vessels prone to spasm are conducting vessels, where a large decrease in diameter does not significantly diminish flow. Voldby et al. (196) have shown that decreases in regional CBF are closely correlated with the degree of angiographic vasospasm. Only when intraluminal diameter is reduced by 50% or more is CBF significantly affected. Lesser degrees of vasospasm produce no decrease in CBF (196). This view, that large arteries are primarily conduit vessels and that small arteries and arterioles regulate vascular resistance, has been a widely accepted one in vascular physiology. A growing body of evidence, however, suggests that large arteries may play a significant role in regulating vascular resistance, especially in the cerebral circulation, where the long length of these "conducting vessels" makes their contribution to the precapillary resistance greater than in most other vascular beds (31).

Anatomical location of constricted vessels and the adequacy of collateral circulation are additional factors which determine whether vasospasm leads to ischemia (80). There may be differential susceptibility of large and small vessels to the insult of SAH. Constriction of large conduit vessels is accompanied by considerable compensatory dilatation of intraparenchymal vessels, resulting in large increases in CBV in regions of severe vasospasm (5, 50). In accordance with autoregulatory mechanisms, this is probably a consequence of severe reductions in perfusion pressure distal to constricted arterial segments. Compensatory increases in OEF in these regions would also mitigate the ischemic effects of vasospasm.

Finally, the large degree of CBF reserve must be considered. Due to the significant difference between normal CBF rates and the electrical failure threshold, a large reduction of CBF is necessary before electrical silence producing clinical deficits ensues.

Despite these considerations, it is clearly possible for critical ischemic thresholds to be exceeded in the face of vasospasm. Disturbed regional CBF autoregulation in the acute stage after SAH has been demonstrated in several experimental studies (79, 104). Impairment of cerebral autoregulation and CO_2 reactivity has been associated with cerebral vasospasm (60, 72, 195). Voldby et al. (195) demonstrated that the degree of impairment of cerebrovascular reactivity correlated closely with the severity and extent of cerebral vasospasm identified angiographically. Patients without vasospasm demonstrated intact pressure autoregulation and CO_2 response (195).

Under vasospastic conditions where cerebrovascular resistance is abnormally elevated, the response of the vessel wall to alterations in transmural pressure is reduced or abolished entirely, depending on the underlying degree of spasm. Consequently, the autoregulatory mechanism which would normally maintain CBF in the face of relative hypotension is impaired. In areas where a reduction in CBF causes focal ischemia, cerebral metabolic acidosis ensues and adversely affects vasomotor responses, ultimately leading to complete vasoparalysis (124, 127). As reflected by increased CSF lactate levels, cerebral metabolic acidosis is commonly found in association with dysautoregulation. In a cat model of focal cerebral ischemia, Symon et al. (182) have shown a correlation between the degree of ischemia and the extent of loss of autoregulation. In areas where CBF was maintained at >40% of baseline, some autoregulation was preserved. Complete loss of autoregulation, however, occurred in regions in which CBF fell to <20% of base-line (182). Similar results were obtained by Dirnagl and Pulsinelli (21) in a rat model of focal ischemia. With complete vasoparalysis, CBF in the ischemic area of the vascular bed becomes passively dependent on CPP. In this setting, reductions in CPP from a variety of causes can have profound ischemic consequences (Table 3.1).

Reduced, although preserved, CBF responses to hyperventilation have been observed in patients with ruptured intracranial aneurysms (72, 75, 79, 104, 131) as well and have been well correlated with the degree of vasospasm (195). While some patients with mild vasospasm had preserved CO_2 reactivity and disturbed autoregulation, so-called "dissociated vasomotor paralysis" (121), more severe vasospasm resulted in dysfunction of both modes of reactivity (195). It is theorized that this dissociation is due to the degree of tissue acidosis incurred. Disturbed autoregulatory mechanisms can be temporarily restored in most patients by hypocapnia, presumably due to the correction of perivascular acidosis (128). Correlation of CSF lactate levels with the degree of vasospasm supports this hypothesis (196).

THERAPEUTIC IMPLICATIONS

The previously noted alterations in the physiology of CBF control in the presence of SAH permit some understanding of general approaches that can be utilized to improve CBF in this setting. Although cerebral vasospasm is the principal cause of cerebral ischemia following SAH, it should be remembered that there are a number of other pathophysiological events amenable to ther-

TABLE 3.1.
Causes of CPP Reduction

Reduction in CPP due to decreased systemic blood pressure
  Arrhythmias
  Myocardial damage
  Reduced effective blood volume due to dehydration
    Inadequate intake
    Use of osmotic diuretic agents
    Diuresis due to renal-dose dopamine
    DI
    Cerebral salt-wasting syndrome
  Antihypertensive medications
  Calcium channel blockers
  Intraoperative hypotension
Reduction in CPP due to increased ICP
  Intracerebral hematoma
  Hydrocephalus
  Cerebral edema

apeutic intervention: arterial injury or compromise during surgical repair of the aneurysm or neuroradiological procedures; increased ICP secondary to acute hydrocephalus, ICH, or edema; thromboembolic events; hypotension; and complications of medical therapy or general anesthesia.

While the avoidance of elevated systemic blood pressure in a patient with an unsecured aneurysm is a prime consideration for the prevention of rehemorrhage, the presence of altered autoregulatory mechanisms in patients with SAH necessitates caution in blood pressure reduction if focal ischemia is to be prevented. It is especially vital to determine the premorbid blood pressure history of the patient, in order to avoid producing ischemia by overzealous blood pressure reduction in someone whose autoregulatory curve has been "shifted to the right" due to hypertension.

Therapy aimed at preventing cerebral vasospasm has centered around the use of hypervolemia, hypertension, and hemodilution to optimize CBF and oxygen delivery to the brain. The use of aggressive hypervolemia and hypertension is relatively contraindicated if a ruptured aneurysm remains unsecured. Although the importance of blood viscosity in the routine regulation of CBF remains controversial (40, 49, 62, 69, 101, 157, 188, 210), under ischemic conditions even small alterations in the rheological properties of blood may have significant functional relevance (49, 83, 125, 154, 189). This selective contribution to the regulation of CBF under impaired flow conditions can be explained by certain properties of blood. Due largely to the effect of erythrocyte deformability and aggregation, blood behaves as a non-Newtonian fluid. As such, its viscosity is inconstant and dependent upon shear rate, which is proportional to velocity and inversely proportional to vessel radius (210). At low shear rates blood viscosity increases, while at higher shear rates viscosity is decreased. Therefore, the relationship between blood flow and viscosity is imprecisely described by the Hagen-Poiseuille equation, especially at low shear rates. In "low-flow" states seen with incomplete vascular occlusion (as in vasospasm), perfusion pressure is reduced and compensatory vasodilatation of the microcirculation occurs. Under these conditions average shear rates are quite low, and blood flow is further reduced by an increase in viscosity. Viscous resistance may become so high that blood flow stops completely (15, 20). Thus, under ischemic conditions an intricate relationship exists between vasomotor compensatory mechanisms and blood viscosity, and even small alterations in the rheological properties of blood have significant functional relevance.

Perhaps the most important determinant of blood viscosity is the hematocrit value, especially when shear rates are low (Fig. 3.2). The steep portion of the hematocrit-viscosity curve falls within the physiological range of hematocrit values. Decreases in shear rate shift the curve to the left. Thus, reductions

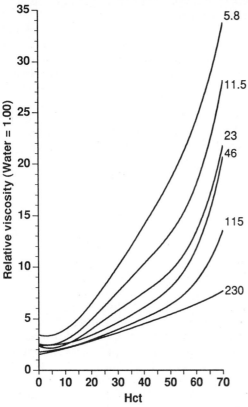

Figure 3.2. Influence of hematocrit value (Hct) on viscosity at varying rates of shear (expressed in sec^{-1} to the right of each curve). (Modified from Stone, H. O., Thompson, H. K., and Schmid-Nielson, K. Influence of erythrocytes on blood viscosity. *Am. J. Physiol. 214:* 913–918, 1968.)

in hematocrit values within the physiological range significantly reduce blood viscosity, and this effect is most marked at low shear rates, as is seen in focal cerebral ischemia.

Experimental studies have shown augmentation of diminished CBF following the acute reduction of hematocrit by infusion of low-molecular weight dextran or autologous plasma (191, 211). Although reduction of hematocrit values (and thus hemoglobin content) reduces the oxygen content of blood, relative oxygen transport capacity has been calculated to increase due to improved CBF with hematocrit reductions to approximately 30% (210). Below this hematocrit level, the decrease in blood oxygen content overrides the beneficial effect of decreased viscosity on CBF in the microcirculation. This is consistent with several studies that indicate a hematocrit range of 30–32% as optimal for tissue oxygen delivery (66, 106, 210). As discussed in subsequent chapters, on the basis of these considerations hemodilution has been advocated in the treatment of delayed ischemia after SAH.

Balloon angioplasty for dilatation of vasospastic intracranial arteries has been shown to be a rapid and effective means of reestablishing adequate CBF and reversing ischemic deficits (63, 116). The threshold for performing cerebral angiography and, if necessary, angioplasty should be low when a patient has evidence of vasospasm either by transcranial Doppler or clinical assessment.

In many instances, though, it is not possible to improve flow such that the brain is not all risk for infarction. Therapies designed to alter the events in the ischemic cascade, as outlined in the previous sections of this chapter, may be utilized in this setting. Thus, agents which block calcium entry into cells, those which can modulate the effects of the release of excitatory neurotransmitters, and those which alter lipid peroxidation and the generation of free radicals during ischemia may prove effective alone or in combination. Modulation of the NO pathway may also become important in future therapeutic endeavors. It is hoped that the results of trials designed to evaluate such therapies will reveal solutions for the devastating mortality and morbidity associated with aneurysmal SAH.

REFERENCES

1. Astrup, J., Rehncrona, S., and Siesjö, B. K. The increase in extracellular potassium concentration in the ischemic brain in relation to the preischemic functional activity and cerebral metabolic rate. Brain Res. *199:* 161–171, 1980.
2. Astrup, J., Siesjö, B., and Symon, L. Thresholds in cerebral ischemia: the ischemic penumbra. Stroke *12:* 723–725, 1981.
3. Astrup, J., Symon, L., Branston, N. M., *et al.* Extracellular potassium activity, evoked potential and tissue blood flow: relationship during progressive ischaemia in baboon cerebral cortex. J. Neurol. Sci. *32:* 305–321, 1977.
4. Barton, E., and Tudor, J. Subdural haematoma in association with intracranial aneurysm. Neuroradiology *23:* 157–160, 1982.
5. Bergvall, U., Steiner, L., and Forster, D. M. C. Early pattern of cerebral circulatory disturbances following subarachnoid hemorrhage. Neuroradiology *5:* 24–32, 1973.
6. Black, P. M. Hydrocephalus and vasospasm after subarachnoid hemorrhage from ruptured intracranial aneurysms. Neurosurgery *18:* 12–16, 1986.
7. Black, P. M., Tzouras, A., and Foley, L. Cerebrospinal fluid dynamics and hydrocephalus after experimental subarachnoid hemorrhage. Neurosurgery *17:* 57–62, 1985.
8. Branston, N. M., Strong, A. J., and Symon, L. Different flow thresholds for failure of evoked response and increase in extracellular potassium activity during progressive ischaemia in cerebral cortex. J. Physiol. *263:* 139P–140P, 1976.
9. Branston, N. M., Symon, L., Crockard, H. A., *et al.* Relationship between the cortical evoked potential and local cortical blood flow following acute middle cerebral artery occlusion in the baboon. Exp. Neurol. *45:* 195–208, 1974.
10. Brawley, B. W., Strandess, D. E. J., and Kelly, W. A. The biphasic response of cerebral vasospasm in experimental subarachnoid hemorrhage. J. Neurosurg. *28:* 1–8, 1968.
11. Brayden, J. E., and Bevan, J. A. Acetylcholine and vasoactive intestinal polypeptide in the cerebral circulation: histochemical and biochemical indices of innervation. In: *Neural Regulation of Brain Circulation*, edited by C. Owman and J. E. Hardebo, pp. 371–381. Elsevier, Amsterdam, 1986.
12. Bredt, D. S., Hwang, P. M., and Snyder, S. H. Localization of nitric oxide synthase indicating a neural role for nitric oxide. Nature *347:* 768–770, 1990.
13. Britton, S. L., Lutherer, L. O., and Davies, D. G. Effect of cerebral extracellular fluid acidity on total and regional cerebral blood flow. J. Appl. Physiol. *47:* 818–826, 1979.
14. Chan, P. H., and Fishman, R. A. Transient formation of superoxide radicals in polyunsaturated fatty acid-induced brain swelling. J. Neurochem. *35:* 1004–1007, 1980.
15. Chien, S., Vsami, S., Taylor, H. M., *et al.* Effects of hematocrit and plasma proteins on human blood rheology at low shear rates. J. Appl. Physiol. *21:* 81–87, 1966.
16. Choi, D. W., Maulucci-Gedde, M. A., and Kriegstein, A. R. Glutamate neurotoxicity in cortical cell culture. J. Neurosci. *7:* 357–368, 1987.
17. Compton, M. R. Intracerebral haematoma complicating ruptured cerebral berry aneurysm. J. Neurol. Neurosurg. Psychiatry *25:* 378–386, 1962.
18. Conner, R. C. Heart damage associated with intracranial lesions. Br. Med. J. *3:* 29–31, 1968.
19. Deshpande, J. K., Siesjö, B. K., and Wieloch, T. Calcium accumulation and neuronal damage in the rat hippocampus following cerebral ischemia. J. Cereb. Blood Flow Metab. *7:* 89–95, 1987.
20. Dinterfass, L. *Blood Microrheology: Viscosity Factors in Blood Flow, Ischemia, and Thrombosis.* Appleton-Century-Crofts, New York, 1971.
21. Dirnagl, U., and Pulsinelli, W. Autoregulation of cerebral blood flow in experimental focal brain ischemia. J. Cereb. Blood Flow Metab. *10:* 327–336, 1990.
22. Dóczi, T., Bende, J., Huszka, E., *et al.* Syndrome of inappropriate secretion of antidiuretic hormone after subarachnoid hemorrhage. Neurosurgery *9:* 394–397, 1981.
23. Doshi, R., and Neil-Dwyer, G. A clinicopathological study of patients following a subarachnoid hemorrhage. J. Neurosurg. *52:* 295–301, 1980.
24. Ducker, T. B., and Simmons, R. L. Increased intracranial pressure and pulmonary oedema. 2. The hemodynamic response of dogs and monkeys to increased intracranial pressure. J. Neurosurg. *28:* 118–123, 1968.
25. Ecker, A., and Reimenschneider, P. A. Arteriographic demonstration of spasm of the intracranial arteries with special reference to saccular arterial aneurysm. J. Neurosurg. *8:* 660–667, 1951.
26. Eichlin, F. Experimental vasospasm, acute and chronic, due to blood in the subarachnoid space. J. Neurosurg. *35:* 646–656, 1971.
27. Eichlin, F. A. Spasm of basilar and vertebral arteries caused by experimental subarachnoid hemorrhage. J. Neurosurg. *23:* 1–11, 1965.
28. Fabinyi, G., Hunt, D., and McKinley, L. Myocardial creatine kinase isoenzyme in serum after subarachnoid hemorrhage. J. Neurol. Neurosurg. Psychiatry *40:* 818–820, 1977.
29. Faraci, F. M. Role of nitric oxide in regulation of basilar artery tone *in vivo.* Am. J. Physiol. *259:* H1216–H1221, 1990.
30. Faraci, F. M. Role of endothelium-derived relaxing factor in cerebral circulation: large arteries vs. microcirculation. Am. J. Physiol. *261:* H1038–H1042, 1991.
31. Faraci, F. M., and Heistad, D. D. Regulation of large cerebral arteries and cerebral microvascular pressure. Circ. Res. *66:* 8–17, 1990.
32. Findlay, J. M., Weir, B. K., Kassell, N. F., *et al.* Intracisternal recombinant tissue plasminogen activator after aneurysmal subarachnoid hem-

orrhage. J. Neurosurg. *75:* 181–188, 1991.

33. Findlay, J. M., Weir, B. K. A., Kanamaru, K., *et al.* Arterial wall changes in cerebral vasospasm. Neurosurgery *25:* 736–746, 1989.

34. Fishman, R. A. Brain edema. Physiol. Med. *293:* 706–711, 1975.

35. Flamm, E. S., Demopoulos, H. B., Seligman, M. L., *et al.* Free radicals in cerebral ischemia. Stroke *9:* 445–447, 1978.

36. Fox, J. L., Falik, J. L., and Shalhoub, R. J. Neurosurgical hyponatremia: the role of inappropriate antidiuresis. J. Neurosurg. *34:* 506–514, 1971.

37. Fraser, R. A. R., Stein, B. M., Barret, R. E., *et al.* Noradrenergic mediation of experimental cerebrovascular spasm. Stroke *1:* 356–362, 1970.

38. Fujita, Y., Shingu, T., Yamada, K., *et al.* Noxious free radicals derived from oxyhemoglobin as a cause of prolonged vasospasm. Neurol. Med. Chir. (Tokyo) *20:* 137–144, 1980.

39. Furchgott, R. F., and Zawadzky, J. V. The obligatory role of endothelial cells in the relaxation of arterial smooth muscle by acetylcholine. Nature *288:* 373–376, 1980.

40. Gaehtgens, P., and Marx, P. Hemorheological aspects of the pathophysiology of cerebral ischemia. J. Cereb. Blood Flow Metab. *7:* 259–265, 1987.

41. Garcia-Uria, J., Hoff, J. T., Miranda, S., *et al.* Experimental neurogenic pulmonary edema. 2. The role of cardiopulmonary pressure changes. J. Neurosurg. *54:* 632–636, 1981.

42. Gardiner, S. M., Compton, A. M., Bennett, T., *et al.* Control of regional blood flow by endothelium-derived nitric oxide. Hypertension *15:* 486–492, 1990.

43. Garthwaite, J. Glutamate, nitric oxide and cell-cell signalling in the nervous system. Trends Neurosci. *14:* 60–67, 1991.

44. Garthwaite, J., Charles, S. L., and Chess-Williams, R. Endothelium-derived relaxing factor release on activation of NMDA receptors suggests role as intercellular messenger in the brain. Nature *336:* 385–388, 1988.

45. Gastaut, H., Roger, J., Ouahchi, S., *et al.* Generalized convulsive seizures without local onset. In: *Handbook of Clinical Neurology,* edited by P. J. Vinken and G. W. Bruyn, pp. 107–129. American Elsevier, New York, 1974.

46. Gibbs, J. M., Wise, R. J. S., Leenders, K. L., *et al.* Cerebral haemodynamics in occlusive carotid-artery disease. Lancet *1:* 933–934, 1985.

47. Graff-Radford, N. R., Torner, J., Adams, H. P., Jr., *et al.* Factors associated with hydrocephalus after subarachnoid hemorrhage: a report of the Cooperative Aneurysm Study. Arch. Neurol. *46:* 744–752, 1989.

48. Greenberg, J., Hand, P., Sylvestro, A., *et al.* Localized metabolic-flow couple during functional activity. Acta. Neurol. Scand. *72:* 12–13, 1979.

49. Grotta, J., Ackerman, R., Correia, J., *et al.* Whole blood viscosity parameters and cerebral blood flow. Stroke *13:* 296–301, 1982.

50. Grubb, R. L., Jr., Raichle, M. E., Eichling, J. O., *et al.* Effects of subarachnoid hemorrhage on cerebral blood volume, blood flow, and oxygen utilization in humans. J. Neurosurg. *46:* 446–453, 1977.

51. Haining, J. L., Clower, B. R., Honma, Y., *et al.* Accumulation of intimal platelets in cerebral arteries following experimental subarachnoid hemorrhage in cats. Stroke *19:* 898–902, 1988.

52. Hansen, A. J. Extracellular potassium concentration in juvenile and adult rat brain cortex during anoxia. Acta Physiol. Scand. *99:* 412–420, 1977.

53. Hansen, A. J. Effects of anoxia on ion distribution in the brain. Physiol. Rev. *65:* 101–148, 1985.

54. Harada, T., and Mayberg, M. R. Inhibition of delayed arterial narrowing by the iron-chelating agent deferoxamine. J. Neurosurg. *77:* 763–767, 1992.

55. Harper, A. M. Autoregulation of cerebral blood flow: influence of the arterial blood pressure on the blood flow through the cerebral cortex. J. Neurol. Neurosurg. Psychiatry *29:* 398–403, 1966.

56. Harries, A. D. Subarachnoid hemorrhage and the electrocardiogram: a review. Postgrad. Med. J. *57:* 294–296, 1981.

57. Hart, R. G., Byer, J. A., Slaughter, J. R., *et al.* Occurrence and implications of seizures in subarachnoid hemorrhage due to ruptured intracranial aneurysms. Neurosurgery *8:* 417–421, 1981.

58. Hasan, D., Vermeulen, M., Wijdicks, E. F., *et al.* Management problems in acute hydrocephalus after subarachnoid hemorrhage. Stroke *20:* 747–753, 1989.

59. Hasan, K., and Tanghe, H. L. Distribution of cisternal blood in patients with acute hydrocephalus after subarachnoid hemorrhage. Ann. Neurol. *31:* 374–378, 1992.

60. Heilbrun, M., Olesen, and Lassen, N. Regional cerebral blood flow studies in subarachnoid hemorrhage. J. Neurosurg. *37:* 36–44, 1972.

61. Heiss, W. D., Hayakawa, T., and Waltz, A. G. Cortical neuronal function during ischaemia. Arch. Neurol. *33:* 813–820, 1976.

62. Henriksen, L., Paulson, O. B., and Smith, R. J. Cerebral blood flow following normovolemic hemodilution in patients with high hematocrit. Ann. Neurol. *9:* 454–457, 1981.

63. Higashida, R. T., Halbach, V. V., Dowd, C. F., *et al.* Intravascular balloon dilatation therapy for intracranial arterial vasospasm: patient selection, technique, and clinical results. Neurosurg. Rev. *15:* 89–95, 1992.

64. Hillered, L., Smith, M.-L., and Siesjö, B. K. Lactic acidosis and recovery of mitochondrial function following forebrain ischemia in the rat. J. Cereb. Blood Flow Metab. *5:* 259–266, 1985.

65. Hino, A., Mizukawa, N., Tenjin, H., *et al.* Postoperative hemodynamic and metabolic changes in patients with subarachnoid hemorrhage. Stroke *20:* 1504–1510, 1989.

66. Hint, H. The pharmacology of dextran and the physiological background for the clinical use of Rheomacrodex. Acta Anaesthesiol. Belg. *19:* 119–138, 1968.

67. Hossmann, K. A., Sakaki, S., and Zimmerman, V. Cation activities in reversible ischemia of the cat brain. Stroke 8: 77–81, 1977.

68. Hughes, J. T., and Schianchi, P. M. Cerebral arterial spasm: a histologic study at necropsy of the blood vessels in cases of subarachnoid hemorrhage. J. Neurosurg. 48: 515–525, 1978.

69. Humphrey, P. R. D., DuBoulay, G. H., Marshall, J., et al. Cerebral blood flow and viscosity in relative polycythaemia. Lancet 2: 873–878, 1979.

70. Hunt, W. E., and Hess, R. M. Surgical risks as related to time of intervention in the repair of intracranial aneurysms. J. Neurosurg. 28: 14–20, 1968.

71. Irvine, R. F. Calcium transients: mobilization of intracellular Ca^{2+}. Br. Med. Bull. 42: 369–374, 1986.

72. Ishii, R. Regional cerebral blood flow in patients with ruptured intracranial aneurysms. J. Neurosurg. 50: 587–594, 1979.

73. Ito, U., Spatz, M., Walker, J. J., et al. Experimental cerebral ischemia in Mongolian gerbils. I. Light microscopic observations. Acta Neuropathol. 32: 209–223, 1975.

74. Jackson, J. H. Case of tumour of the middle lobe of the cerebellum: rigidity in cerebellar attitude. Br. Med. J. 2: 528–529, 1871.

75. Jakubowski, J., Bell, B. A., Symon, L., et al. A primate model of subarachnoid hemorrhage: change in regional cerebral blood flow, autoregulation, carbon dioxide reactivity, and central conduction time. Stroke 13: 601–611, 1982.

76. Jones, T. H., Morawetz, R. B., Crowell, R. M., et al. Thresholds of focal cerebral ischemia in awake monkeys. J. Neurosurg. 54: 773–782, 1981.

77. Kågström, E., Smith, M.-L., and Siesjö, B. K. Recirculation in rat brain following incomplete ischemia. J. Cereb. Blood Flow Metab. 3: 183–192, 1983.

78. Kalimo, H., Rehncrona, S., Söderfeldt, B., et al. Brain lactic acidosis and ischemic cell damage. 2. Histopathology. J. Cereb. Blood Flow Metab. 1: 313–327, 1981.

79. Kamiya, K., Kuyama, H., and Symon, L. An experimental study of the acute stage of subarachnoid hemorrhage. J. Neurosurg. 59: 917–924, 1983.

80. Kassel, N. F., Saski, T., Colohan, A. R. T., et al. Cerebral vasospasm following aneurysmal subarachnoid hemorrhage. Stroke 16: 562–572, 1985.

81. Kassel, N. F., Torner, J. C., Haley, E. C., et al. The International Cooperative Study on the Timing of Aneurysm Surgery. I. Overall management results. J. Neurosurg. 73: 18–36, 1990.

82. Kassel, N. F., Torner, J. C., Jane, J. A., et al. The International Cooperative Study on the Timing of Aneurysm Surgery. II. Surgical results. J. Neurosurg. 73: 37–47, 1990.

83. Kee, D. B., Jr., and Wood, J. H. Blood viscosity and cerebral blood flow. In: Cerebrovascular Diseases: 14th Princeton-Williamsburg Conference, edited by F. Plum and W. A. Pulsinelli, pp. 107–177. Raven Press, New York, 1985.

84. Kibler, R. F., Couch, R. S. C., and Crompton, M. R. Hydrocephalus in the adult following spontaneous subarachnoid haemorrhage. Brain 84: 45–61, 1961.

85. Kirino, T. Delayed neuronal death in gerbil hippocampus following ischemia. Brain Res. 239: 57–69, 1982.

86. Klahr, S., and Rodriguez, H. J. Natriuretic hormone. Nephron 15: 387–408, 1975.

87. Knowles, R. G., Palacios, M. R., Palmer, M. J., et al. Formation of nitric oxide from L-arginine in the central nervous system: a transduction mechanism for stimulation of the soluble guanylate cyclase. Proc. Natl. Acad. Sci. USA 86: 5159–5162, 1989.

88. Knudsen, F., Jensen, H. P., and Peterson, P. L. Neurogenic pulmonary edema: treatment with dobutamine. Neurosurgery 29: 269–270, 1991.

89. Kolin, A., and Norris, J. Myocardial damage from acute cerebral lesions. Stroke 15: 990–993, 1984.

90. Koskelo, P., Punsar, S., and Sipila, W. Subendocardial haemorrhage and ECG changes in intracranial bleeding. Br. Med. J. 1: 1479–1480, 1964.

91. Kosteljanetz, M. CSF dynamics in patients with subarachnoid and/or intraventricular hemorrhage. J. Neurosurg. 60: 940–946, 1984.

92. Kozniewska, E., Oseka, M., and Stys, T. Effects of endothelium-derived nitric oxide on cerebral circulation during normoxia and hypoxia in the rat. J. Cereb. Blood Flow Metab. 12: 311–317, 1992.

93. Lagerkranser, M., Pehrsson, K., and Sylvén, C. Neurogenic pulmonary oedema: a review of the pathophysiology with clinical and therapeutic implications. Acta Med. Scand. 212: 267–271, 1982.

94. Lassen, N. A. Cerebral blood flow and oxygen consumption in man. Physiol. Rev. 39: 183–238, 1959.

95. Lebrun-Grandié, P., Baron, J. C., Soussaline, F., et al. Coupling between regional blood flow and oxygen utilization in the normal human brain: a study with positron tomography and oxygen 15. Arch. Neurol. 40: 230–236, 1983.

96. Little, J. R., Blomquist, G. A. J., and Ethier, R. Intraventricular hemorrhage in adults. Surg. Neurol. 8: 143–149, 1977.

97. Lundberg, N. Continuous recording and control of ventricular fluid pressure in neurosurgical practice. Acta Psychiatr. Scand. Suppl. 149: 1–193, 1960.

98. Macdonald, R. L., and Weir, B. K. A review of hemoglobin and the pathogenesis of cerebral vasospasm. Stroke 22: 971–982, 1991.

99. Macdonald, R. L., Weir, B. K., Grace, M. G., et al. Morphometric analysis of monkey cerebral arteries exposed in vivo to whole blood, oxyhemoglobin, methemoglobin, and bilirubin. Blood Vessels, 28: 498–510, 1991.

100. Marion, D. W., Segal, R., and Thompson, M. E. Subarachnoid hemorrhage and the heart. Neurosurgery 18: 101–106, 1986.

101. Marshall, J. The viscosity factor in cerebral ischemia. Cereb. Blood Flow Metab. *2*(suppl. 1): S47–S49, 1982.

102. Marshall, J. J., and Kontos, H. A. Endothelium-derived relaxing factors: a perspective from *in vivo* data. Hypertension *16:* 371–386, 1990.

103. Martin, W. R. W., Baker, R. P., Grubb, R. L., Jr., et al. Cerebral blood volume, blood flow, and oxygen metabolism in cerebral ischemia and subarachnoid hemorrhage: an *in vivo* study using positron emission tomography. Acta Neurochir. (Wien) *70:* 3–9, 1984.

104. Mendelow, A. D., McCalden, T. A., Hattingh, J., et al. Cerebrovascular reactivity and metabolism after subarachnoid hemorrhage in baboons. Stroke *12:* 58–65, 1981.

105. Merwarth, H. R., and Freiman, I. S. Hydrocephalus following subarachnoid hemorrhage: report of a case with pathologic study. Brooklyn Hosp. J. *1:* 149–157, 1939.

106. Messmer, K., Gornandt, L., Jesch, F., et al. Oxygen transport and tissue oxygenation during hemodilution and dextran. Adv. Exp. Med. Biol. *37:* 669–680, 1973.

107. Milhorat, T. H. Acute hydrocephalus after aneurysmal subarachnoid hemorrhage. Neurosurgery *20:* 15–20, 1987.

108. Mohr, G., Ferguson, G., Khan, M., et al. Intraventricular hemorrhage from ruptured aneurysm: retrospective analysis of 91 cases. J. Neurosurg. *58:* 482–487, 1983.

109. Moncada, S., Palmer, R. M. J., and Higgs, E. A. The discovery of nitric oxide as endogenous nitrovasodilator. Hypertension *12:* 365–372, 1988.

110. Morawetz, R. B., Crowell, R. H., DeGirolami, U., et al. Regional cerebral blood flow thresholds during cerebral ischemia. Fed. Proc. *38:* 2493–2494, 1979.

111. Morawetz, R. B., DeGirolami, U., Ojemann, R. G., et al. Cerebral blood flow determined by hydrogen clearance during middle cerebral artery occlusion in unanesthetized monkeys. Stroke *9:* 143–149, 1978.

112. Murphy, S., Minor, R. L. J., Welk, G., et al. Evidence for an astrocyte derived vasorelaxing factor with properties similar to nitric oxide. J. Neurochem. *55:* 349–351, 1990.

113. Nagy, Z., Szabo, M., and Huttner, I. Blood-brain barrier impairment by low buffer perfusion via the internal carotid artery in rat. Acta Neuropathol. (Berl.) *68:* 160–163, 1985.

114. Nelson, P. B., Seif, S. M., Maroon, J. C., et al. Hyponatremia in intracranial disease: perhaps not the syndrome of inappropriate secretion of antidiuretic hormone (SIADH). J. Neurosurg. *55:* 938–941, 1981.

115. Nelson, P. B., Seif, S. M., Robinson, A. G., et al. Increased secretion of antidiuretic hormone in patients with intracranial aneurysms. Stroke *8:* 13, 1977.

116. Newell, D. W., Eskridge, J., Mayberg, M., et al. Endovascular treatment of intracranial aneurysms and cerebral vasospasm. Clin. Neurosurg. *39:* 348–360, 1992.

117. Norenberg, M. D., Leslie, K. O., and Robertson, A. S. Association between rise in serum sodium and CPM. Ann. Neurol. *11:* 128–135, 1982.

118. Okamoto, S. Experimental study of cerebral vasospasm: biochemical analysis of vasoconstrictor in the red blood cell hemolysate and the mechanism of action. Arch. Jpn. Chir. *51:* 93–103, 1982.

119. Oldendorf, W., Braun, L., and Cornford, E. pH dependence of blood-brain barrier permeability to lactate and nicotine. Stroke *10:* 577–581, 1979.

120. Olesen, J. Quantitative evaluation of normal and pathologic cerebral blood flow regulation to perfusion pressure. Arch. Neurol. *28:* 143–149, 1973.

121. Olesen, J. *Cerebral Blood Flow, Methods for Measurement, Regulation, Effects of Drugs and Changes in Disease.* Copenhagen, Foreningen af danske Laegestuderendes Forlag, 1974.

122. Olney, J. W., Ho, O. L., and Rhee, V. Cytotoxic effects of acidic and sulfur containing amino acids on the infant mouse central nervous system. Exp. Brain Res. *14:* 61–76, 1971.

123. Olney, J. W., Rhee, V., and Ho, O. L. Kainic acid: a powerful neurotoxic analogue of glutamate. Brain Res. *77:* 507–512, 1974.

124. Olsen, T. S., Larsen, B., Herning, M., et al. Blood flow and vascular reactivity in collaterally perfused brain tissue: evidence of an ischemic penumbra in patients with acute stroke. Stroke *14:* 332–341, 1983.

125. Ott, E. O., Ladurner, G., and Elchner, H. Relationship between disturbed rheological properties and cerebral hemodynamics in recent cerebral infarction. Prog. Biochem. Pharmacol. *13:* 349–371, 1982.

126. Park, B. E. Spontaneous subarachnoid hemorrhage complicated by communicating hydrocephalus: ϵ-amino caproic acid as a possible predisposing factor. Surg. Neurol. *11:* 73–80, 1979.

127. Paulson, O. B. Pathogenesis, pathophysiology and therapy as illustrated by regional blood flow measurements in the brain. Stroke *2:* 327–360, 1971.

128. Paulson, O. B., Olesen, J., and Christensen, M. S. Restoration of autoregulation of cerebral blood flow by hypocapnia. Neurology *22:* 286–293, 1972.

129. Peerless, S. J., and Yasargil, M. G. Adrenergic innervation of the cerebral blood vessels in the rabbit. J. Neurosurg. *35:* 148–154, 1971.

130. Peters, J. P., Welt, L. G., Sims, E. A. H., et al. A salt-wasting syndrome associated with cerebral disease. Trans. Assoc. Am. Physicians *63:* 57–64, 1950.

131. Petruck, K. C., Weir, B. K., Overton, T. R., et al. The effect of graded hypocapnia and hypercapnia on regional cerebral blood flow and cerebral vessel caliber in the rhesus monkey: study of cerebral hemodynamics following subarachnoid hemorrhage and traumatic internal carotid spasm. Stroke *5:* 230–246, 1974.

132. Phillips, L. H., II, Whisnant, J. P., O'Fallon, W.

M., *et al.* The unchanging pattern of subarachnoid hemorrhage in a community. Neurology *30:* 1034–1040, 1980.

133. Pollick, C., Bibiana, C., Parker, S., *et al.* Left ventricular wall motion abnormalities in subarachnoid hemorrhage: an echocardiographic study. J. Am. Coll. Cardiol. *12:* 600–605, 1988.

134. Powers, W. J. Cerebral hemodynamics in ischemic cerebrovascular disease. Ann. Neurol. *29:* 231–240, 1991.

135. Powers, W. J., Grubb, R. L., Jr., Baker, R. P., *et al.* Regional cerebral blood flow and metabolism in reversible ischemia due to vasospasm. J. Neurosurg. *62:* 539–546, 1985.

136. Powers, W. J., and Raichle, M. E. Positron emission tomography and its application to the study of cerebrovascular disease in man. Stroke *16:* 361–376, 1985.

137. Powers, W. J., Raichle, M. E., and Grubb, R. L., Jr. Positron emission tomography to assess cerebral perfusion. Lancet *1:* 102–103, 1985.

138. Prado, R., Watson, B. D., Kuluz, J., *et al.* Endothelium-derived nitric oxide synthase inhibition: effects on cerebral blood flow, pial artery diameter and vascular morphology in rats. Stroke *23:* 1118–1124, 1992.

139. Pulsinelli, W. A., and Brierley, J. B. A new model for bilateral hemispheric ischemia in an unanesthetized rat. Stroke *10:* 267–272, 1979.

140. Pulsinelli, W. A., Brierley, J. B., and Plum, F. Temporal profile of neuronal damage in a model of transient forebrain ischemia. Ann. Neurol. *11:* 499–509, 1982.

141. Pulsinelli, W. A., Waldman, S., Rawlinson, D., *et al.* Moderate hyperglycemia augments ischemic brain damage: a neuropathological study in the rat. Neurology *32:* 1239–1246, 1982.

142. Raichle, M. E. The pathophysiology of brain ischemia. Ann. Neurol. *13:* 2–10, 1983.

143. Reis, D. J. Central neural control of cerebral circulation and metabolism. In: *Neurotransmitters and the Cerebral Circulation*, edited by E. T. MacKenzie, J. Seylaz, and A. Best, pp. 91–119. Raven Press, New York, 1984.

144. Reis, D. J., and Iadecola, C. Central neurogenic regulation of cerebral blood flow. In: *Neurotransmission and Cerebrovascular Function II*, edited by J. Seylaz and R. Sercombe, pp. 369–390. Elsevier, Amsterdam, 1989.

145. Reis, D. J., Iadecola, C., and Nakai, M. Control of cerebral blood flow and metabolism by intrinsic neural systems in brain. In: *Cerebrovascular Diseases: 14th Princeton-Williamsburg Conference*, edited by F. Plum and W. A. Pulsinelli, pp. 1–22. Raven Press, New York, 1985.

146. Reynolds, A. F., and Shaw, C. M. Bleeding patterns from ruptured intracranial aneurysms: an autopsy series of 205 patients. Surg. Neurol. *15:* 232–235, 1981.

147. Reynolds, R. W. Pulmonary edema as a consequence of hypothalamic lesions in rats. Science *141:* 930–932, 1963.

148. Richardson, J. C., and Hyland, H. H. Intracranial aneurysms: a clinical and pathological study of subarachnoid hemorrhage and intracerebral hemorrhage caused by berry aneurysms. Medicine *20:* 1–83, 1941.

149. Robertson, E. G. Cerebral lesions due to intracranial aneurysms. Brain *72:* 150–161, 1949.

150. Rose, C. F., and Sarner, M. Epilepsy after ruptured intracranial aneurysm. Br. Med. J. *1:* 18–21, 1965.

151. Rosenberg, G. A., Kyner, W. T., and Estrada, E. Bulk flow of brain interstitial fluid under normal and hyperosmolar conditions. Am. J. Physiol. *238:* F42–F49, 1980.

152. Rosenblum, W. I., Nishimura, H., and Nelson, G. H. Endothelium-dependent L-Arg and L-NMMA-sensitive mechanisms regulate tone of brain microvessels. Am. J. Physiol. *259:* H1396–H1401, 1990.

153. Sakaki, S., Ohta, S., Nakamura, H., *et al.* Free radical reaction and biological defense mechanism in the pathogenesis of prolonged vasospasm in experimental subarachnoid hemorrhage. J. Cereb. Blood Flow Metab. *8:* 1–8, 1988.

154. Sakuta, S. Blood filterability in cerebrovascular disorders, with special reference to erythrocyte deformability and ATP content. Stroke *12:* 824–827, 1981.

155. Sano, K., Asano, T., Tanishima, T., *et al.* Lipid peroxidation as a cause of cerebral vasospasm. Neurol. Res. *2:* 253–272, 1980.

156. Sasaki, T., Asano, T., and Sano, K. Cerebral vasospasm and free radical reactions. Neurol. Med. Chir. (Tokyo) *20:* 145–153, 1980.

157. Schmid-Schönbein, H. Macrorheology and microrheology of blood in cerebrovascular insufficiency. Eur. Neurol. *6:* 242–246, 1983.

158. Schmidt, D. F., and Pierson, J. C. The intrinsic regulation of the blood vessels of the medulla oblongata. Am. J. Physiol. *108:* 241–263, 1934.

159. Schneck, S. A. On the relationship between ruptured intracranial aneurysm and cerebral infarction. Neurology *14:* 691–702, 1964.

160. Schousboe, A. Transport and metabolism of glutamate and GABA in neurons and glial cells. Int. Rev. Neurobiol. *22:* 1–45, 1981.

161. Seylaz, J., Hara, H., Pinard, E., *et al.* Effect of stimulation of the sphenopalatine ganglion on cortical blood flow in the rat. J. Cereb. Blood Flow Metab. *8:* 875–878, 1988.

162. Siesjö, B. K. Cell damage in the brain: a speculative synthesis. J. Cereb. Blood Flow Metab. *1:* 155–185, 1981.

163. Siesjö, B. K. Cerebral circulation and metabolism. J. Neurosurg. *60:* 883–908, 1984.

164. Siesjö, B. K. Influence of acidosis in lipid peroxidation in brain tissue *in vitro*. J. Cereb. Blood Flow Metab. *5:* 253–258, 1985.

165. Siesjö, B. K. Acidosis and ischemic brain damage. Neurochem. Pathol. *9:* 31–88, 1988.

166. Siesjö, B. K. Historical overview: calcium, ischemia, and death of brain cells. Ann. NY Acad. Sci. *522:* 638–661, 1988.

167. Siesjö, B. K. Pathophysiology and treatment of focal cerebral ischemia. I. Pathophysiology. J. Neurosurg. *77:* 169–184, 1992.

168. Siesjö, B. K. Pathophysiology and treatment of

focal ischemia. II. Mechanisms of damage and treatment. J. Neurosurg. *77:* 337–354, 1992.

169. Siesjö, B. K., and Bengtsson, F. Calcium fluxes, calcium antagonists, and calcium-related pathology in brain ischemia, hypoglycemia, and spreading depression: a unifying hypothesis. J. Cereb. Blood Flow Metab. *9:* 127–140, 1989.

170. Siesjö, B. K., and Wieloch, T. Cerebral metabolism in ischemia: neurochemical basis for therapy. Br. J. Anaesth. *57:* 47–62, 1985.

171. Sinar, E. J., Mendelow, A. D., Graham, D. I., *et al.* Experimental intracerebral haemorrhage: effects of a temporary mass lesion. J. Neurosurg. *66:* 568–576, 1987.

172. Smith, R. R., Clower, B. R., Grotendorst, G. M., *et al.* Arterial wall changes in early human vasospasm. Neurosurgery *16:* 171–176, 1985.

173. Spallone, A., and Gagliardi, F. M. Hydrocephalus following aneurysmal SAH. Zentralbl. Neurochir. *44:* 141–150, 1983.

174. Stavraky, G. W. Response of cerebral blood vessels to electrical stimulation of the thalamus and hypothalamic regions. Arch. Neurol. Psychiatry *35:* 1002–1028, 1936.

175. Steele, J. A., Stockbridge, N., Malijkovic, G., *et al.* Free radicals mediate actions of oxyhemoglobin on cerebrovascular smooth muscle cells. Circ. Res. *68:* 416–423, 1991.

176. Stehbens, W. E. Aneurysms and anatomical variations of cerebral arteries. Arch. Pathol. *75:* 45–64, 1963.

177. Strandgaard, S., Olesen, J., Shinhoj, E., *et al.* Autoregulation of brain circulation in severe arterial hypertension. Br. Med. J. *1:* 507–510, 1973.

178. Strang, R. R., Tovi, D., and Hugosson, R. Subdural hematomas resulting from the rupture of intracranial arterial aneurysms. Acta Chir. Scand. *121:* 345–350, 1961.

179. Sundaram, M. B. M., and Chow, F. Seizures associated with spontaneous subarachnoid hemorrhage. Can. J. Neurol. Sci. *13:* 229–231, 1986.

180. Sutton, L. N., McLaughlin, A. C., Dante, S., *et al.* Cerebral venous oxygen content as a measure of brain energy metabolism with increased intracranial pressure and hyperventilation. J. Neurosurg. *73:* 927–932, 1990.

181. Suzuki, J. Cerebral vasospasm: prediction, prevention and protection. In: *Cerebral Aneurysms. Advances in Diagnosis and Therapy*, edited by H. W. Pia, C. Langmaid, and J. Zierski, pp. 155–161. Springer, Berlin, 1979.

182. Symon, L., Branston, N. M., and Strong, A. J. Autoregulation in acute focal ischemia: an experimental study. Stroke *7:* 547–554, 1976.

183. Symon, L., Pasztor, E., and Branston, N. M. The distribution and density of reduced cerebral blood flow following acute middle cerebral artery occlusion: an experimental study by the technique of hydrogen clearance in baboons. Stroke *5:* 355–364, 1974.

184. Szabo, M. D., Crosby, G., Hurford, W. E., *et al.* Myocardial perfusion following acute subarachnoid hemorrhage in patients with an abnormal electrocardiogram. Anesth. Analg. *76:* 253–258, 1993.

185. Takaku, A., Tanaka, S., Mori, T., *et al.* Postoperative complications in 1,000 cases of intracranial aneurysms. Surg. Neurol. *12:* 137–144, 1979.

186. Takei, F., Shapiro, K., Hirano, A., *et al.* Influence of the rate of ventricular enlargement on the ultrastructural morphology of the white matter in experimental hydrocephalus. Neurosurgery *21:* 645–650, 1987.

187. Theodore, J., and Robin, E. D. Speculations on neurogenic pulmonary edema. Am. Rev. Respir. Dis. *113:* 405–411, 1976.

188. Thomas, D. J. Whole blood viscosity and cerebral blood flow. Stroke *13:* 285–287, 1982.

189. Thomas, D. J., DuBoulay, G. H., Marshall, J., *et al.* Effect of haematocrit on cerebral blood flow in man. Lancet *2:* 941–943, 1977.

190. Toda, N., and Okamura, T. Mechanism underlying the response to vasodilator nerve stimulation in isolated dog and monkey cerebral arteries. Am. J. Physiol. *259:* H1511–H1517, 1990.

191. Tu, Y. K., Heros, R. C., Candia, G., *et al.* Isovolemic hemodilution in experimental focal cerebral ischemia. 2. Effects on regional cerebral blood flow and size of infarction. J. Neurosurg. *69:* 72–81, 1988.

192. Tuor, U. I., Kelly, P. A. T., Tatemoto, K., *et al.* Neuropeptide Y and the cerebral circulation. In: *Neural Regulation of Brain Circulation*, edited by C. Owman and J. E. Hardebo, pp. 333–354. Elsevier, Amsterdam, 1986.

193. Van Gijn, J., Hijdra, A., Wijdicks, E. F. M., *et al.* Acute hydrocephalus after aneurysmal subarachnoid hemorrhage. J. Neurosurg. *63:* 355–362, 1985.

194. Van Gilder, J. C., and Torner, J. C. Subarachnoid hemorrhage: patients with severe neurologic deficit. In: *Aneurysmal Subarachnoid Hemorrhage: Report of the Cooperative Study*, edited by A. L. Sahs, D. W. Nibbelink, and J. C. Torner, pp. 349–361. Urban and Schwarzenberg, Baltimore, 1981.

195. Voldby, B., Enevoldsen, E. M., and Jensen, F. T. Cerebrovascular reactivity in patients with ruptured intracranial aneurysms. J. Neurosurg. *62:* 59–67, 1985.

196. Voldby, B., Enevoldsen, E. M., and Jensen, F. T. Regional CBF, intraventricular pressure and cerebral metabolism in patients with ruptured intracranial aneurysms. J. Neurosurg. *62:* 48–58, 1985.

197. von Santha, K., and Cipriani, A. Focal alterations in subcortical circulation resulting from stimulation of the cerebral cortex. Res. Publ. Assoc. Nerv. Ment. Dis. *18:* 346–357, 1937.

198. Wahl, M., Deetjen, P., Thurau, K., *et al.* Micropuncture evaluation of the importance of perivascular pH for the arteriolar diameter on the brain surface. Pfleugers Arch. *316:* 152–163, 1970.

199. Walton, J. N. The electroencephalographic sequelae of spontaneous subarachnoid haemor-

rhage. Electroencephalogr. Clin. Neurophysiol. *5:* 41–52, 1953.

200. Watson, B. D., and Ginsberg, M. D. Ischemic injury in the brain: role of oxygen radical-mediated processes. Ann. NY Acad. Sci. *559:* 269–281, 1989.

201. Weir, B. The effect of clot removal on cerebral vasospasm. Neurosurg. Clin. N. Am. *1:* 377–385, 1990.

202. Weir, B., Menon, D., and Overton, T. Regional cerebral blood flow in patients with aneurysms: estimation by xenon-133 inhalation. Can. J. Neurol. Sci. *5:* 301–305, 1978.

203. Weir, B., Myules, T., Kahn, M., *et al.* Management of acute subdural hematomas from aneurysmal rupture. Can. J. Neurol. Sci. *11:* 371–376, 1984.

204. Weir, B., Rothberg, C., Grace, M., *et al.* Relative prognostic significance of vasospasm following subarachnoid hemorrhage. Can. J. Neurol. Sci. *2:* 109–114, 1975.

205. Weir, B. K. Pulmonary edema following fatal aneurysm rupture. J. Neurosurg. *49:* 502–507, 1978.

206. Whittam, R. The dependence of the respiration of brain cortex on active cation transport. Biochem. J. *82:* 205–212, 1962.

207. Wieloch, T., and Siesjö, B. K. Ischemic brain injury: the importance of calcium, lipolytic activities, and free fatty acids. Pathol. Biol. (Paris) *30:* 269–277, 1982.

208. Wilkins, R. H., and Levitt, P. Intracranial arterial spasm in the dog: a chronic experimental model. J. Neurosurg. *29:* 121–134, 1970.

209. Wise, B. L. Syndrome of inappropriate antidiuretic hormone secretion after spontaneous subarachnoid hemorrhage: a reversible cause of clinical deterioration. Neurosurgery *3:* 412–414, 1978.

210. Wood, J. H., and Kee, D. B., Jr. Hemorheology of the cerebral circulation in stroke. Stroke *16:* 765–772, 1985.

211. Wood, J. H., Simeone, F. A., Fink, E. A., *et al.* Hypervolemic hemodilution in experimental focal cerebral ischemia: elevation of cardiac output, regional cortical blood flow, and ICP after intravascular volume expansion and low molecular weight dextran. J. Neurosurg. *59:* 500–509, 1983.

212. Yoshida, S., Ikeda, M., Busto, R., *et al.* Cerebral phosphoinositide, triacylglycerol, and energy metabolism in reversible ischemia: origin and fate of free fatty acids. J. Neurochem. *47:* 744–757, 1986.

Timing of Operation for Ruptured Aneurysms: Early Surgery

H. HUNT BATJER, M.D.

INTRODUCTION

Despite decades of clinical experience with subarachnoid hemorrhage (SAH) in which accurate diagnosis was possible during life and >20 years of work during which microsurgical techniques have been applied to aneurysm patients, persistent uncertainty and controversy continue to surround the issue of surgical timing following SAH. Over the years the relative importance of rebleeding and delayed ischemia, as well as the other common complications of aneurysm rupture, has been studied carefully and the chief issues well clarified. Yet, despite the availability of this accurate epidemiological and pathophysiological information, no clear optimal medical and surgical strategy for individual patients has emerged and we continue to lose more than one half of the victims of this catastrophic form of cerebrovascular disease. The societal importance of this problem is magnified by the fact that the peak incidence of SAH is substantially earlier in life than that of thrombo-occlusive stroke, thus eliminating many productive years from the lives of these unfortunate people.

Perhaps the persistent disagreement among neurosurgeons regarding whether early or late surgery is most beneficial relates in large measure to the profound heterogeneity of the SAH population. Marked clinical diversity is the rule in terms of the medical and neurological condition of the patients, in addition to the substantial im-

pact of age, particularly regarding the very young or very elderly. Anatomic diversity is also common with all severities of SAH, including the frequent presence of intraventricular or intraparenchymal hematoma. The offending aneurysm is also of paramount importance. Substantially more brain retraction and dissection are required for superiorly or posteriorly projecting anterior communicating artery aneurysms and distal basilar artery aneurysms than for proximal carotid or vertebral-pica artery aneurysms. Similarly, the technical problems are very different in treating a giant, calcific, and partially thrombotic aneurysm, compared to a 7-mm thin-walled lesion. Finally, it remains unknown whether the use of temporary arterial occlusion and resultant transient cerebral ischemia is more hazardous at any given interval after SAH.

Due to these uncertainties and in the absence of definitive information, decisions regarding the timing of intervention remain dependent on the philosophy of the individual surgeon, his own results, and a rather subjective or intuitive analysis at the bedside of individual patients and their particular circumstances. In this chapter, no attempt is made to render definitive recommendations for the timing of operation for SAH in general. Rather, existing knowledge is reviewed and individual factors and parameters which influence the decision-making process for this surgeon are discussed. It should be stated at the outset that I favor early operation (within 72 hours) for the majority of patients suffering SAH, and I attempt to offer justification for this bias when possible.

Natural History

Patients who survive their initial ictus and reach medical care after SAH face many critical days during which neurological and medical events can occur which jeopardize their survival. The most striking and dangerous of these complications include irreversible damage from the initial effects of SAH, rebleeding, and delayed ischemia from vasospasm. Since the initial damage from the hemorrhage itself cannot currently be modified, the issues of rebleeding and vasospasm are discussed in more detail. It is clear from early work with SAH that roughly 50% of aneurysms rebleed during the first 6 months, after which the rate of rebleeding drops to 3%/year (10).

Considerable prognostic information can be obtained from simply examining the patient after resuscitation. The International Cooperative Aneurysm Study demonstrated that mortality increased sharply with decreasing level of consciousness. For alert patients an 11% mortality rate was noted, while these statistics worsened for each subsequent grade: 27% for drowsy patients, 44.5% for stuporous patients, and 71.3% for comatose patients (1). In addition, the computerized tomography (CT) scan obtained on admission was found to be extremely predictive of outcome. A 5.8% mortality rate was noted when the CT scan was normal, and the risk increased to 10.3% when a local thin collection of subarachnoid blood was seen. Diffuse subarachnoid blood carried a 32.8% mortality rate and was similar in significance to local thick collections. An approximately 45% mortality rate was noted when intracerebral or intraventricular hematoma was seen, and the presence of mass effect was associated with a 42% mortality rate (1).

Rebleeding

Historically, aneurysm rebleeding was the most feared complication for SAH patients, because it carried a >50% mortality rate. The International Cooperative Aneurysm Study has clarified the risk periods for rebleeding.

morrhage. The peak risk of recurrent bleeding was found to be within the first 24 hours, when a 4.1% incidence was seen (15). After 48 hours the risk had decreased to 1.5%/day and slowly declined from that point on. The cumulative risk was 19% at day 14. When subgroups that either did or did not receive antifibrinolytic therapy were analyzed, significant findings were noted. For those not receiving antifibrinolytic agents the average daily rebleeding risk was 1.5%/day, with a cumulative 14-day risk of 26.5%. For those patients receiving antifibrinolytic agents the daily risk was 0.8% and the cumulative 14-day risk was 14.1% (15). When the final data were tabulated, however, no clear favorable impact on morbidity or mortality rates was found for the antifibrinolytic agents due to an increase in ischemic complications and, except for unique circumstances, they appear to have no definite prophylactic value in the care of SAH patients (23). The findings of the Cooperative Study regarding the incidence of rebleeding in the very early period and the failure of medical agents to modify outcome have fundamental implications for the treating surgeon.

Vasospasm

Arterial vasospasm leading to delayed cerebral ischemia remains the most significant cause of death and disability for those suffering SAH and is responsible for 14% of such adverse occurrences, while rebleeding is currently responsible for only 7% of patient loss (13). Using careful angiographic measurements in a large number of studies, Weir et al. (24) found that vasospasm had its onset at about day 3 after SAH, was maximal at days 6–8, and usually resolved by day 12. Another angiographic study showed a distinct difference between patients suffering a single SAH and those with a probable earlier first bleed. For those with a single hemorrhage the appearance of spasm was most frequently seen between days 10 and 17, with only 4.2% incidence at day 3. During the peak period 49% of patients developed vasospasm. When a history of prior hemorrhage was present, vasospasm within the first 3 days of the most recent hemorrhage was seen in 38.7% of cases and was noted in only 20% between days 10 and 17 (18).

Fisher *et al.* (6) in 1980 made a key observation of clear clinical relevance regarding the predictive importance of the initial CT scan. When the CT scan failed to demonstrate blood or only a thin layer was noted, clinical symptoms of ischemia failed to develop in any of 18 patients. When subarachnoid clots larger than 5×3 mm or cisternal layers of 1 mm or more were seen, severe angiographic spasm and clinical deficits followed in nearly every case (23 of 24 patients). Intracerebral or intraventricular blood appeared to carry no threat of delayed ischemic sequelae (6). These observations have been confirmed by numerous other investigators. Therefore, a second piece of vital information is available to the clinician, who can now quite accurately predict who will develop ischemic symptoms in the days following SAH. The types of therapy available to modify this ischemia have immediate importance for the issue of surgical timing.

The Questions Regarding Surgical Timing

In a landmark report, Hunt and Hess (8) suggested categorizing patients neurologically on admission. Early surgery in alert patients resulted in excellent results, with only 14% mortality rate. Fourteen of 15 nonsurgical deaths in good-grade patients resulted from rebleeding. Interestingly, of patients initially considered grade III, a policy of delayed surgery showed that 55% improved to a normal level of consciousness, 34% deteriorated, and only 11% remained grade III. The authors concluded that good-grade patients should be operated upon early to minimize rebleeding and that delayed surgery should be performed for those with neurological deficit, to allow time for improvement (8).

Following early pioneering efforts in which early surgery was most often emphasized, surgeons particularly in North America became disillusioned with early operation due to high surgical morbidity. It is likely that some morbidity initially attributed to the operation itself was actually due to vasospasm. As more surgeons gained expertise with microsurgical technology, however, enthusiasm returned for early operation. While surgical risk was clearly lower in patients undergoing late operation, a large number of the overall population were lost to rebleeding or vasospasm before being offered a protective procedure. Increasing emphasis on management morbidity and mortality rates, as opposed to surgical results, led to reopening of the issue of early operation both in North America and around the world (11). Kassell and Drake (11) articulated the major issues well when they stated that early operation had the following advantages: prevention of rebleeding, potential amelioration of vasospasm by removal of blood, optimization of treatment for vasospasm, ease of operation, prevention of medical complications, elimination of the psychological stress of waiting, and shorter hospital stays. Their arguments in favor of delayed surgery also had merit and included improved brain slackness, ease of dissection, opportunity to observe and study patients, flexible scheduling, and well documented excellent surgical results (11). With the goal of settling this issue, the International Cooperative Study on Timing of Aneurysm Surgery was undertaken (14, 16). While this study was essentially epidemiological in nature, because it did not require randomization to early or late surgery, it did yield a wealth of important information. Important insights gained included the importance of the initial CT scan, the pattern of rebleeding, the role of antifibrinolytic agents, and the persistent high morbidity under current treatment standards, with only 56% of patients having favorable outcomes (16). Unfortunately, neither early nor late surgery emerged as being clearly preferable. It is important, however, that early surgery did not appear to be more dangerous to the patient than late surgery, as had been passionately argued in the past.

Perhaps as a natural evolution with increasing numbers of well trained microsurgeons being in practice or as a response to the Cooperative Study, progressively more units adopted the strategy of early operation. Ljunggren *et al.* (20) reported 99 grade I-III patients who underwent acute operation; 76% recovered without neurological deficit and only 4% died. Similar results had been reported earlier from the same center, with a suggestion that early surgery with evacuation of blood from the cisterns might decrease the risk of vasospasm (19).

Disney *et al.* (5) compared the outcome of patients operated upon prior to 1978, during a policy of delayed surgery, with outcomes obtained after 1978, when early surgery was the rule. With early surgery, overall management mortality rates decreased from 47% to 38% and rates for good-grade patients decreased from 17% to 10%. In addition, patients operated upon between days 0 and 3 had better outcomes than did those operated upon later, in both periods. The authors concluded that early surgery had made a significant contribution to decreasing morbidity and mortality rates (5).

An Argument for Early Operation

The preceding discussion has considered certain disease-specific issues which argue somewhat in favor of early operation: rebleeding can be minimized and vasospasm may be modified by removal of hematoma. The following discussion considers a number of patient-specific, aneurysm-specific, and unit-specific issues that I feel are important in selecting patients who will benefit from having their aneurysm secured as early as possible after SAH.

Prevention of Rebleeding

Given that the best evidence suggests that the highest risk of rebleeding occurs in the first 48 hours and that the chances for meaningful survival after a second hemorrhage are small, the obvious conclusion would be that patients should be surgically treated within that crucial early period. In practice, however, logistics frequently preclude accomplishing this goal. Many physicians continue to feel that patients should be "stabilized" for several days before being referred to a neurosurgical center, thus preventing the neurosurgeon from having the chance to intervene early. Another critical variable, which is discussed below, concerns the local environment. In many centers weekend personnel in the neuroradiology facility and the operating room are not of the highest level, and surgeons are reluctant to subject a patient to an involved procedure without the availability of the "first team." This reluctance is absolutely justified in my opinion, because the added risk of a suboptimal procedure is much greater than the few percentage points of risk involved in waiting for 2 or 3 days. It is clear that we should better educate primary care physicians about the value of early referral and make every attempt to improve our own local environment so that early operation is a feasible option for appropriate patients.

In addition to the generalities expressed above, I believe that there are a number of circumstances that mandate every effort to secure the aneurysm early.

1. The patient with a "sentinel leak" or very minor SAH with little or no CT-evident blood has nothing to gain and everything to lose by delay in diagnosis and operation.

2. The patient, even if of poor grade, who has demonstrated repetitive SAH has a disease which, in my opinion, has declared its malignancy. These are very high-risk patients by any criteria, but a policy of waiting offers little benefit to the patient, particularly if he has a straight forward aneurysm.

3. The patient who has severe meningeal signs and is agitated by either pain or confusion has a large and dangerous catecholamine response to his illness, and the resultant hypertensive episodes can precipitate rebleeding. I feel that these patients are far better off under controlled general anesthesia than being restrained in the intensive care unit.

4. The severely hypertensive patient is at high risk for early rebleeding. Obviously every attempt should be made to control the pressure medically, but if these efforts are unsuccessful general anesthesia and aneurysm clipping may be the safest option.

5. Many "poor-grade" patients have an altered level of consciousness due to severe hydrocephalus. This complication, if severe enough to warrant early ventricular drainage, may represent an argument for early operation. The decompression associated with ventricu-

lar drainage risks de-tamponade and alteration of the transmural gradient, which may precipitate rebleeding. On the other hand, the hydrocephalus can be used operatively to gain additional space. Intraoperative ventricular puncture allows access to the basal cistern without retraction (22). Therefore, the symptomatic hydrocephalic patient may be best served by early surgical intervention.

Vasospasm

As mentioned previously, it is now possible simply to study the CT scan obtained on admission and determine quickly whether the patient is or is not at high risk for developing delayed ischemia between day 4 and day 10 after SAH (6). Once ischemic symptoms develop, the most effective treatment to date involves hyperdynamic therapy with increasing intravascular volume and arterial pressure (12, 17). Nearly three fourths of all symptomatic patients may improve with this regimen (12). The addition of hemodilution to this regimen is probably also beneficial. I have seen no convincing evidence, either published or in my personal experience, which suggests that calcium channel blockers alter the course of this disease. There is hope that endovascular techniques with angioplasty will be of benefit to some patients, but certainly hyperdynamic therapy is the first line of therapy at this time. It is not known how far these measures can be taken in a patient with an unsecured aneurysm, but I am reluctant to elevate the systolic blood pressure above 160–170 torr in that setting. Clearly, it is preferable to have the offending aneurysm secured prior to the onset of any deficit necessitating hyperdynamic therapy, thus suggesting that surgery within the first 72 hours should be performed.

Considerable work is in progress which offers substantial hope that it may be possible to prevent vasospasm by eliminating the offending spasmogens in the extravasated blood soon after SAH. Excellent documentation has been obtained, especially by Mizukami *et al.* (21), showing that surgical evacuation of the subarachnoid space at the time of aneurysm clipping prevented vasospasm (angiographic and clinical) in those targeted sites. It is clear that, to be effective, this maneuver must be accomplished by day 4. Unfortunately, it is not feasible or particularly safe to evacuate contralateral or distal sylvian cisterns. It should be mentioned, however, that conflicting opinions exist regarding the effectiveness of this aggressive approach (9).

Current hopes for prevention of vasospasm center around the efforts of Weir and his investigations with recombinant tissue plasminogen activator, which are detailed in Chap. 6C. This important emerging body of information may prove to be extremely important for those high-risk patients seen early after SAH. If further studies reinforce these initial ones, it will become difficult to justify delayed surgery.

Patient-Specific Factors

Fortunately, most of the information which is of significant benefit to the surgeon making a decision regarding surgical timing is available at the patient's bedside. Only part of this key information relates to the neurological status.

Good Grade

There are very few circumstances, in my opinion, in which the alert patient is well served by delaying surgery. Exceptions might be that very elderly patients or those in whom serious cardiac, pulmonary, renal, or hepatic disease is present should have appropriate medical consultations. This practice is certainly worthwhile for assisting these patients through their anesthesia. Of extreme pertinence is the correction of any coagulopathy as soon as possible, because of the risk of spontaneous rebleeding as well as the obvious problems at craniotomy. Similar delay is occasionally advisable for patients with complex, thrombotic, giant aneurysms, as discussed below. For otherwise medically well patients with typical anterior circulation or vertebral-pica artery aneurysms however, I strongly favor operation at the earliest time that the surgeon and team can be assembled.

Poor Grade

Poor-grade patients are much more difficult to manage, and treatment remains controversial. Winn *et al.* (26) reported results on the early surgical management of poor-grade patients, including diligent and aggressive perioperative care, which appear to represent an improvement over the natural history. Mortality rates by neurological grades in this series were as follows: grade III, 13%; grade IV, 35%; and grade V, 41%. Disney *et al.* (4) reviewed the Edmonton, Alberta, Canada, experience with poor-grade patients and found that the management mortality rate for days 0–3 was 38% and for the entire series at all times was 49%. Thus, the patients operated upon earlier tended to fare better.

My personal philosophy is that not all patients and not all aneurysms are alike and therefore I do not have a universal approach to poor-grade patients. Early operation for a posterior carotid artery wall aneurysm, an antero-inferiorly projecting anterior communicating artery aneurysm, or a pica artery aneurysm in a grade III-IV patient is an entirely different matter, compared with treatment of a difficult postero-superiorly projecting anterior communicating artery aneurysm, a basilar artery aneurysm, or a lesion at the vertebral confluens. The degree of retraction and dissection is markedly greater in the latter lesions. The lesions of the middle cerebral bifurcation or the carotid bifurcation are intermediate in difficulty between the other two groups. In general, I push to operate on the technically easy aneurysms in the very early period and wait for neurological improvement with the more difficult lesions. In general, however, I try to have the aneurysm secured in all grade III-IV patients prior to their peak risk of vasospasm, to facilitate the medical management of cerebral ischemic complications.

Extreme Youth

Very young patients present a difficult challenge, partly because so many productive years are at stake. In general, they are ideal candidates for anesthesia and they seem to recover from any given neurological insult more completely than their older cohorts. I usually try to operate upon the young patients as early as possible, even if they are of grade III or IV.

Extreme Age

Very elderly patients also present unique challenges, because they are frequently medically fragile and often have associated problems in other organ systems. It is critically important that they are fully evaluated medically and fully hydrated prior to induction of anesthesia. The demands of an aneurysm neuroanesthetic in this group of patients require a highly skilled neuroanesthesiologist or else the risk of fatal cardiac or pulmonary complications is inordinately high. In my experience, elderly fragile patients with difficult posterior circulation aneurysms have a chance for a favorable outcome only if all aspects of their anesthetic and operative procedures are flawless. For that reason, I take great care to ensure that "all bases are touched" prior to their arrival in the operating room.

The Aneurysm Itself

While all aneurysms are unique, there are certain circumstances which cause me to re-evaluate the philosophy of early surgery. As we have reported previously, distal basilar artery aneurysms, by their location, broad base, and intimate association with critical thalmoperforating arteries, are often not well served by an urgent operation (2). For the smaller lesions of the basilar bifurcation I do operate early but, if a subtemporal or half-and-half exposure is required, I am more aggressive in temporal lobe resection than I have been previously. The degree of retraction necessary is substantial and there is no morbidity associated with resection of the temporal tip or the inferior temporal gyrus. Leaving this damaged tissue behind risks postoperative swelling or hematoma. For thrombotic giant sacs in more typical locations which require significant temporary occlusion, my tendency has been to let a few days pass to optimize the surgical environment but still to offer surgery prior to the peak vasospasm risk period. This strategy is not scientifically based, however, and one could argue equally well that earlier surgery or much delayed surgery has a more rational basis to maximize hemodynamic reserve. I can only rely on my experience that the degree of brain tightness seems to dissipate somewhat within 3 or 4 days of SAH. Unfortunately, we still do not have data regarding whether temporary arterial occlusion is safer at any given time interval following hemorrhage. This information would be of great help in eliminating some of the empiricism from these management decisions in more complex aneurysms.

Intracerebral Hematoma

While neurological grading scales have been of great benefit to the clinician in assisting with decision-making for patients with diffuse SAH, the presence of a large hematoma renders these scales of questionable value. The recent Cooperative Study has demonstrated that the presence of intraparenchymal hematoma increases the management mortality rate to 43.6% (1). An interesting prospective randomized trial was conducted in this patient subgroup by Heiskanen et al. (7). Thirty patients were studied and 15 underwent emergency craniotomy. Overall, the mortality rate was 80% for the conservatively treated patients and only 27% in the surgical arm. Wheelock et al. (25) reviewed 132 patients with aneurysmal intracerebral hemorrhage and found that only 9% left the hospital without significant deficit. Of this series, 41% had evidence of herniation syndromes. In this herniation subgroup, 21% of those operated upon early survived, while all unoperated patients died. In their review, when urgent craniotomy for hematoma evacuation was performed without aneurysm clipping, 75% died. If the aneurysm was secured, however, the mortality rate dropped to 29%.

Our own experience suggests that emergency operation is indicated in this situation as long as some evidence of brainstem function remains (3). All patients rendered comatose by the hemorrhage will die if it is not decompressed. In our review, we were surprised at the actual delay imposed by preoperative evaluation and angiography. The delay for angiography may be eliminated in some cases in favor of urgent decompression and microsurgical exploration of the appropriate subarachnoid space.

Surgical Environment

Neurovascular surgery in general and aneurysm surgery in particular are critically dependent on a well coordinated and experienced team. Vital components in addition to the surgeon include neuroanesthesiology, neuroradiology, the scrub nurse, the circulating nurse, and an accomplished critical care environment. A suboptimal component in this large group gravely jeopardizes the patient's chances for a successful outcome. Therefore, the ability of any given unit to perform urgent or early surgery is not dependent solely on the surgeon. He is, however, responsible for ensuring that each component of the team is appropriately skilled (and rested) before the patient is brought to the operating room. Only for the patient *in extremis* with life-threatening hematoma should this requirement be bypassed. For most surgeons who perform early surgery, the operations are performed on the first day that the appropriate support personnel can be assembled. In our unit, a typical patient admitted Friday evening is usually operated upon Saturday morning. The surgeon must be well aware of his own functional status; particularly for the difficult aneurysm, a rested surgeon offers the patient a better chance for recovery, despite the added risk of a few hours delay, than one who is fatigued after a long day's work.

Conclusion

Despite one's individual bias or passionate philosophy regarding early, late, or intermediate surgery, our collective goal is to offer each patient the best possible chance for recovery from this catastrophic illness. I have attempted to discuss several individual considerations (although the list was certainly not complete) which I feel should be evaluated before a final decision is made. As in most aspects of neurosurgery, there are no steadfast rules or pieces of laboratory data which can make these decisions for us. In my opinion, careful study of the patient's neurological and medical status followed by review of appropriate radiographic studies and finally appraisal of the surgical environment provide the best basis for an admittedly somewhat intuitive decision.

Early aneurysm surgery is feasible and safe in skilled hands. There is little doubt in my mind that early operation is the best alternative for good- to moderate-grade patients with straightforward aneurysms. It is not overly simplistic to reason that early operation minimizes the risk of rebleeding and maximizes our capacity to prevent or treat delayed ischemia from vasospasm. The decision-making process becomes much more difficult and subjective as the status of the patient deteriorates and the complexity of the aneurysm increases.

REFERENCES

1. Adams, H. P., Kassell, M. F., and Torner, J. C. Usefulness of computed tomography in predicting outcome after aneurysmal subarachnoid hemorrhage: a preliminary report of the Cooperative Aneurysm Study. Neurology 35:1263–1267, 1985.
2. Batjer, H. H., and Samson, D. S. Causes of morbidity and mortality from surgery of aneurysms of distal basilar artery. Neurosurgery 25:904–916, 1989.
3. Batjer, H. H., and Samson, D. S. Emergent aneurysm surgery without cerebral angiography for the comatose patient. Neurosurgery 28:283–287, 1991.
4. Disney, L., Weir, B., Grace, M., and the Canadian Nimodipine Study Group. Factors influencing the outcome of aneurysm rupture in poor grade patients: a prospective series. Neurosurgery 23:1–9, 1988.
5. Disney, L., Weir, B., and Petruk, K. Effect on management mortality of a deliberate policy of early operation on supratentorial aneurysms. Neurosurgery 20:695–701, 1987.
6. Fisher, C. M., Kistler, J. P., and Davis, J. M. Relation of cerebral vasospasm to subarachnoid hemorrhage visualized by computerized tomographic scanning. Neurosurgery 6:1–9, 1980.
7. Heiskanen, O., Poranen, A., Kuurne, T., et al. Acute surgery for intracerebral hematomas caused by rupture of an intracranial arterial aneurysm: a prospective randomized study. Acta Neurochir. (Wien) 90:81–83, 1988.
8. Hunt, W. E., and Hess, R. M. Surgical risk as related to time of intervention in the repair of intracranial aneurysms. J. Neurosurg. 28:14–20, 1968.
9. Inagawa, T., Yamamoto, M., and Kamiya, K. Effect of clot removal on cerebral vasospasm. J. Neurosurg. 72:224–230, 1990.
10. Jane, J. A., Kassell, N. F., Torner, J. C., and Winn, H. R. The natural history of aneurysms and arteriovenous malformations. J. Neurosurg. 62:321–323, 1985.
11. Kassell, N. F., and Drake, C. G. Timing of aneurysm surgery. Neurosurgery 10:514–519, 1982.
12. Kassell, N. F., Peerless, S. J., Durward, Q. J., et al. Treatment of ischemic deficits from vasospasm with intravascular volume expansion and induced arterial hypertension. Neurosurgery 11:337–343, 1982.
13. Kassell, N. F., Sasaki, T., Colohan, A. R. T., and Nazar, G. Cerebral vasospasm following aneurysmal subarachnoid hemorrhage. Stroke 16:562–572, 1985.
14. Kassell, N. F., and Torner, J. C. The International Cooperative Study on Timing of Aneurysm Surgery. Acta Neurochir. (Wien) 63:119–123, 1982.
15. Kassell, N. F., and Torner, J. C. Aneurysmal rebleeding: a preliminary report from the Cooperative Aneurysm Study. Neurosurgery 13:479–481, 1983.
16. Kassell, N. F., and Torner, J. C. The International Cooperative Study on Timing of Aneurysm Surgery: an update. Stroke 15:566–570, 1984.
17. Kosnik, E. J., and Hunt, W. E. Postoperative hypertension in the management of patients with intracranial arterial aneurysms. J. Neurosurg. 45:148–154, 1976.
18. Kwak, R., Niizuma, H., Ohi, T., and Suzuki, J. Angiographic study of cerebral vasospasm following rupture of intracranial aneurysms. 1. Time of the appearance. Surg. Neurol. 11:257–262, 1979.
19. Ljunggren, B., Brandt, L., Kagstrom, E., and Sundbarg, G. Results of early operations for ruptured aneurysms. J. Neurosurg. 54:473–479, 1981.
20. Ljunggren, B., Saveland, H., Brandt, L., and Zygmunt, S. Early operation and overall outcome in aneurysmal subarachnoid hemorrhage. J. Neurosurg. 62:547–551, 1985.
21. Mizukami, M., Kawase, T., Usami, T., and Tazawa, T. Prevention of vasospasm by early operation with removal of subarachnoid blood. Neurosurgery 10:301–307, 1982.
22. Paine, J. T., Batjer, H. H., and Samson, D. S. Intraoperative ventricular puncture. Neurosurgery 22:1107–1109, 1988.
23. Weir, B. Antifibrinolytics in subarachnoid hemorrhage: do they have a role? No. Arch. Neurol. 44:116–118, 1987.
24. Weir, B., Grace, M., Hansen, J., and Rothberg, C. Time course of vasospasm in man. J. Neurosurg. 18:173–178, 1978.
25. Wheelock, B., Weir, B., Watts, R., et al. Timing of surgery for intracerebral hematomas due to aneurysm rupture. J. Neurosurg. 58:476–481, 1983.
26. Winn, H. R., Newell, D. W., Mayberg, M. R., et al. Early surgical management of poor grade patients with intracranial aneurysms. Clin. Neurosurg. 36:289–298, 1990.

Timing of Operation for Ruptured Aneurysms: Delayed Surgery

WILLIAM SHUCART, M.D., JULIAN WU, M.D.

INTRODUCTION

After Dandy's historic operation, in which he eliminated a posterior communicating artery aneurysm with a silver clip (3), neurosurgeons believed it was important to treat ruptured aneurysms as soon after a hemorrhage as possible, to prevent another bleed. Unfortunately, these pioneering neurosurgeons encountered very high patient mortality and morbidity rates. Clinical studies dealing with these issues showed that waiting 10 days or more following hemorrhage to perform surgery allowed patients to recover from the trauma of the hemorrhage and was associated with much lower mortality and morbidity rates (8, 14). Delayed surgery became fairly standard treatment for ruptured intracranial aneurysms in the late 1960s and early 1970s.

There were several likely reasons why delayed surgery improved operative results: the patient's medical condition could be stabilized; brain swelling was reduced; vasospasm, if ever present, had usually subsided; and there was decreased blood in the subarachnoid space, which facilitated surgical dissection. There were also technical advances in aneurysm surgery developed during that same time: the use of the operating microscope became fairly standard; there were significant improvements in microsurgical technique and instrumentation; and there was increased sophistication in anesthesia and available anesthetic agents. The concurrence of these advances and delaying surgery until patients were in ideal medical condition produced excellent operative results.

In the late 1970s the issue was revisited, looking at the overall rather than strictly operative management of patients with ruptured intracranial aneurysms. It was clear that patients who were operated on in a delayed fashion did extremely well, but the overall case management mortality rates for patients with ruptured aneurysms remained high. There were a number of reasons for the latter observation, including the fact that many patients never recovered well enough to be considered surgical candidates and were ultimately lost and that there were patients who, as they were recovering, rebled and died. Many drugs were evaluated during that time, with the hope of finding one which would allow the surgeon to wait a meaningful period of time after the hemorrhage with the assurance that there would not be a rehemorrhage, but none of these proved adequate (18, 20).

A major cause of poor outcomes was and is the appearance of ischemic deficits. Increasing evidence suggested that surgery in the presence of angiographic vasospasm was probably related to an increased incidence of ischemic deficits (7). It was also found that angiographic vasospasm rarely occurred prior to the third post-hemorrhage day (19). While there is no uniformly successful treatment for the prevention or treatment of delayed ischemic deficits, several techniques have been helpful, including increasing blood pressure and increasing fluid volume (16). A major concern with these therapies is that they are felt to be risky in the presence of an unclipped aneurysm.

It was postulated that early surgery, within 3 days after the hemorrhage, would address several issues. It would eliminate the aneurysm and the risk of rebleeding; it would decrease the risk of some of the anti-ischemic treatments; and it would avoid surgery when angiographic spasm was present. In many series overall mortality rates were improved. The remaining issue then became the quality of patient survival, which is still being investigated. Suffice it to say that each surgeon is biased by personal experience and there is no clear consensus on the timing of surgery for all patients with ruptured aneurysms.

Here we outline our approach to treating ruptured aneurysms and, in particular, when we consider delaying surgery. We try to correlate the studies reported in the literature, with particular emphasis on the more recent literature. We do this with the underlying assumption that there is a high quality of surgical skill being brought to bear on the treatment of intracranial aneurysms throughout the world at the present time.

INTRODUCTION

The surgeon has a say in regard to the timing of surgery only after the patient reaches the hospital. In some centers the majority of patients are admitted within minutes to hours after a hemorrhage, whereas in some referral centers patients do not reach the hospital until the second, third, or later posthemorrhage day. Our approach is that, for patients admitted within the first 3 days after a hemorrhage, the decision to operate is dependent primarily on the patient's clinical grade. If the patient's status is grade I, grade II, or grade III without significant alteration in the level of consciousness, surgery is done early. If the patient's status is poor grade III or worse, surgery is delayed until the patient clinically improves.

If the patient is admitted after the third posthemorrhage day, we use the criteria described above as well as the arteriographic findings. If there is significant vasospasm present angiographically (>50% narrowing of the lumina of major vessels), surgery is delayed regardless of the patient's clinical grade. The patient is treated with bed rest, sedation, and other standard treatments for patients with ruptured aneurysms. The arteriogram is repeated in 5–7 days. As soon as the vasospasm shows signs of subsiding, the patient is operated upon.

Preoperative Grade

The preoperative grade of the patient following subarachnoid hemorrhage is the single most important factor for us in determining the time of surgery. We rely heavily on it because it is clear that, if patients are categorized based on their level of consciousness, the presence or absence of signs of meningeal irritation, and neurological deficit, the overall case and management outcomes can be predicted (11, 12). The grading system we use is the five-tier one devised by Hunt and Hess (9) (Table 4B.1). Generally, patients of preoperative grade I or II have the most favorable outcomes following, sur-

TABLE 4B.1
Hunt and Hess Grading System for Classification of Patients with Intracranial Aneurysms According to Surgical Risk

Category[a]	Criteria
Grade I	Asymptomatic, or minimal headache and slight nuchal rigidity
Grade II	Moderate to severe headache, nuchal rigidity, and no neurological deficit other than cranial nerve palsy
Grade III	Drowsiness, confusion, or mild focal deficit
Grade IV	Stupor, moderate to severe hemiparesis, and possibly early decerebrate rigidity and vegetative disturbances
Grade V	Deep coma, decerebrate rigidity, and moribund appearance

[a] Serious systemic diseases such as hypertension, diabetes, severe arteriosclerosis, or chronic pulmonary disease, or severe vasospasm seen on arteriography, result in placement of the patient in the next less favorable category.

gery. Results from the International Cooperative Study on the timing of aneurysm surgery show that patients who are alert upon admission and undergo surgery within 2–3 days have the best overall outcomes (11, 12). Sporadic reports from independent neurosurgeons also support this conclusion (4, 10, 13). We also operate on grade I or II patients with ruptured aneurysms within the first 3 days after the subarachnoid hemorrhage. If for some reason a grade I or II patient is not seen until 3 or more days following the hemorrhage, the decision as to the time of surgery is based on the results of the arteriogram, as discussed above.

Poor grade III patients who have significant alterations in the level of consciousness are, we think, generally candidates for delayed surgery. These patients have clearly sustained significant brain insult from the hemorrhage. Our concern is that operation in the face of this compromise will add more trauma and lessen the likelihood of a complete recovery. When the patient improves surgery is performed. The International Cooperative Study showed that good recovery and improved mortality rates, as evaluated at 6-month follow-up were more likely with delayed surgery in this group (12). This advantage, however, was not statistically significant. Occasionally, patients of grade III or worse respond dramatically to cerebrospinal fluid drainage and rapidly improve to grade I or II. They are then treated as any other grade I or II patient.

Patients of clinical grade IV or V have very likely sustained irreversible brain damage and as a group have poor outcomes, with >50% mortality rates reported (11, 12). Occasionally, one of these patients has a dramatic recovery and an excellent long-term outcome. As discussed above, there may be a subgroup of these patients with acute elevation of intracranial pressure who improve with ventricular drainage. An algorithm for managing these patients based primarily on radiographic criteria was suggested by one group; it resulted in 66% fair to good outcomes at 3 months and may hold promise (1). The conflict which neurosurgeons face in these cases is the possibility of prolonging a vegetative existence, as opposed to saving someone who might have a good outcome.

Aneurysm Size

The size of the aneurysm is not a factor in determining the timing of surgery unless it is >25 mm in diameter. Aneurysms that are 25 mm in diameter or larger can pose several technical problems, including the size itself, which make the surgical dissection more difficult. In these situations there is a frequent association of intraluminal clot, which may be a problem, and the aneurysm neck can be broad-based, with important arterial branches partially incorporated into the neck or base of the dome of the aneurysm.

Eliminating these aneurysms usually requires greater than usual manipulation of the parent vessel, and long periods of temporary occlusion of involved vessels may be necessary. In these difficult large aneurysms significant brain retraction may be required, and occasionally special techniques such as arterial graft bypass, hypothermia, and less commonly extracorporeal bypass with cardiac standstill are used (17, 20). We think all of these measures are best done in an elective situation with the patient's overall medical status being as good as possible. The potential for compromise of either the brain itself or its blood supply when giant aneurysms are treated is so great that it seems best to allow the brain to recover as much as possible before definitive surgery is performed.

Location of the Aneurysm

Aneurysm location is usually irrelevant in making a decision as to the timing of surgery. A personal bias of one of the authors is related to anterior communicating artery aneurysms. If patients with anterior communicating artery aneurysms appear to be of grade I or II except for a memory deficit, the surgeon is reluctant to perform early surgery. It has been his experience that these patients tend to have a more severe and persistent memory deficit than if given several days to allow for some degree of recovery after the initial insult. If there is no memory deficit associated with an anterior communicating artery aneurysm, surgery is decided upon as with any other patient. This is clearly a personal bias, rather than being based on an objective study, but it is one which we indulge.

Angiographic Vasospasm

Clinical correlation of angiographic vasospasm may be helpful but is less than perfect (2). It has been our experience that patients of grade I may have severe angiographic vasospasm and patients of grade IV may have no vasospasm. The literature suggests that all patients with severe vasospasm are in poor condition clinically, but this has not been our experience (6). It is clear, however, that if there is significant vasospasm evident on the arteriogram at the time of surgery patients often do not do as well as they otherwise might (2). The definition of significant vasospasm is variable, but we define it as >50% narrowing of one of the major vessels, such as the anterior, middle, or posterior cerebral arteries, the internal carotid artery, or the basilar artery. It is likely that blood vessels in this state do not respond well to further manipulation. Many patients found to have postoperative angiographic vasospasm when they were not doing well probably had vasospasm present at the time of surgery. Both mechanical irrigation and agents such as tissue plasminogen activator to eliminate the blood and blood products in the cisterns, in the hope of decreasing the severity of the vasospasm, are being evaluated (5, 20).

Intracerebral Hematoma

Occasionally when an aneurysm ruptures a sizable intracerebral hematoma develops. Generally the presence of a clot is a small factor in the overall clinical condition, but if it is causing clinical problems or significant deterioration the patient is operated upon urgently. At the time the clot is removed the aneurysm is eliminated (21).

Rehemorrhage

The risk of a second hemorrhage from a ruptured aneurysm is the most compelling argument for early aneurysm surgery. The risk of rebleeding in the first few weeks following the initial hemorrhage has been estimated to be 0.2–2.1% (15). With each rehemorrhage there is a greater likelihood of the patient dying. In our practice, if there is a rebleed prior to planned surgery the decision as to whether to proceed with surgery is based on clinical grade. As soon as the patient improves to grade I or II, surgery is performed, providing there is no significant arteriographic vasospasm. If the patient's status deteriorates, standard supportive treatment is given and delayed surgery is carried out as outlined above.

Medical Complications

Occasionally, medical problems occur which make it reasonable to delay surgery until they are corrected. These include serious cardiac problems, difficulty with blood pressure control, and significant aberrations in fluid and electrolyte balance or pulmonary function. In a large study the presence of significant medical problems and hypertension were associated with unfavorable outcomes (11).

Summary

There is no simple answer to the question of which patients should have early surgery and which delayed surgery for a ruptured intracranial aneurysm. We have suggested that some patients do better with delayed surgery, admittedly assuming the risk of another hemorrhage while waiting. Our concern is with overall outcome, rather than just mortality rate. There is little question that for patients of good grade early surgery is best, and these patients have the best overall results. However, patients of poor clinical grade and those with significant arteriographic vasospasm, giant aneurysms, medical complications, or uncontrolled hypertension do better if allowed to improve and stabilize prior to surgery.

REFERENCES

1. Bailes, J. E., Spetzler, R. F., Hadley, M. N., and Baldwin, H. Z. Management morbidity and mortality of poor-grade aneurysm patients. J. Neurosurg. 72:559–566, 1990.
2. Cooper, P. R., Shucart, W. A., Tenner, M., and Hussain, S. Preoperative arteriographic spasm and outcome from aneurysm surgery. Neurosurgery 7:587–592, 1980.
3. Dandy, W. E. Intracranial aneurysm of the internal carotid artery: cured by operation. Ann. Surg. 107:654–659, 1938.

4. Disney, L., Weir, B., and Patruk, K. Effect on management mortality of a deliberate policy of early operation on supratentorial aneurysms. Neurosurgery 20:695–701, 1987.

5. Findlay, J. M., Weir, B. K. A., Steinke, D., et al. Effect of intrathecal thrombolytic therapy on subarachnoid clot and chronic vasospasm in a primate model of SAH. J. Neurosurg. 69:723–735, 1988.

6. Fisher, C. M., Roberson, G. H., and Ojemann, R. G. Cerebral vasospasm with ruptured saccular aneurysm: the clinical manifestations. Neurosurgery 1:245–248, 1977.

7. Fleischer, A. S., and Tindall, G. T. Cerebral vasospasm following aneurysm rupture: a protocol for therapy and prophylaxis. J. Neurosurg. 52:149–152, 1980.

8. Graf, J. C., and Nibbelink, D. W. Cooperative study of intracranial aneurysms and subarachnoid hemorrhage: report on a randomized treatment study. III. Intracranial surgery. Stroke 5:559–601, 1974.

9. Hunt, W. E., and Hess, R. M. Surgical risk as related to time of intervention in the repair of intracranial aneurysms. J. Neurosurg. 28:14–19, 1968.

10. Kassell, N. F., and Drake, C. G. Timing of aneurysm surgery. Neurosurgery 10:514–519, 1982.

11. Kassell, N. F., Torner, J. C., Haley, C., et al. The International Cooperative Study on the Timing of Aneurysm Surgery. 1. Overall management results. J. Neurosurg. 73:18–36, 1990.

12. Kassell, N. F., Torner, J. C., Jane, J. A., et al. The International Cooperative Study on the Timing of Aneurysm Surgery. 2. Surgical results. J. Neurosurg. 73:37–47, 1990.

13. Ljunggren, B., Saveland, H., and Brandt, L. Causes of unfavorable outcomes after early aneurysm operation. Neurosurgery 13:629–633, 1983.

14. Norlen, G., and Olivecrona, H. The treatment of aneurysms of the circle of Willis. J. Neurosurg. 10:404–415, 1953.

15. Rosenorn, J., Eskesen, V., Schmidt, K., and Ronde, F. The risk of rebleeding from ruptured intracranial aneurysms. J. Neurosurg. 67:329–332, 1987.

16. Solomon, R. A., Fink, M. E., and Lennihan, L. Prophylactic volume expansion therapy for the prevention of delayed cerebral ischemia after early aneurysm surgery: results of a preliminary trial. Arch. Neurol. 45:325–332, 1988.

17. Sundt, T. M., and Piepgras, D. G. Surgical approach to giant intracranial aneurysms: operative experience with 80 cases. J. Neurosurg. 51:731–742, 1979.

18. Vermeulen, M., Lindsay, K. W., Cheah, M. F., et al. Antifibrinolytic treatment in subarachnoid hemorrhage. N. Engl. J. Med. 311:432–437, 1984.

19. Weir, B., Grace, M., Hansen, J., and Rothberg, C. Time course of vasospasm in man. J. Neurosurg. 48:173–178, 1978.

20. Weir, B. Aneurysms Affecting the Nervous System. Williams and Wilkins, Baltimore, 1987.

21. Wheelock, B., Weir, B., Watts, R., et al. Timing of surgery for intracranial hematomas due to aneurysm rupture. J. Neurosurg. 58:476–481, 1983.

Principles of Management of Subarachnoid Hemorrhage: General Management

ROBERT M. CROWELL, M.D., DARYL R. GRESS, M.D.,
CHRISTOPHER S. OGILVY, M.D., J. PHILIP KISTLER, M.D.

INTRODUCTION

The leading cause of nontraumatic subarachnoid hemorrhage (SAH) is intracranial aneurysm. The approximately 28,000 cases of aneurysmal SAH encountered annually in the United States make this a significant public health problem (56). As many as a third of the patients die from the initial injury. With the remainder, the principal task is prompt diagnosis and prevention of complications of this complex and devastating illness (see Table 5A.1).

The main preventable complication is rebleeding, which is often disabling or fatal (27, 32, 42, 63). Thus, a major aim of treatment is the obliteration of the aneurysm to prevent rebleeding. Although initial experience with prompt surgery for this purpose produced discouraging results, recent experience has demonstrated an advantage for early operation (3, 4, 23, 29, 40, 41, 71). Microsurgery has become the main technique for obliteration of intracranial aneurysms, and the results have been impressively good (55, 70, 86). Recent information indicates that endovascular treatment with detachable coil technology may offer another effective means for treatment (22). Because obliteration of the aneurysm is a crucial goal, the initial phases of management are designed to quickly stabilize the patient for obliteration (24, 39, 54).

Other neurological complications of SAH must also be prevented and treated. These include cerebrovascular vasospasm, hydro-

cephalus, and seizures. Complications are generally diagnosed by the correlation of clinical deterioration with findings on imaging studies such as computerized tomographic (CT) scan. Transcranial Doppler can suggest vasospasm, but angiography remains the gold standard for this diagnosis. To prevent ischemia from vasospasm, hypervolemia is warranted (52). Once vasospasm becomes symptomatic, hypertensive therapy can minimize infarction (31).

Treatment of neurological complications may include decompression of an intracranial mass, either by evacuation of an intracerebral hematoma or insertion of a ventriculostomy to relieve hydrocephalus (5). Hyperventilation, steroid therapy, and diuretic therapy are also used for treatment of neurological deterioration related to elevated intracranial pressure (ICP).

Systemic complications may also play a role in clinical neurological deterioration. These include pneumonia, hypotension, and electrolyte abnormalities. Nursing observations are important in detection of these changes. A range of clinical data must be monitored systematically, including pulse, blood pressure, temperature, intake and output, and in some cases central venous pressure and ICP. Management is aided by periodic determinations of arterial blood gases and electrolytes, as well as hematological, biochemical, and bacteriological data.

Weir (79) has emphasized the goal of preservation of neurological function by preven-

TABLE 5A.1.
Goals for the Management of SAH

1. Patient stabilization (neurological, cardiac, and pulmonary)
2. Prevention of rebleeding
   A. Early surgery (or endovascular treatment)
   B. Control of hypertension
   C. Antifibrinolytic agents[a]
3. Vasospasm
   A. Prevention
      1. Hypervolemia and hemodilution
      2. Vasodilators
      3. Calcium channel blockers
      4. Phlebotomy[a]
   B. Therapy
      1. Hypertension
      2. Angioplasty[a]
4. Treatment of symptomatic hydrocephalus
   A. Ventriculostomy
   B. Ventriculo-peritoneal shunt[a]
5. Prevention of seizures and systemic complications

[a] In selected cases.

tion of systemic complications. In a series of 100 aneurysms, he noted respiratory complications in 54%, cardiovascular complications in 23%, genito-urinary complications in 26%, and gastrointestinal complications in 3%. Other systemic complications include electrolyte and endocrine complications, as well as renal and hematological abnormalities. On the basis of available data, we attempt to prevent complications after SAH with the admission protocol shown in Table 5A.2.

Rebleeding

Bleeding from an intracranial aneurysm generally occurs from the dome of the lesion (often from a daughter lobule), although sometimes from the neck. This event is often followed by increased ICP, and a thrombin-fibrin plug may then seal the point of rup-

TABLE 5A.2.
Protocol for the Emergency Management of SAH

Problem	Management
Evaluation	Airway, breathing, and circulation
	Glasgow Coma Scale
	Hunt and Hess Grading (1–5)
Monitoring	Complete blood count
	PT/PTT/platelets
	Glucose
	Liver function tests
	Electrolytes/omsolarity
Airway protection	Pulse oximetry
	Arterial blood gases
	Arterial blood pressure
	Intake and output (every hour)
	Electrolytes/osm (every 8 hours)
	Transcranial Doppler daily
	Nimodipine
	Endotracheal Intubation Ventilation[a]
Blood pressure stabilization	Intravenous fluids[b]
	Neosynephrine[a]
	Nitroprusside[a]
Agitation	Phenobarbital[a]
Pain	Codeine[a]
Seizures	Phenytoin or phenobarbital
Vomiting/aspiration	Nasogastric suction (grade 3–5)
Vasospasm	Hypervolemia/hemodilution

[a] If indicated.
[b] 5% dextrose in 0.9% normal saline solution.

ture. This seal is tenuous, and recurrent bleeding is common (Fig. 5A.1). Kassell and Torner (32) have reported a maximum rebleeding rate of 4%/day for day 0 and then

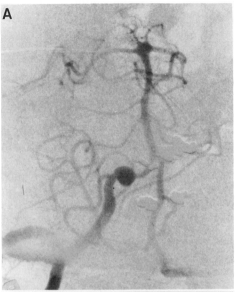

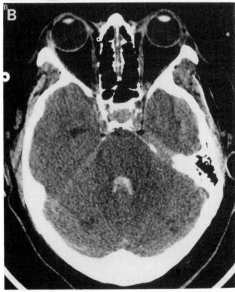

Figure 5A.1. Rebleeding. (*A*) A 55-year-old woman of grade 2 after SAH, transferred for therapy of a right vertebral artery aneurysm. En route to the operating room on day 7, she experienced headache and then coma. (*B*) CT scan showed fresh SAH with extension to IV ventricle, together with cerebellar swelling. Fatal outcome despite maximum medical therapy.

1.5%/day to a total of 27% bleeding in 2 weeks. Rebleeding rates of up to 52% have been reported overall (53). Torner *et al.* (73) noted that the likelihood of rebleeding appears to be greater in poor-grade patients, those with hypertension, and the elderly. Moreover, in patients with multiple SAHs the likelihood of further SAH and death is markedly elevated.

Microsurgical clipping is the best proven means of prevention of recurrent hemorrhage (55, 70, 86). In the presence of an unsecured aneurysm, it is logical to reduce the systemic blood pressure, especially if it is in the hypertensive range (see *Hypertension*) (66). However, induced hypotension does not reliably prevent rebleeding, and it can aggravate ischemia caused by cerebrovascular vasospasm. Early clipping obviates the need for induced hypotension (79).

Endovascular treatment has been utilized to obliterate aneurysms. Parent vessel balloon occlusion is effective for certain lesions. Intra-aneurysmal balloon treatment is difficult to perform and may not be reliable. More promising is the Guglielmi detachable coil (GDC) for aneurysm obliteration, but more data are needed (22).

Antifibrinolytic therapy is another logical measure to prevent lysis of the fibrin platelet seal and thus to prevent recurrent hemorrhage. Mullan and Dawley (47) initially suggested this approach, which was widely used for a time. However, several studies have demonstrated that ϵ-aminocaproic acid does not result in overall improvement of outcome because of increased complications from ischemia and hydrocephalus (33, 58, 75). There may be a place for this therapy when surgery cannot be performed promptly and little or no blood is seen in the subarachnoid space, suggesting a low likelihood of vasospasm (79). Endovascular treatment might be used in this setting as well.

Surgical Management
Microsurgical Clipping

Microsurgical clipping of an intracranial aneurysm is the keystone of treatment, to prevent rebleeding and to set the stage for other therapy. The basic principle is total obliteration of the aneurysm with preservation of all native vessels. It is now possible to achieve these goals with low morbidity and mortality rates.

For poor-grade patients (grades 4 and 5), up to 50% may make a good recovery. Recently an algorithm has been established which suggests that, if ICP can be brought under 30 mm Hg with a ventriculostomy, immediate operation may be followed by good results (5). This is especially useful if the patient shows neurological improvement in relation to ventriculostomy. For patients of grade 4 or 5 in whom ICP cannot be brought under control, operative intervention is not offered, because the results of aggressive treatment are dismal.

To prevent early rebleeding, surgery is performed as soon as possible (see Table 5A.3). Practically speaking, SAH patients only occasionally come to a center that is prepared to treat them in the first 24 hours. Because of the peak incidence of rehemorrhage in the first 24 hours (about 4%) (32), we perform emergency angiography and surgery for patients admitted in the first 24 hours. In addition, patients with more than one SAH are known to have a higher risk of further bleeding (32), and therefore these patients are also operated upon as an emergency. Otherwise, the rate of rebleeding is approximately 1%/day for the first 3 weeks after bleeding and, in view of the slightly elevated hazard of night-time surgery with less familiar support personnel, we prefer day-time surgery as soon as practically possible. These recommendations apply to

good-grade patients (Hunt and Hess grades 1–3) (25).

Early surgery helps set the stage for other prevention and treatment strategies. Although, it was once thought that operation increased the complications from vasospasm, modern data do not confirm this impression (4, 79). In fact, early operation improves the situation for vasospasm prevention and treatment in several ways. Most importantly, when the aneurysm is secured, blood pressure can confidently be elevated as high as 200 torr to improve perfusion (31) (Fig. 5A.2). In addition, craniotomy makes possible removal of hematoma in the subarachnoid space or in the brain, which may be helpful to the patient. Of great promise is intracisternal tissue plasminogen activator, which can lyse subarachnoid clot and help prevent spasm if administered early (16) (Fig. 5A.3). When hydrocephalus is present,

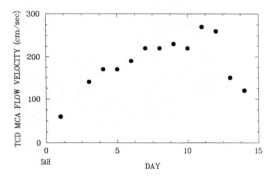

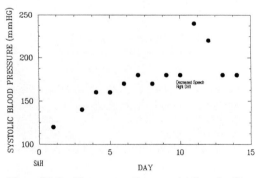

Figure 5A.2. Vasospasm. Transcranial Doppler Scan of left middle cerebral artery (MCA) flow velocity (*above*) and systolic blood pressure (*below*) after SAH and middle cerebral artery aneurysm clipping on day 1. Blood pressure was elevated as treatment. Neurological symptoms appeared on day 10 and resolved with further increase in blood pressure. Excellent outcome.

TABLE 5A.3.
Timing of Surgery

Emergency
 1. Hematoma evacuation and aneurysm obliteration, for deterioration from hematoma (even without angiography)
 2. Angiography and obliteration
    A. For SAH <24 hours earlier
    B. For two or more SAHs
 3. Ventriculostomy (external ventricular drainage), for grade 4 or 5 with hydrocephalus
Urgent (within 24 hours)
 4. Angiography and obliteration
    A. For grade 1–3
    B. For grade 4 or 5 improved by external ventricular drainage

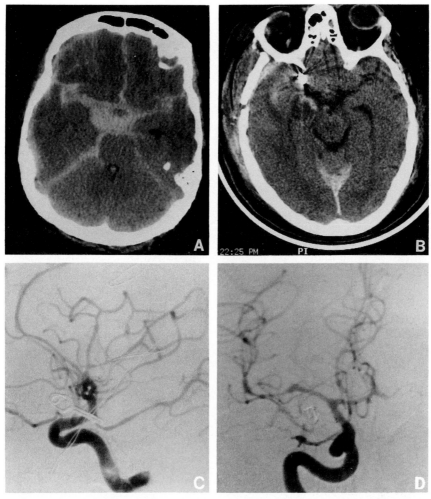

Figure 5A.3. Use of tissue plasminogen activator against vasospasm. (*A*) CT scan from 55-year-old woman of grade 3 after severe SAH. (*B*) CT scan 2 days after craniotomy to clip right ICA aneurysm, with instillation of subarachnoid tissue plasminogen activator; note diminished basal clot. Lateral (*C*) and anterior-posterior (*D*) angiograms 10 days postoperatively show obliterated aneurysm, with moderate vasospasm. Good outcome.

a ventriculostomy can be placed at the time of surgery if needed. This maneuver facilitates brain relaxation. We do not believe that surgery is more difficult, for the experienced aneurysm surgeon, in the early phase after SAH.

Other Procedures

Occasionally, evacuation of an intracerebral hematoma is indicated. If a patient is deteriorating despite medical therapy and harbors a hematoma that is producing symptoms of a mass lesion, craniotomy to evac-

uate the clot may be life-saving. Particularly in cases of carotid and middle cerebral artery aneurysms, emergency clot evacuation, even without angiography, may pave the way for clipping of the aneurysm in the same session.

Ventriculostomy may be required in cases of ventricular dilatation with deterioration. If the patient does not tolerate clamping of the ventricular drain, a ventriculo-peritoneal shunt may be needed after the blood is cleared from the ventricular cerebrospinal fluid. Most patients with moderate ventriculomegaly do not develop significant symptoms, and ventricular size gradually returns to normal; ventriculostomy is not indicated for these patients.

Endovascular Treatment

Percutaneous transvascular obliteration of aneurysms has been reported sporadically since the mid-1970s. However, many cases cannot be treated with endovascular balloons, and significant complications and recurrences have been reported. Recently experience with GDCs has given more encouraging results (22). The technique appears best suited to aneurysms with narrow necks, from 5 mm to giant size, particularly on the internal carotid artery (ICA), middle cerebral artery, and basilar artery circulations. Treatment can be done under local or general anesthesia but requires an experienced, highly skilled, neurointerventionist. To date, GDC therapy has been confined to a few investigational centers, but general availability is likely in the near future. While coil therapy may now be considered an alternative for inoperable aneurysms the long-term results are not known, specifically with regard to recurrence at the area of the aneurysmal neck (the most difficult zone to treat). Further data are needed to define the role of GDC therapy. Nonetheless, endovascular treatment may be considered in certain cases with 1) medical contraindications to general anesthesia and neurosurgery or 2) very risky and inoperable intracranial aneurysms.

Postoperative Care

The surgeon must be alert to the development of early or late postoperative complications. Our protocol is intended to minimize such complications (Table 5A.4). In most patients, a postoperative angiogram is warranted to ensure complete obliteration. If there is an aneurysm remnant, reoperation may be justified. In disabled patients, angiography may be postponed.

Vasospasm

Pathophysiology

After SAH, blood may be caked around basal arteries. Sometimes this clot lyses naturally, but in other cases the clot persists. Much work has gone into the identification of the mechanism whereby this clot causes intense local vasospasm and, in severe cases, downstream ischemia leading to infarction and permanent neurological deficit. Recent evidence suggests that hemoglobin breakdown products play an important role (79). In addition, the clot may produce important changes by occluding access of endothelium-derived relaxing factor to the muscularis, with resultant loss of normal vasodilatation.

Clinical Features and Diagnosis

Thick basal clot has been correlated on the CT scan with the eventual development of delayed vasospasm and neurological deficit, (17, 35). Along with the damage caused by the primary SAH, brain damage due to vasospasm is an important cause of morbidity and mortality after SAH. After SAH, 14–36% of patients may experience disability or death secondary to vasospasm (18, 61). Clinical signs of vasospasm are evident in about one third of patients after SAH, while angiographic studies reveal spasm in up to 70% of the cases.

When the condition of a patient deteriorates 3–14 days after SAH, vasospasm should be considered a possible cause. A CT scan should be performed promptly to rule Serum electrolytes and arterial blood gases should be checked to exclude abnormalities as a cause for deterioration. A decline in serum sodium level (sometimes precipitous) may presage symptomatic vasospasm. Serial transcranial Doppler examinations can detect progressive increase of cerebral blood flow velocity, an effect of vasospasm. In questionable cases, direct confirmation of vasospasm may be obtained by cerebral angiographic study, which remains the gold standard for diagnosis.

Management

Prevention of vasospasm may be achieved by maintaining cerebral perfusion through induction of moderate hypervolemia and hemodilution at normotension (52). The common practice of dehydration for neurosurgical patients is to be discouraged, unless increased ICP requires osmotherapy. Administration of hyposmolar fluids, such as Ringer's lactate (or 5% dextrose in 0.5% normal saline solution), beginning at admis-

TABLE 5A.4
Protocol for Post-Clipping Management

1. General monitoring

Neurological checks
ABG[a]
Hematocrit/hemoglobin
Glucose
Blood pressure
Pulse oximetry
Electrolytes/osmolarity
Intake and output

2. Prevention of complications

Complication	Detection	Prevention	Therapy
Seizures		Phenytoin	
Deep vein thrombosis/pulmonary embolism	Ventilation/perfusion lung scan (or PA[b])	Boots, mobilization	Inferior vena cava filter
Vasospasm	TCD[c], angiogram	Hypervolemia/hemodilution	Triple H[d]
Infarction	CT	Hypervolemia/hemodilution Nimodipine	

3. Management of neurological deterioration

Diagnosis	Evaluation	Treatment
Pneumonia (chest x-ray)	ABG	Antibiotics
Pulmonary embolus		Pulmonary angiography IVC filter
Na+/osmolarity	Electrolytes	Intravenous fluids or restriction
Hydrocephalus	CT	External ventricular drainage
Subdural hematoma		Evacuate
Increased ICP		Hyperventilation, mannitol

4. Ongoing management

Problem	Management	Timing
Nutrition	Oral/tube feeds/total parenteral nutrition	As soon as possible
Mobilization	Physical therapy/rehabilitation	2–3 days
Total obliteration	Angiography (for most)	7 days

[a] ABG, arterial blood gases.
[b] PA, Pulmonary angiogram.
[c] TCD, transcranial Doppler.
[d] Triple H, hypervolemia/hemodilution/hypertension.

sion can gradually achieve hypervolemic hemodilution. In most cases, careful intake and output records and serum electrolyte values can guide therapy, with an aim of giving 2–3 liters of excess input over the initial 24 hours. There is an impression that symptomatic vasospasm has become less common since hypervolemia has been used routinely in SAH cases. As described elsewhere, vasospasm may be prevented by injection of tissue plasminogen activator into the basal cisterns, but this method is still in the investigational phase (16).

For treatment of established symptomatic vasospasm, hypertensive hypervolemic hemodilution ("triple-H therapy") is usually indicated (52) (Figs. 5A.2 and 5A.3). In essence, hypertension is added to hypervolemia and hemodilution. The central venous pressure is raised to 8–12 cm or the pulmonary artery wedge pressure to 14–18 mm in an effort to increase systemic blood pressure and cerebral blood flow. Pressors are used to elevate the blood pressure to 160–170 torr in patients with unsecured aneurysms or more vigorously, up to 200 torr in patients with secured aneurysms. Phenylephrine, dopamine, or dobutamine infusions are titrated to elevate blood pressure, with careful monitoring of arterial pressure. Extra caution is warranted in patients with cardiac, pulmonary, or renal dysfunction. Central venous pressure monitoring is often helpful in these cases, and some patients will need pulmonary artery catheters to guide therapy. At times, measurement of ICP and cerebral perfusion pressure has been useful to guide therapy, especially in the presence of hydrocephalus. The optimum hematocrit value is 30–33%, and occasionally phlebotomy is added to hydration to achieve this level. One must watch carefully for pulmonary edema, electrolyte abnormalities, and cerebral edema in such complex patients.

Mannitol has also been shown to increase cerebral blood flow in the setting of vasospasm, with improvement in neurological function (7, 26). Recently the calcium channel blocker nimodipine has been shown to have a beneficial effect on stroke after SAH, and a beneficial effect on blood flow is suspected; nimodipine is without documented effect upon angiographic spasm (57).

Recently, experience with balloon angioplasty has suggested a beneficial effect in selected cases treated early (89). Numerous failures have been observed with angioplasty, and the indications for this form of treatment are not yet established. In practice, when severe deficit persists for 2 hours despite maximal medical therapy, we consider angioplasty of clinically relevant proximal intracranial arteries (internal carotid artery, middle cerebral artery, anterior cerebral artery, vertebral and basilar arteries, and posterior cerebral artery).

Several recent reports indicated that intraarterial papaverine may be of benefit in dilating distal intracranial arteries, but controlled data are lacking. A host of other treatments have not been shown to provide a benefit, including trinitroglycerin, nitroprusside, aminophylline, isoproterenol, and reserpine/kanamycin. On the basis of available data on vasospasm, we have instituted the protocol detailed in Table 5A.5.

Hydrocephalus

Acute hydrocephalus after SAH can lead to rapid decline and death (83). More often, gradually increasing hydrocephalus produces a diminished level of alertness and increased ICP. The condition can be diagnosed by careful clinical observation and correlation with a CT scan showing enlarged ventricles (Fig. 5A.4).

When a patient arrives deeply comatose after SAH (grade 4 or 5) and the CT scan confirms hydrocephalus, it is worthwhile to insert a ventriculostomy. In a significant number, ICP can be brought to normal levels and the clinical picture improved. There is a chance for useful recovery. Angiography and surgery appear warranted in these cases (5).

In other cases with progressive deterioration, a ventricular drain provides both decompression and monitoring. With an unsecured aneurysm, one should avoid overdrainage by gradually lowering the pressure to 15–30 cm. In most cases, the drain may be weaned over a few days and removed.

TABLE 5A.5.
Protocol for Vasospasm Treatment

1. Maintain central venous pressure at 10–12 cm with albumin, blood, and fluids.
2. In selected patients with cardiopulmonary problems, monitor with pulmonary artery catheter. Maintain wedge pressure at 14–18 torr using albumin, blood, or fresh frozen plasma.
3. Maintain blood glucose level at 100–150 mg/liter.
4. Elevate systolic blood pressure to 160–180 torr if aneurysm is secured, using phenylephrine or dopamine. If no improvement, increase blood pressure to 200 torr unless there is a cardiac complication or other contraindication.
5. If no improvement after maximal medical therapy, consider angioplasty.

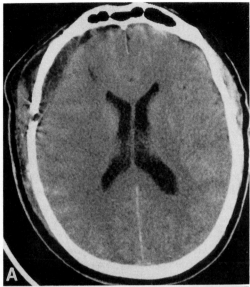

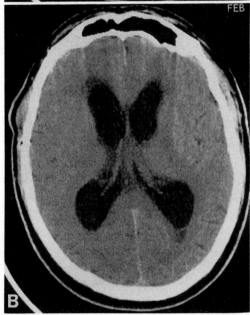

Figure 5A.4. Hydrocephalus. (*A*) CT scan 1 day after clipping of right ICA aneurysm. (*B*) CT scan 10 days later shows development of marked hydrocephalus requiring VP shunt.

Only a few patients eventually require a shunt. At times, ventricular drainage helps maintain cerebral perfusion pressure at appropriate levels during the treatment of vasospasm. In such instances, it may be necessary to change the site of the ventricular drain to permit drainage for prolonged periods of time.

Increased ICP

This common complication of SAH results from (re)bleeding, intracranial hematoma, hydrocephalus, and cerebral edema or ischemia related to vasospasm (50). Increased ICP can lead to impairment of cerebral perfusion with exacerbation of ischemia and concomitant edema. Pressure gradients and intracranial comparmentalization may lead to transtentorial herniation and brainstem injury. Level of consciousness is the best clinical measure of ICP. Progressive stupor suggests critically elevated ICP. Increased ICP is not a major concern in alert patients with minimal deficit.

Measures to lower ICP include moderate restriction of free water, elevation of the head of the bed, avoidance of hypoventilation and hypercarbia, and control of agitation and pain. Hyperventilation is a temporarily effective method to lower ICP in a patient developing signs of herniation. In patients without cerebral ischemia, pCO_2 can be safely lowered to 30 torr, but further reduction can cause ischemia. The effects of hyperventilation, by reducing intracranial intravascular volume, are immediate but short lived. Hyperventilation should be supplemented with mannitol (0.5 mg/kg in a 20% solution, given over 20 min). Mannitol is an osmotic agent that extracts water from normal brain. Effects begin in 20 min and persist for 4–6 hours. Additional doses of mannitol (0.25 mg/kg) can be given every 4–6 hours as needed. Monitoring of fluid status must go on serially, with serum osmolarity not to exceed 310 mOsm. Monitoring of ICP with a subdural transducer or ventricular catheter facilitates management. Drainage of cerebrospinal fluid may help control ICP. Other diuretic agents include furosemide and Diamox. Rarely, pentobarbital coma is warranted for management of refractory elevated ICP.

Medical management is often of limited value in long-term control of elevated ICP. Ventricular drainage for hydrocephalus and surgical evacuation of intraparenchymal or subdural hematomas can be life-saving in some instances.

Seizures

Seizures are not uncommon after SAH, occurring in up to 13% of cases (62, 77). Seizures appear to be considerably more common in middle cerebral artery aneurysms (up to 30% of middle cerebral artery aneurysms with intracerebral hematoma). When there is a neurological deficit, seizure can occur in up to 41% of cases. Seizures generally occur within 18 months if they will ever occur. Fits may be generalized, focal, or complex partial. In a study of 53 cases, 83% had fewer than three seizures, indicating that these are usually not difficult to treat (60).

Following SAH, EEG changes are common, including slow waves and even spikes (85). EEG has been used as a guide to therapy. Richardson and Uttley (60) recommended that, even without seizures, patients with ICA or anterior communicating artery aneurysms should be treated for 6–12 months but patients with middle cerebral artery aneurysms, a neurological deficit, or intracerebral hemorrhage should be treated for 2–3 years. Dilantin levels should be monitored.

For the occasional case of status epilepticus, valium (10 mg, intravenously, over 5–10 min) is recommended, with repetition as required (up to 80 mg). Patients must be observed carefully for respiratory depression. Phenytoin loading at the same time is recommended, with 1 g (or 15 mg/kg) given slowly (no more than 50 mg/min intravenously), with 100 mg every 8 hours and adjustment of dosage according to serum concentration determinations (51).

On the basis of available data, we treat all aneurysmal SAH patients with anticonvulsants for 3 months after obliteration and then taper the medication. If there are seizures, extended therapy and EEG monitoring are used. If rash or other reaction occurs, phenytoin is replaced with phenobarbital (usual loading dose of 1000 mg or 20 mg/kg, with 30–60 mg every 6–8 hours).

Psychiatric Alterations

Psychiatric alterations are common after SAH (12, 36, 45, 65, 68, 69, 83). Storey (69) reported that 45% of patients showed no abnormality, while 24% had mild alteration, 18% moderate, 10% severe, and 3% very severe. Abnormal neurological signs were associated with psychiatric alterations in 45%.

The most common changes are personality alteration, psychological symptoms, diminished intelligence quotient, anxiety, and depression. Other alterations include akinetic mutism and its lesser cousin hypomania, which can be treated with lithium. Sengupta et al. (65) reported loss of interest and diminished initiative and energy, which did not seem to be more pronounced with early operation. After anterior communicating artery aneurysm surgery, Kodama et al. (30) reported that 9% of patients had difficulties with activities of daily living, but 60% had a full recovery. Personality changes, amnesia, and other such alterations seem to be more common in anterior communicating artery aneurysms. All of these alterations appear to diminish over time.

Electrolyte Abnormalities

For some time hyponatremia has been thought to be due to the syndrome of inappropriate antidiuretic hormone secretion (11, 28, 83). This syndrome was initially identified after bleeding from an anterior communicating artery aneurysm, and fluid restriction was found to be effective treatment. Fox et al. (19) suggested that the diagnosis be confirmed when urinary sodium is greater than 25 milliequivalents/liter. More recently it has been thought that this syndrome might be related to a salt-wasting syndrome (49), possibly caused by centrally elaborated atrial natriuretic factor (10, 82). With declining sodium levels, there may be declining blood pressure and increases in hematocrit values. These tend to occur 3–15 days after SAH and may last 2 weeks. Free water restriction is usually an effective treatment, but when the sodium level falls below 115 milliequivalents/liter 3% saline solution may be given (Fig. 5A.5).

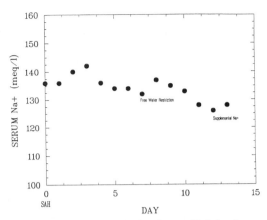

Figure 5A.5. Hyponatremia. Serum Na⁺ levels recorded following SAH. Note gradual decline, with response to interventions.

The latter must be carefully considered in patients with heart disease, advanced age, or hypertension. Note that hyponatremia and vasospasm have similar time courses. Therapy for the former could exacerbate the latter and therefore, to maintain intravascular volume, albumin should be administered to avert hypovolemia from fluid restriction.

Hypernatremia may also occur, especially after anterior communicating artery aneurysm surgery (38, 46). A diagnosis of diabetes insipidus may be entertained when the hourly urine output is in excess of 250 ml/hour for 2 successive hours. Antidiuretic hormone (vasopressin) (5–10 units intramuscularly, every 4–6 hours) may be given. One should beware of early postoperative mobilization of intraoperative intravenous fluids, which may pose as diabetes insipidus. The diagnosis of diabetes insipidus should be suspected with polyuria, polydipsia, and hypernatremia, in the presence of serum osmolarity of 320–330 mOsm (milliosmols) and urine osmolarity of <1. These patients are not thirsty.

Cardiac Complications

A variety of cardiac complications can occur after SAH. In a recent review (30), congestive heart failure was noted in 1%, angina in 1%, myocardial infarction in 1%, (significant) arrhythmia in 2%, and hypertension in 16%. Occasionally, cardiac problems are so significant that hypotension may occur (34).

The frequency of significant cardiac injury has been debated. In some series, proven myocardial infarction has been documented in as high as 12% of patients (67). The rate of diagnosis will, of course, be a function of the care with which patients are observed for cardiac abnormalities. According to Estanol *et al.* (13) in a study with careful electrocardiograph (EKG) monitoring of 15 cases with SAH, 20% had runs of ventricular tachycardia and 60% showed long QT intervals. In a continuous EKG study by Vidal *et al.* (76), 100% of the patients with SAH had arrhythmias in the first 48 hours, the time frame most common for arrhythmia. These same workers noticed that all EKGs had returned to normal after 10 days. In another study by Marion *et al.* (44), 50% of all patients with SAH were found to have EKG abnormalities. Thirty-seven percent had increased QT intervals, T-wave changes were seen in 47%, and ST changes were noted in 30%. There were prominent U-waves in 25% and rhythm disturbances in 35%.

Myocardial infarction documented with enzyme and serial EKG changes were demonstrated in 12% of fatal intracranial hemorrhages by Smith and Tomlinson (67). Thallium persantine studies in our unit have shown scanning abnormalities in the majority of patients with SAH. Evidence suggests that these EKG and cardiac abnormalities are related to subendocardial ischemia caused by increased levels of local and/or circulating norepinephrine. These catecholamine disturbances are presumed to be secondary to the SAH, with attendant alteration in the hypothalamus. While subendocardial ischemia may be modest and reversible in most cases, pathological studies have shown myocardial hemorrhage, focal necrosis, and even overt myocardial infarction, which can occasionally be fatal.

Therapy for these conditions has logically focused on the use of β-blockers such as propranolol (44). It has been shown that β-blockade prevents ventricular arrythmia and subendocardial lesions (8, 48).

Often the question arises as to whether patients with EKG abnormalities are stable enough to undergo general anesthesia and surgery. In consultation with our neuroanesthesia and cardiology colleagues, we have come to the conclusion that in the great majority of these cases treatment can proceed, despite EKG changes, to procedures including angiography and surgery. We take this approach even when there has been a small enzyme leak. Obviously these decisions must be individualized, and rarely a patient with clear-cut dramatic evidence of myocardial infarction may be better served by deferring anesthesia and surgery.

Pulmonary Complications

Pulmonary complications are extremely common in patients with SAH (79). Obtunded patients are vulnerable to respiratory obstruction and hypoxia, as well as atelectasis, aspiration, and pneumonia. The resulting hypoxemia, hypercarbia, and acidosis may all contribute significantly to intracranial complications, including cerebral ischemia, cerebral edema, and increased ICP.

Therefore, prompt intubation and ventilation are indicated for all patients with SAH who are obtunded or seem likely to become so. Controlled ventilation is indicated with the aim of maintaining satisfactory oxygenation. Positive end-expiratory pressure is warranted for patients with a history of asthma, bronchitis, or emphysema. Positive end-expiratory pressure does not have an adverse effect on ICP if peak pressure is maintained below 10 cm of water (21). In many patients with increased ICP, ventilation aimed to achieve hypocarbia in the range of 30–35 torr is appropriate. More extreme degrees of hypocarbia, however, may bring unwanted cerebral ischemia and should be avoided. For comatose patients, frequent suctioning and chest physical therapy are helpful to keep the bronchial tree free of secretions.

Pulmonary care for SAH patients is a team efforts. It is important to involve the nursing staff as well as the respiratory therapy service in the ongoing complex pulmonary care of these patients. Frequent monitoring of tidal volume and arterial blood gases permits the physician to tailor the best pulmonary program for each patient.

In unconscious patients, pneumonia is a common complication after SAH. Kassell and Boarini (30) recently reported pneumonia in 8% of patients with SAH. Frequent evaluation of 1) sputum by Gram stain and culture and 2) pulmonary status by chest X-ray permits early diagnosis of symptomatic pneumonia and specific treatment with antibiotics selected according to sensitivity. A high index of suspicion should be maintained and infectious disease consultation obtained at the earliest hint of trouble. If comatose patients can awaken, then the ability to fight off intercurrent pneumonitis is much improved.

Pulmonary edema is a relatively common complication after SAH. This problem is particularly common in poor-grade patients and those with increased ICP (80). Neurogenic pulmonary edema can be delayed in onset. It appears to be related to increased levels of circulating catecholamines. Management requires intubation and positive end-expiratory pressure. Frequent suctioning is needed to clear the bronchial passages. Lasix and morphine sulfate are also helpful. Usually pulmonary edema is a transient phenomenon in patients with SAH. When neurogenic pulmonary edema is severe, efforts to obliterate the aneurysm may have to be postponed. Pulmonary edema can also be iatrogenic in patients receiving hypervolemic hemodilution therapy.

Hypertension

Moderate levels of hypertension are common following SAH. In the setting of increased ICP and vasospasm, hypertension is a homeostatic response by the body to maintain cerebral perfusion. Probably such a hypertensive response is related to increased catecholamines intracranially and systemically. With an unsecured aneurysm, elevation of the blood pressure can lead to increased transmural ("bursting") pressure, with concomitant recurrent and potentially fatal SAH. Management must be cautiously calculated to avoid both recurrent bleeding and hypoperfusion after SAH.

Often sedation and bed rest are followed by gradual normalization of blood pressure (54, 79). Analgesia should also be offered to alert patients. When moderate hypertension persists, gentle therapy with hydrochlorothiazide or Lasix and propranolol may be all that is required to normalize blood pressure. In some cases, intravenous labetalol or oral nifedipine are appropriate. One should make every effort to avoid hypotension.

In a few cases, marked hypertension is encountered, with blood pressures of 200 torr or above. In view of the threat of recurrent SAH, such hypertension should be treated promptly. In many such cases, intravenous nitroprusside is needed, along with an intra-arterial catheter for continuous monitoring of blood pressure. Obviously, hypotension is to be avoided, because this can lead to ischemia and neurological deficit. In some instances a ventricular catheter, by lowering increased ICP, can lead to reduction of hypertension. This is particularly true in poor-grade patients (15).

In the fluid management of patients with SAH, it has been suggested that volume expansion is helpful in avoiding delayed ischemic deficits. Obviously this measure would tend to counteract efforts to lower blood pressure. A study has been performed in which the impact of volume expansion on blood pressure was evaluated (64). In one group, volume expansion was administered along with vasodilator and central antihypertensive drugs; another group was treated exactly the same way but without volume expansion. All patients had blood pressures in excess of 150/95 torr and were monitored with pulmonary artery catheters. Hydralazine and methydolpate were administered, and a few patients needed nitroprusside as well. A significantly greater proportion of the patients receiving volume expansion survived long term, and therefore volume expansion along with control of blood pressure was recommended in the setting of aneurysmal SAH.

Infection

The infectious complications are essentially those of postoperative patients and comatose patients. Because they are so common, infections must be assiduously sought from the time of admission. Infection may occur in relation to a craniotomy wound or ventricular catheter, intravenous or intra-arterial catheters, a bladder catheter, the broncho-pulmonary tree, or pressure sores. The clinician should also be alert to the emergence of rashes, which may indicate infection or medication reactions. The common use of steroids often complicates the situation, by masking infection.

After SAH, patients are often confined to bed for a time and in the perioperative period are subject to a wide variety of infections. When a patient in this situation is found to have a fever, a careful evaluation including inspection of the wound, evaluation of pressure sores and rashes, and a careful review of medications should be carried out. In-lying vascular catheters must be evaluated and frequently cultured and changed. The urine should be subjected to urinalysis and culture. Sputum samples should be subjected to Gram staining and culture and sensitivity testing, and a chest X-ray should be performed. If there is an in-lying ventriculostomy, this source should be sampled for cell count as well as cultured. Infection of a ventriculostomy is relatively common (7% in one series) (43) and therefore an antibiotic regimen of intravenous ampicillin during maintenance of a ventriculostomy has been recommended (84). When there is no ventriculostomy, a judgment is made as to the appropriateness of spinal puncture, which is safe in the postoperative period in the absence of intracranial mass effect.

When there is concern about infection, it is wise to consult an infectious disease specialist. This consultant may assist in evaluation and in the selection of antibiotic therapy, should that become appropriate. One must be alert to the possibility of both Gram-positive and Gram-negative bacterial infection (and even fungal infection) in persistently comatose patients (14).

When meningitis is diagnosed, the antibiotic should be selected on the basis of sensitivities (14). For *Staphylococcus aureus*, nafcillin, Chloromycetin, or vancomycin is generally effective. For *Streptococcus pneumoniae* or *pyogenes*, penicillin G or Chloromycetin is effective. For Gram-negative organisms such as *Escherichia coli*, effective treatment is ampicillin, Chloromycetin, or gentamicin given intravenously (and in some cases intraventricularly).

Venous Thrombosis and Thrombo-Embolism

Deep venous thrombosis is very common in patients with stroke and paralysis (up to 60%, according to the study of Warlow *et al.*) (78). About 2% of patients with aneurysmal SAH have deep venous thrombosis and pulmonary embolus.

Efforts to prevent these complications are mandatory. The basic regimen involves pneumatic compression thigh-high stockings and early mobilization. While these measures diminish the frequency of deep venous thrombosis, they do not prevent pulmonary embolus from pelvic venous sources (72).

There is evidence that subcutaneous heparin given in doses of 5000 units every 12 hours ("mini-heparin") effectively reduces the frequency of pulmonary embolus in general surgical patients and orthopedic surgical patients. While neurosurgeons have shied away from this form of treatment for patients undergoing intracranial surgery, it is clear that full heparinization is safe 6 days after craniotomy (9), and recent data from our unit indicate that mini-heparinization as described can be instituted the day after neurosurgical operations (20). A controlled study is now underway to determine whether this approach is effective in reducing the frequency of pulmonary embolus in patients with SAH and other neurosurgical conditions.

Endocrine Abnormalities

Hypopituitarism is not uncommon in relation to giant aneurysms that compress the hypothalamic-pituitary axis (6, 37, 74, 81, 87). Hypopituitarism, usually of a mild form, can also appear following SAH. This is usually more pronounced with anterior communicating artery aneurysms, poor-grade patients, vasospasm, and hydrocephalus.

Diabetes insipidus may also be seen in patients with SAH. This usually occurs in relation to direct manipulation of the hypothalamic-pituitary axis. Diabetes insipidus can also occur in the setting of massive brain injury from SAH, increased ICP, and a pre-terminal state. Management includes careful input and output measurements of fluids, monitoring of serum and urine electrolytes, and judicious administration of arginine-vasopressin subcutaneously (not in oil). Sometimes desmopressin acetate is useful, and only rarely is 3% hypertonic saline solution appropriate (serum sodium levels below 115 milliequivalents/liter).

Iatrogenic Addison's syndrome may be induced by the abrupt withdrawal of steroid supplements in patients who have been receiving this type of medication for some weeks.

It should be recalled that diabetes mellitus is exaggerated in the presence of corticosteroid therapy. Careful monitoring of blood sugar levels is required, with a sliding scale of insulin therapy as needed.

Gastrointestinal Complications

Hemorrhagic and ulcerative gastric mucosal abnormalities are common after SAH. Such abnormalities were observed in 83% of 29 fatal cases of anterior communicating artery aneurysm (59). These problems are exacerbated by administration of steroids and aspirin-containing compounds. The clinician should be alert to abdominal pain and distention with ileus, anemia, and hypotension. Hematemesis and melena are more dramatic signs, but gastrointestinal (GI) bleeding may be painless.

To prevent significant GI bleeding, prophylaxis with antacids or H$_2$ blockers is recommended. Treatment of ongoing GI bleeding begins with nasogastric suction. Saline lavage may be utilized as required, along with intravenous fluids and blood transfusion. Sometimes endoscopic coagulation of ulcerated bleeding sites may be useful, and occasionally laparotomy is needed. In rare cases, vagotomy and partial gastrectomy may be required.

Kassell and Boarini (30) reported documented GI hemorrhage in 4% of patients with aneurysmal SAH. This was more common in comatose patients. In patients with serious GI bleeding after SAH there may be a prior history of GI bleeding. There may be a delay of 7 days following SAH before a problem occurs.

Genito-Urinary Complications

Genito-urinary complications consist primarily of infections in obtunded patients. Initial treatment with antibiotics and continuous Foley catheter drainage is recommended. Once the patient reaches stable status, intermittent catheterization is probably a better approach.

Rarely there may be more complex problems. Andrew *et al.* (2) reported six patients with anterior communicating artery aneurysms who developed incontinence, priapism, or impotence after SAH.

Rehabilitation

A stroke or SAH is a catastrophe for the patient and the family. Rehabilitation is the key to maximizing the remainder of the patient's lifetime. The physician should plan with the family, as soon as possible, a realistic program of physical, mental, and social rehabilitation (1). A positive attitude by the principal physician is important in achieving the best outcome. Since depression is extremely common in patients following SAH, special attention should be given to this problem. The surgeon should dispel undue fears of rebleeding for patients with satisfactory clipping of an aneurysm. A team of specialists, including a physiatrist, occupational therapist, physical therapist, and psychologist, to assist in the rehabilitation of these patients is desirable. When there is a significant disability, an inpatient program of rehabilitation is usually indicated. For lesser deficits, outpatient treatment frequently suffices. Some common problems can easily be overlooked, such as a frozen shoulder or urinary tract infection.

REFERENCES

1. Alekseeva, V. S., Karaseva, A., Naidin, V. L., and Shtamberg, N. A. Social and medical rehabilitation of patients subjected to surgery on account of aneurysms of the anterior connecting artery. Zh. Nevropatol. Psikhiatr. *77*:1329–1333, 1977.

2. Andrew, J., Nathan, P. W., and Spanos, N. C. Disturbances of micturition and defecation due to aneurysms of anterior communicating or anterior cerebral arteries. J. Neurosurg. *24*:1–10, 1966.

3. Auer, I. M. Acute surgery of cerebral aneurysms and prevention of symptomatic vasospasm. Acta Neurochir. (Wien.) *69*:273–281, 1983.

4. Ausman, J. I., Diaz, E. G., Malik, G. M. *et al.* Current management of cerebral aneurysms: is it based on facts or myths? Surg. Neurol. *24*:625–635, 1985.

5. Bailes, J. E., Spetzler, R. F., Hadley, M. N., and Baldwin, H. Z. Management morbidity and mortality of poor-grade aneurysm patients. J. Neurosurg. *72*:559–566, 1990.

6. Bramwell, B. Clinical and pathologic memoranda. XII. Two enormous intra-cranial aneurisms. Edin. Med. J. *32*:911–922, 1887.

7. Brown, E. D., Hanlon, K., and Mullan, S. Treatment of aneurysmal hemiplegia with dopamine and mannitol. J. Neurosurg. *49*:525–529, 1978.

8. Cruickshank, J. M., Neil-Dwyer, G., and Lange, J. The effect of oral propranolol upon ECG changes occurring in SAH. Cardiovasc. Res. *9*:236–245, 1975.

9. DiRicco, G., Marini, C., Rindi, M., *et al.* Pulmonary embolism in neurosurgical patients: diagnosis and treatment. J. Neurosurg. *60*:972–975, 1984.

10. Diringer, M., Landenson, P., Stern, B., *et al.* Plasma atrial natriuretic factor and subarachnoid hemorrhage. Stroke *19*:1119–1124, 1988.

11. Doczi, T., Bende, J., Huszka, E., and Kiss, J. Syndrome of inappropriate secretion of antidiuretic hormone after subarachnoid hemorrhage. Neurosurgery *9*:394–397, 1981.

12. Editorial. Psychological effects of subarachnoid haemorrhage. Lancet *1*:644–645, 1970.

13. Estanol, B. V., Dergal, E. B., Cesarman, E., *et al.* Cardiac arrhythmias associated with subarachnoid hemorrhage: prospective study. Neurosurgery *5*:675–680, 1969.

14. Everett, E. D., and Strausbaugh, I. J. Antimicrobial agents and the central nervous system. Neurosurgery *6*:691–714, 1980.

15. Feibel, J. H., Baldwin, C. A., and Joynt, R. J. Catecholamine-associated refractory hypertension following acute intracranial hemorrhage: control with propranolol. Ann. Neurol. *9*:340–343, 1981.

16. Findlay, J. M., Weir, B. K., Kassell, N. F., *et al.* Intracisternal recombinant tissue plasminogen activator after aneurysmal subarachnoid hemorrhage. J. Neurosurg. *75*:181–188, 1991.

17. Fisher, C. M., Kistler, J. P., and Davis, J. M. Relation of cerebral vasospasm to subarachnoid hemorrhage visualized by computerized tomographic scanning. Neurosurgery *6*:1–9, 1980.

18. Fisher, C. M., Robertson, G. H., and Ojemann, R. G. Cerebral vasospasm with ruptured saccular aneurysm: the clinical manifestations. Neurosurgery *1*:245–248, 1977.

19. Fox, J. L., Falik, J. L., and Shalhoub, R. J. Neurosurgical hyponatremia: the role of inappro-

priate antidiuresis. J. Neurosurg. *34:*506–514, 1971.

20. Frim, D. M., Barker, E. G., III, Poletti, C. E., and Hamilton, A. J. Postoperative low-dose heparin decreases thromboembolic complications in neurosurgical patients. Neurosurgery *30:*830–833, 1992.

21. Frost, E. A. Effects of P. E. E. P. on ICP and compliance in brain injured patients. J. Neurosurg. *47:*195–200, 1977.

22. Guglielmi, G., Vinuela, E., Dion, J., and Duckwiler, G. Electrothrombosis of saccular aneurysms via endovascular approach. 2. Preliminary clinical experience. J. Neurosurg. *75:*8–14, 1991.

23. Haley, E. C., Jr., Kassell, N. E., Torner, J. C., *et al.* The International Cooperative Study on the Timing of Aneurysm Surgery: the North American Experience. Stroke *23:*205–214, 1992.

24. Holmes, J. M. The medical management of subarachnoid haemorrhage. Br. Med. J. [Clin. Res.] *1:*788–790, 1958.

25. Hunt, W. E., and Hess, R. M. Surgical risk as related to time of intervention in the repair of intracranial aneurysms. J. Neurosurg. *28:*14–20, 1968.

26. Jafar, J. J., Johns, L. M., and Mullan, S. F. The effect of mannitol on cerebral blood flow. J. Neurosurg. *64:*754–759, 1984.

27. Jane, J. A., Winn, R. H., and Richardson, A. E. The natural history of intracranial aneurysms: rebleeding rates during the acute and long term period and implication for surgical management. Clin. Neurosurg. *24:*176–184, 1976.

28. Joynt, R. I., Afifi, A., and Harbison, J. Hyponatremia in subarachnoid hemorrhage. Arch. Neurol. *13:*633–638, 1965.

29. Kassell, N. E., Boarini, D. J., Adams, H. P., *et al.* Overall management of ruptured aneurysms: comparison of early and later operation. Neurosurgery *9:*120–128, 1981.

30. Kassell, N. E., and Boarini, D. J. Perioperative care of the aneurysm patient. Contemp. Neurosurg. *6:*1–6, 1984.

31. Kassell, N. E., Peerless, S. J., Durward, O. J., *et al.* Treatment of ischemic deficits from vasospasm with intravascular volume expansion and induced arterial hypertension. Neurosurgery *11:*337–343, 1982.

32. Kassell, N. K., and Torner, J. C. Aneurysmal rebleeding: a preliminary report from the Cooperative Aneurysm Study. Neurosurgery *13:*479–481, 1983.

33. Kassell, N. E., Torner, J. C., and Adams, H. P. Jr. Antifibrinolytic therapy in the acute period following aneurysmal subarachnoid hemorrhage: preliminary observations from the Cooperative Aneurysm Study. J. Neurosurg. *61:*225–230, 1984.

34. Kataoka, K., and Taneda, M. Aneurysmal subarachnoid hemorrhage causing arterial hypotension. Neurol. Med. Chir. (Tokyo) *23:*203–210, 1983.

35. Kistler, J. P., Crowell, R. M., Davis, K. R., *et al.* The relation of cerebral vasospasm to the extent and location of subarachnoid blood visualized by CT scan: a prospective study. Neurology *33:*424–436, 1983.

36. Kodama, T., Uemura, S., Nonaka, N., *et al.* The quantitative analysis of psychiatric sequelae after direct surgery of anterior communicating aneurysms: follow-up study. Neurol. Med. Chir. (Tokyo) *17:*327–333, 1977.

37. Kuwayama, A., Ikada, C., Takanohashi, M., *et al.* Endocrine function in post-operative patients with anterior communicating aneurysm. Neurol. Med. Chir. (Tokyo) *17:*209–217, 1977.

38. Landolt, A. M., Yasargil, M. G., and Krayenbuhl, H. Disturbances of the serum electrolytes after surgery of intracranial arterial aneurysms. J. Neurosurg. *37:*210–218, 1972.

39. Langfitt, T. W. Conservative care of intracranial hemorrhage. Adv. Neurol. *16:*169–180, 1977.

40. Ljunggren, B., Brandt, L., Sundbarg, G., *et al.* Early management of aneurysmal subarachnoid hemorrhage. Neurosurgery *11:*412–418, 1982.

41. Ljunggren, B., Saveland, H., Brandt, K., and Zygmont, S. Early operation and overall outcome in aneurysmal subarachnoid hemorrhage. J. Neurosurg. *62:*547–551, 1985.

42. Locksley, H. B. Report on the Cooperative Study of Intracranial Aneurysms and SAH. Section V. II. Natural history of SAH, intracranial aneurysms and AVM: based on 6368 cases in the Cooperative Study. J. Neurosurg. *25:*321–368, 1966.

43. Lundberg, N. Continuous recording and control of ventricular fluid pressure in neurosurgical practice. Acta Psychiatr. Scand. *36*(suppl.)*:*146–149, 1960.

44. Marion, D. W., Segal, P., and Thompson, M. E. Subarachnoid hemorrhage and the heart. Neurosurgery *18:*101–106, 1986.

45. May, R. G., and Kaelbling, R. Coma of over a year's duration with favorable outcome. Dis. Nerv. Syst. *29:*837–840, 1968.

46. Mineta, T., Tsutsumi, E., Suzuki, H., and Kasai, M. Clinical and experimental studies on cerebral hypernatremia. Tohoku J. Exp. Med. *104:*233–249, 1971.

47. Mullan, S., and Dawley, J. Antifibrinolytic therapy for intracranial aneurysms. J. Neurosurg. *28:*21–23, 1968.

48. Neil-Dwyer, G., Walter, P., and Cruickshank, J. M. *Beta*-blockade benefits patients following a subarachnoid hemorrhage. Eur. J. Clin. Pharmacol. *28*(suppl. 1)*:*25–29, 1985.

49. Nelson, P. B., Seif, S. M., Maroon, J. C., *et al.* Hyponatremia in intracranial disease: perhaps not the syndrome of inappropriate secretion of antidiuretic hormone (SIADH). J. Neurosurg. *65:*938–941, 1981.

50. Nornes, H., and Magnaes, B. Intracranial pressure in patients with ruptured saccular aneurysm. J. Neurosurg. *36:*536–547, 1972.

51. Olanow, C. W., and Finn, A. L. Phenytoin: pharmacokinetics and clinical therapeutics. Neurosurgery *8:*112–117, 1981.

52. Origitano, T. C., Wascher, T. M., Reichman, O. H., and Anderson, D. E. Sustained increased cerebral blood flow with prophylactic hyperten-

sive hypervolemic hemodilution ("Triple-H" therapy) after subarachnoid hemorrhage. Neurosurgery 27:729–740, 1990.

53. Pakarinen, S. Incidence, aetiology, and prognosis of primary subarachnoid hemorrhage: a study based on 589 cases diagnosed in a defined urban population during a defined period. Acta Neurol. Scand. 43(suppl. 29):1–128, 1967.

54. Peerless, S. J. Pre- and post-operative management of cerebral aneurysms. Clin. Neurosurg. 26:209–231, 1978.

55. Peerless, S. J., and Drake, C. G. Posterior circulation aneurysm. In: Neurosurgery edited by P. H. Wilkins and S. S. Rengachary, Vol. 2, pp. 1167–1917. McGraw-Hill, New York, 1985.

56. Phillips, L. H., Whisnant, J. P., O'Fallon, W. M. et al. The unchanging pattern of subarachnoid hemorrhage in a community. Neurology 30:1034–1046, 1980.

57. Pickard, J. D., Murray, G. D., Illingworth, R., et al. Effect of oral nimodipine on cerebral infarction and outcome after subarachnoid hemorrhage: British Aneurysm Nimodipine Trial. Br. Med. J. [Clin., Res.] 298:636–642, 1989.

58. Ramirez-Lassepas, M. Antifibrinolytic therapy in subarachnoid hemorrhage caused by ruptured intracranial aneurysm. Neurology 31:316–322, 1981.

59. Redondo, A., Hanau, J., Creissard, P., and Le Beau, J. Complications gastro-duodenales des rupture anevrismales du systeme communicant anterieur. Neurochirurgie 16:471–488, 1970.

60. Richardson, A. E., and Uttley, D. Prevention of postoperative epilepsy. Lancet 1:650, 1980.

61. Ropper, A. H., and Zervas, N. T. Outcome one year after subarachnoid hemorrhage from cerebral aneurysm. J. Neurosurg. 60:909–915, 1984.

62. Rose, F. C., and Sarnen, M. Epilepsy after ruptured intracranial aneurysm. Br. Med. J. [Clin. Res.] 1:18–21, 1965.

63. Rosenhorn, J., Eskesen, V., Schmidt, K., and Ronde, F. The risk of rebleeding from ruptured intracranial aneurysms. J. Neurosurg. 67:329–332, 1987.

64. Rosenwasser, R. H., Delgado, T. F., Buchheit, W. A., and Freed, M. H. Control of hypertension and prophylaxis against vasospasm in cases of subarachnoid hemorrhage: a preliminary report. Neurosurgery 12:658–661, 1983.

65. Sengupta, R. P., Chiu, J. S. P., and Brierley, H. Quality of survival following direct surgery for anterior communicating artery aneurysm. J. Neurosurg. 43:58–64, 1975.

66. Slosberg, P. G. The current status of medical treatment of intracranial aneurysms. Prog. Neurol. Surg. 3:230–248, 1969.

67. Smith, R. B., and Tomlinson, B. E. Subendocardial haemorrhages associated with intracranial lesions. J. Pathol. 68:327–334, 1954.

68. Sours, J. A. Akentic mutism simulating catatonic schizophrenia. Am. J. Psychiatry 119:451–455, 1962.

69. Storey, R. B. Psychiatric sequelae of subarachnoid haemorrhage. Br. Med. J. [Clin. Res.] 3:261–266, 1967.

70. Sundt, T. M., Jr., Kobayashi, S., Fode, N. C., and Whisnant, J. P. Results and complications of surgical management of 809 intracranial aneurysms in 722 cases. J. Neurosurg. 56:753–765, 1982.

71. Suzuki, J., Onuma, T., and Yoshimoto, T. Results of early operations on cerebral aneurysms. Surg. Neurol. 11:407–412, 1979.

72. Swann, K. W., and Black, P. M. Deep vein thrombosis and pulmonary emboli in neurosurgical patients. J. Neurosurg. 61:1055–1062, 1984.

73. Torner, J. C., Kassell, N. E., Wallace, P. B., and Adams, H. B., Jr. Preoperative prognostic factors for rebleeding and survival in aneurysm patients receiving antifibrinolytic therapy: report of the Cooperative Aneurysm Study. Neurosurgery 9:506–511, 1981.

74. Van, T., Hoff, W., Hornabrook, R. W., and Marks, V. Hypopituitarism associated with intracranial aneurysms. Br. Med. J. [Clin. Res.] 2:1190–1193, 1961.

75. Vermeulen, M., Lindsay, K. W., Cheah, M. E., et al. Antifibrinolytic treatment in subarachnoid hemorrhage. N. Engl. J. Med. 311:432–437, 1984.

76. Vidal, B. E., Dergal, E. B., Cesarman, E., et al. Cardiac arrhythmias associated with subarachnoid hemorrhage: prospective study. Neurosurgery 5:675–680, 1979.

77. Walton, J. N. The electroencephalographic sequelae of spontaneous subarachnoid haemorrhage. Electroencephalogr. Clin. Neurophysiol. 5:41–52, 1953.

78. Warlow, C., Ogston, D., and Douglas, A. S. Venous thrombosis, following strokes. Lancet 1:1305–1306, 1972.

79. Weir, B. K. Aneurysms Affecting the Nervous System. Williams & Wilkins, Baltimore, 1987.

80. Weisman, S. J. Edema and congestion of the lungs resulting from intracranial hemorrhage. Surgery 6:722–729, 1939.

81. White, J. C., and Ballantine, H. T., Jr. Intrasellar aneurysms simulating hypophyseal tumours. J. Neurosurg. 18:34–50, 1961.

82. Wijdicks, E. E. M., Ropper, A. H., Hunnicutt, E. J., et al. Atrial natriuretic factor and salt wasting after aneurysmal subarachnoid hemorrhage. Stroke 22:1519–1524, 1991.

83. Wise, B. L. Syndrome of inappropriate antidiuretic hormone secretion after spontaneous SAH: a reversible cause of clinical deterioration. Neurosurgery 3:412–414, 1978.

84. Wyler, A. R., and Kelly, W. A. Use of antibiotics with external ventriculostomies. J. Neurosurg. 37:185–187, 1972.

85. Yamamoto, T., Nagasawa, S., Soto, S., et al. Electroencephalogram study of 52 cases following subarachnoid hemorrhage. Neurol. Surg. 6:341–346, 1978.

86. Yasargil, M. G., and Smith, R. D. Management of aneurysms of anterior circulation by intracranial procedures. In: Neurological Surgery: A Comprehensive Reference Guide to the Diagnosis and Management of Neurosurgical Problems. edited by J. R. Youmans, Vol. 3, pp. 1663–1696.

W. B. Saunders, Philadelphia, 1982.

87. Yoshimoto, H., and Uozumi, T. Anterior pituitary function in cerebrovascular disease: ruptured cerebral aneurysm cases. Neurol. Med. Chir. (Tokyo) 25:433–439, 1985.

88. Youmans, J. Special problems associated with sub-

arachnoid hemorrhage. Neurol. Surg. 53:1807–1820, 1982.

89. Zubkov, Y. N., Nikifovov, B. M., and Shustin, V. A. Balloon catheter technique for dilation of constricted cerebral arteries after aneurysmal S. A. H. Acta Neurochir. (Wien.) 70:65–79, 1984.

Principles of Management of Subarachnoid Hemorrhage: Steroids

SUN HO LEE, M.D., ROBERTO C. HEROS, M.D.

Glucocorticoid Steroids

Glucocorticoids have been employed in the management of a variety of disorders in the central nervous system (CNS). Although their effectiveness in the treatment of perifocal vasogenic edema from an intrinsic mass lesion, such as a malignant glioma, metastatic brain tumor, or brain abscess, is well established (19, 52), they have not been clearly proven to have protective effects in the wake of an ischemic insult to the CNS. The use of steroids for the treatment of ischemic stroke dates to the 1950s. Despite extensive clinical and experimental studies, considerable uncertainty still exists regarding the effectiveness of glucocorticoids in the management of cerebral ischemia. In spite of the controversy, the actual use of glucocorticoids for this purpose in clinical practice seems to be substantial.

In the clinical setting of perioperative management of subarachnoid hemorrhage (SAH), many clinicians include dexamethasone as a part of their routine medication regime. In patients with significant neurological deficits or with clinical or radiographic evidence of increased intracranial pressure (ICP) or mass effect, glucocorticoid treatment is frequently used to reduce edema and ICP as well as to increase cerebral perfusion (33, 36). Besides this popular indication, the use of high-dose glucocorticoids has drawn recent attention for the treatment and prevention of vasospasm in the wake of SAH. The use of glucocorticoids in the management of SAH is based on putative effects that are only partially proven. The first is the presumed cellular protective effect after acute ischemia. The second is the effect on edema following an ischemic insult. The third is the presumed inhibitory role in the development of chronic vasospasm. The final effect, relates to possible decrease in the development of delayed hydrocephalus after SAH. The authors have reviewed the experimental and clinical literature concerning the effectiveness of steroids in SAH and summarize the results here.

Brain-Protective Effect in the Early Stages of Ischemia after SAH

In the acute phase of SAH it appears that the increase in ICP and the consequent decrease of cerebral blood flow, the presence of the blood in the subarachnoid spaces, and the decrease in cerebral energy potential are possible factors that trigger a sequence of metabolic events that resembles the brain's response to an anoxic-ischemic insult (23, 67). After experimental SAH, the global hypoxic condition of the brain reduces the delivery of oxygen to neurons and induces a marked dissociation of normally tightly coupled electron-transport chain reactions (51). In this metabolic situation, the production of oxygen free radicals, which enhance lipid peroxidation of cellular and subcellular membrane phospholipids, has been suggested to be the trigger of neuronal damage (14, 53, 61). The pathophysiology and mechanism of cell damage in the wake of cerebral ischemia have not been clearly determined. Energy depletion or failure to maintain adenosine triphosphate (ATP) levels, which is an initial and central step of an ischemic insult, leads to loss of ion homeostasis by limiting the Na^+/K^+ pump, which results in cellular accumulation of Ca^{2+}, Na^+, and Cl^- (51). Another effect of ATP failure is degradation of phospholipids, with the accumulation of breakdown products including free fatty acids (8, 55, 62, 63). Stearic acid and arachidonic acid are preferentially released, and an increase in arachidonic acid may have important consequences in mediating cellular damage; much of this effect is attributed to its conversion to prostaglandins and other oxygenated products, as well as generation of oxygen free radicals (14, 51, 53). This also results in intracellular and extracellular degradation of macromolecules essential to the structural integrity of cells. Siesjö (63) summarized the mechanism of ischemic brain damage into three major phases: first, increases in the cytosolic calcium concentration, which is believed to cause cell damage by overactivation of lipases, proteases, and possibly also endonucleases and by alterations of protein phosphorylation; second, production of free radicals, whose target seems to be the microvasculature, causing microvascular dysfunction and blood-brain barrier (BBB) disruption; and, third, acidosis, which may promote edema formation and prevent recovery of mitochondrial metabolism.

There has been much clinical (4, 15, 42, 54) and experimental (1, 2, 13, 16, 40, 47, 48, 60) work regarding the effectiveness of glucocorticoids in acute ischemia. In some animal studies, glucocorticoids have been shown to be ineffective in altering the course of cerebral ischemia (2, 13, 47, 60). However, there are other reports which provide strong evidence of their effectiveness.

Experimental Studies

The use of glucocorticoids in the management of acute ischemia was initially based on the observation of their effectiveness in the injured cat spinal cord (7, 20). The pathophysiological processes are the same in both physical trauma and ischemic insult,

so that methylprednisolone may have similar therapeutic actions in CNS ischemia and trauma. Regarding actions in the injured spinal cord, large doses of methylprednisolone have been reported to enhance white matter blood flow (71) and to attenuate lipid peroxidation (20). Evidence for this antioxidant effect is seen in the protection of the membrane-bound enzyme Na^+/K^+-ATPase, which is sensitive to lipid peroxidation (7, 50), and the resulting protective effect on CNS membrane functions in cerebral ischemia. It has also been demonstrated that a high dose of methylprednisolone normalizes extracellular calcium ion concentration (71) and inhibits phospholipase A_2 activity, which blocks the production of vasoconstrictor prostaglandins following ischemia (55). In those experiments low-dose glucocorticoids did not show effectiveness, and it has been suggested that many of the therapeutic effects of methylprednisolone in CNS ischemia are probably unrelated to the classic glucocorticoid actions associated with more conventional doses. Glucocorticoids may inhibit lipid peroxidation through a direct antioxidant effect or by making the double bonds of unsaturated membrane lipids less susceptible to free radical attack (14, 66). The dose of methylprednisolone that showed antioxidant effect was in the range of 15–30 mg/kg, and the optimal dose was around 30 mg/kg given intravenously (20, 23).

Hall and Travis (23) demonstrated the effectiveness of glucocorticoids in maintaining CBF in the acute stage of SAH in a cat model. After induction of SAH caudate blood flow decreased 25.1% within 5 min, and between 5 min and 3 hours after injection there was a further and progressive decline in caudate blood flow. The hemorrhage also caused a slow increase in ICP, a decrease in cerebral perfusion pressure, and an increase in caudate vascular resistance. The administration of a single intravenous 30 mg/kg dose of methylprednisolone sodium succinate 30 min after the acute SAH resulted in stabilization of caudate blood flow, suggesting that this effect was a direct effect of the drug on the microvasculature. This may be due to the known effect of high glucocorticoid doses, which antagonize the actions of various vasoconstrictor agents including norepinephrine, epinephrine, serotonin, potassium and calcium chloride, and particularly prostaglandin $F_{2\alpha}$ ($PGF_{2\alpha}$) (55). This inhibitory action on the synthesis and/or release of $PGF_{2\alpha}$, together with a reduction in the cerebral vasoconstrictor response to this prostanoid, could contribute to the beneficial effect of methylprednisolone on CBF (9, 20, 55). Another possible important action of methylprednisolone in ameliorating acute post-SAH hypoperfusion may be an inhibition of SAH-induced microvascular lipid peroxidation (14, 50, 53). The possible molecular mechanism of inhibition of microvascular lipid peroxidation may be direct protection of cerebrovascular smooth muscle and endothelial cell membrane phospholipids from oxygen free radical attack or may be an indirect mechanism through the possible prevention of the formation and release of vasoactive prostaglandins (*e.g.*, $PGF_{2\alpha}$ and thromboxane A_2). It has been reported that glucocorticoids have an early protective "membrane-stabilizing effect" and have additional protective value, including prevention of blood cell aggregation, decrease of the permeability of cerebral microvessels, and inhibition of phospholipase A_2 (56).

Clinical Studies

Clinical studies of glucocorticoid treatment in acute ischemic stroke are rather discouraging (15, 54). Norris and Hachinski (54) showed no clinical evidence of beneficial effects in the treatment of postischemic brain lesions by using high-dose dexamethasone. In clinical use it seems that the time of the initial dose of glucocorticoid might be quite important. It is reasonable to presume that there is only a relatively short window of opportunity for a direct neuronal protective effect after brain ischemia (42).

The side effects of a high dose of glucocorticoids should be also considered in clinical application. A large dose of glucocorticoids may induce gastrointestinal bleeding and diabetes mellitus and mask early signs of infection. Karnik *et al.* (45) suggested that, with the exception of a greater number of urinary tract infections, dexamethasone therapy at high doses carries no increased

risk of medical problems in patients with SAH. However, prophylaxis for stomach ulcer and monitoring of blood sugar and electrolyte levels are deemed necessary.

Effect on Edema Formation after Ischemia

Glucocorticoids are among the most useful drugs in the clinician's armamentarium for treating some forms of cerebral edema. When focal edema is vasogenic in origin, as in tumor and abscess, it may be treated effectively with glucocorticoids. Conversely, steroids have not been shown to be of benefit in post-injury treatment of either focal or diffuse cytotoxic edema (2). During the critical early phase of ischemia, the edema produced is predominantly cytotoxic (49). When edema has been measured, glucocorticoids have had no effect upon its development in ischemic zones (13, 40, 60). However, even though glucocorticoids seem to be effective only in reducing the vasogenic edema which occurs at the late stage of ischemia, several experiments have demonstrated an early effect on edema (5, 16, 56). This may be due to the drug's inhibition of the hemorrhage-initiated vasoconstrictive prostanoid action and microvascular lipid peroxidation.

It is thought that cerebral edema caused by ischemia (often called "ischemic edema") represents a distinct process which is the most serious complication of a stroke. The classification of cerebral edema into vasogenic and cytotoxic types of edema, introduced by Klazo (46), is widely accepted, but neither category is applicable in cerebral ischemia. Edema caused by ischemia overlaps both cytotoxic and vasogenic forms; hence, it should be considered as a separate entity (56). In the early phase of ischemic brain edema, while the BBB is intact, there is a marked increase in tissue sodium and brain water content (49). Some investigators have postulated that, as the cellular sodium pump fails, sodium moves from the brain interstitial fluid into the brain cells, which creates a gradient for the diffusion of sodium from blood to brain interstitial fluid. Other investigators speculate that the active transport of sodium from blood to brain across the brain capillaries is specifically stimulated during the early phase of ischemia (6, 31, 49). As the gradient dissipates, an osmotic gradient develops between blood and the ischemic brain tissue, causing further accumulation of edema fluid. As the ischemic injury progresses, edema fluid accumulates in compliant brain parenchyma (30, 31). Glucocorticoids could reduce brain edema when the BBB is intact by reducing blood to brain sodium transport. The movement of sodium from blood to brain appears to involve Na^+-K^+ ATPase in the brain capillary endothelial cells, and this activity can be reduced *in vitro* by certain steroids (5). Steroids also inhibit production of prostaglandins, which induce cerebral edema in the early stage of cerebral ischemia (8). It has been demonstrated that the use of dexamethasone in cerebral ischemia prevents the accumulation of water, sodium, and calcium in the ischemic brain and reduces BBB permeability; it therefore has therapeutic value in acute cerebral ischemia (5, 16).

Effect on the Development of Vasospasm

Even though extensive experiments have been done to elucidate the pathophysiology of chronic vasospasm, its etiology remains unclear and specific treatment of chronic vasospasm remains elusive. Several factors have been claimed as possibly being involved in the pathogenesis of vasospasm. Adrenergic and serotoninergic pathways, prostaglandins, leukotrienes, and lipid peroxides have been widely investigated (37). Also, there is increasing evidence that chronic cerebral vasospasm may be linked to an inflammatory response of the arterial wall to the presence of blood in the subarachnoid spaces (11, 12). The anti-inflammatory effect of high-dose methylprednisolone may promote the preservation of arterial wall integrity and prevent delayed arterial vasospasm. It is also known that glucocorticoids interfere with prostaglandin synthesis, inhibit complement activation, depress leukocyte migration, and inhibit lymphocyte function (27). Many of these events are known to cause vascular damage.

Fox and Yasargil (18) showed that topically applied soluble glucocorticoids (methylprednisolone and cortisol) had marked vasodilatory effects, possibly through an en-

hancement of the activity of adenyl cyclase, which increases cyclic adenosine monophosphate and results in smooth muscle relaxation. Chyatte *et al.* (11) found that chronic vasospasm could be ameliorated by high-dose methylprednisolone (30 mg/kg intravenously, every 8 hours) and ibuprofen in the canine "double-hemorrhage" model, in which 4 ml of autologous blood were injected twice, 2 days apart. Low-dose methylprednisolone (15 mg/kg intravenously, every 8 hours) was not as effective as high-dose methylprednisolone (30 mg/kg intravenously, every 8 hours) (12). The authors speculated that steroids may be effective because chronic cerebral vasospasm may be linked to an inflammatory response induced by the presence of blood in the subarachnoid space. The time course of chronic vasospasm is consistent with that of an inflammatory reaction, appearing several days after SAH and lasting for days to weeks. Ultrastructural examination of chronically spastic cerebral arteries obtained from humans and experimental animals showed signs of cellular inflammation and damage, most notably necrosis of the arterial media and an inflammatory cell infiltration of the arterial wall.

A clinical study of patients at high risk for vasospasm treated with high-dose methylprednisolone showed reduced incidence and severity of vasospasm and improved morbidity and mortality rates, compared to matched contemporary controls (10). On this basis, high-dose methylprednisolone treatment was recommended for this high-risk group of patients. In that clinical study methylprednisolone was used initially within 72 hours of hemorrhage, at a dose of 30 mg/kg intravenously every 6 hours for 12 doses, then 15 mg/kg intravenously every 6 hours for four doses, then 7.5 mg/kg intravenously every 6 hours for four doses, then 3 mg/kg intravenously every 6 hours for four doses, and then 1.5 mg/kg intravenously every 12 hours for two doses. This treatment produced no side effects such as sepsis, wound complications, or gastrointestinal hemorrhage.

Effect on the Development of Hydrocephalus

Glucocorticoids are employed in clinical medicine on the assumption that their anti-inflammatory effect prevents arachnoiditis, periradicular fibrosis, and aseptic meningitis (41, 43). After SAH, 10–20% of the patients develop hydrocephalus and two thirds of these patients are symptomatic (34). Julow (43) studied the influence of dexamethasone on subarachnoid fibrosis after experimental SAH in dogs, through the scanning electron microscope. Intrathecal dexamethasone seemed to delay the fibrosis somewhat, but statistically there was no significant difference from the control group. It was considered that steroid therapy would only delay the inflammatory process. In that experiment 4 mg of intrathecal dexamethasone were given five or six times at intervals of 2–3 days, beginning 1 or 2 days after SAH or sometimes at the same time. The lack of effect of dexamethasone was explained by the fact that it inhibits the release of plasminogen activator but it does not inhibit the growth of cultured human fibroblasts in guinea pigs; therefore, dexamethasone treatment would not be expected to affect the wound collagen synthesis that results in fibrosis. Physiologically, the wound-healing process is significantly delayed in the subarachnoid space, compared to subcutaneous or intramuscular areas (58). Steroids perhaps increase this delay but do not prevent fibrosis.

Nonglucocorticoid Steroids

Nonglucocorticoid steroids have been developed which have antioxidant activity and improve neurological outcome after experimental spinal cord injury without, at least theoretically, the side effects of glucocorticoids. A nonglucocorticoid analogue of methylprednisolone showed inhibition of lipid peroxidation in experimental head injury and cerebral ischemia (21, 22, 24, 25, 26). One of these compounds is a 21-aminosteroid, U74006F (Fig. 5B.1). It appears that, while the steroid is responsible for the cerebroprotective effect, the 21-amine functional group accounts for the 10,000-fold increased potency and it does not have glucocorticoid receptor activity (26). U74006F has been shown to have considerable effectiveness in inhibiting iron-dependent lipid peroxidation and protecting membranes from the damaging effects of oxygen free

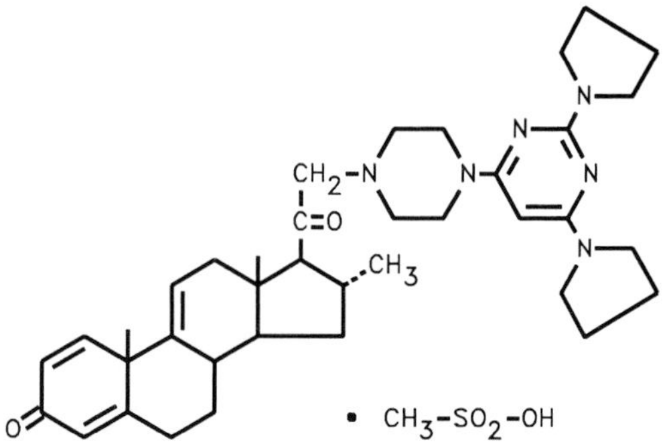

Figure 5B.1. Chemical structure of U74006F, a nonglucocorticoid 21-aminosteroid. (Reproduced with permission from Discovery Research, The Upjohn Company.)

radicals. This compound is thought to inhibit lipid peroxidation via several different actions, including a vitamin E-like membrane antioxidant effect, a superoxide anion-scavenging property, and possibly the ability to chelate iron at the membrane level. Preischemic treatment revealed a sparing of naturally occurring free radical scavenger vitamin E and quicker restoration of extracellular calcium after ischemia (21, 22), with better long-term neuronal survival and improved neurological outcome (57). Postischemic treatment also showed decreased size of infarct (28) and reduced edema in the penumbra zone (72). U74006F also has been shown to attenuate hypoperfusion after 5 min of tourniquet-induced global ischemia in cats (25), to improve survival in gerbils after unilateral carotid ligation (21), and to improve neurological outcome when given just prior to 12 min of complete ischemia in dogs (57). Haraldseth *et al.* (28) studied the effects of preischemic and postischemic treatment with 3 mg/kg U74006F, intravenously, on the recovery of high-energy phosphate and intracellular pH during early reperfusion in an ischemic rat model, using phosphorus-31 nuclear magnetic resonance spectroscopy, and concluded that U74006F led to quicker recovery of high-energy phosphate during early reperfusion; this beneficial effect was also seen with postischemic treatment. An experimental study in cats done by Hall and Travis (24) demonstrated that a 1 mg/kg intravenous dose of U74006F at 30 min after SAH significantly attenuated the progressive brain hypoperfusion which occurs acutely following experimental SAH, as well as the acute spasm that occurs within minutes to hours after SAH. Kanamaru *et al.* (44) reported its effectiveness on chronic cerebral vasospasm using a monkey model. Three dosage groups, of 0.3, 1.0, and 3.0 mg/kg intravenously every 8 hours for 6 days, appeared to have a favorable effect in preventing chronic vasospasm (68). The mechanism by which free radicals might produce arterial luminal narrowing is not presently known. It has been suggested that iron-catalyzed membrane lipid peroxidation associated with arachidonate release enhances the calcium permeability of the membrane and vasoconstrictor prostaglandin synthesis from endoperoxides (53). Hydroperoxides of membrane lipids and oxyhemoglobin also showed vasoconstrictor effect *in vitro* (3).

Mineralocorticoid Steroids

A decrease in plasma volume of >10% occurs in approximately 50% of patients with aneurysmal SAH during the first 6 days. Volume depletion after SAH is likely to be caused by natriuresis due to the release of a natriuretic factor (29, 69, 70). A decrease of plasma volume may lead to an increase in hematocrit, an increase in blood viscosity, and impaired cerebral blood flow, especially in the microcirculation, and leads to an increased risk of cerebral infarction. Fludrocortisone acetate has mineralocorticoid activity and enhances distal tubular sodium reabsorption in the kidney. In a clinical study done by Wijdicks *et al.* (70), it appeared that fludrocortisone acetate was an effective method of decreasing the incidence of volume depletion and negative sodium balance in the first 6 days after SAH. Those authors recommended preventing volume depletion by inhibiting excessive sodium excretion instead of treating volume depletion after signs of cerebral ischemia had already developed. Treatment was started within 48 hours of the hemorrhage, at a dose of 0.2 mg of fludrocortisone intravenously, twice each day. Fludrocortisone may reduce natriuresis and may be of possible therapeutic benefit in the prevention of delayed cerebral ischemia after aneurysmal SAH.

Summary

The authors have tried to summarize the possible beneficial effects of steroids in the treatment and prevention of cerebral ischemia and chronic vasospasm after SAH. The presumed molecular mechanisms of the protective effect of glucocorticoids may be related to their inhibitory action on phospholipase A_2 (38), which is similar to the effect of pentobarbital in inhibiting phospholipase C (32). As a result, production of vasoactive prostaglandins derived from arachidonic acid, which results from phospholipid degradation, is decreased. It is probable that methylprednisolone inhibition of posthemorrhagic hypoperfusion is dependent on some form of antioxidant action on vascular lipid peroxidation, either directly or indirectly, through reduction of $PGF_{2\alpha}$ or thromboxane A_2 formation, or both. There are also some data published which suggest that glucocorticoids reduce the permeability of the BBB through a direct action at the vascular endothelium (73). This diminished permeability of cerebral endothelial cells may also affect the ischemia-induced functional changes in the neurons. The glucocorticoid inhibition of prostaglandin synthesis, inhibition of complement activation, depression of leukocyte migration, and inhibition of lymphocyte function may be beneficial in the prevention of vasospasm.

Clinical Recommendations

There is no definite proof of the effectiveness of steroids in the management of SAH. However, in light of the experimental and clinical data reported, SAH appears to be one form of stroke in which steroids may have a therapeutic role. The use of glucocorticoids in patients with evidence of significantly increased ICP or mass effect is recommended at a rather low dose (4 mg of dexamethasone four times each day). It may be reasonable to consider use of glucocorticoids to prevent chronic vasospasm, on the basis of their anti-inflammatory effects. However, because glucocorticoids have significant side effects and because there are other therapeutic maneuvers that may be of benefit (17, 33, 35–37, 39, 59, 64, 65), these authors do not recommend the routine use of glucocorticoids to treat or prevent vasospasm. Before such treatment can be routinely recommended it will be necessary to perform a large, randomized, controlled clinical trial to evaluate the effectiveness of steroids on chronic vasospasm after SAH. The use of nonglucocorticoid steroids should be considered only after clinical studies have been carried out to demonstrate their effectiveness.

REFERENCES

1. Altman, D. I., Young, R. S. K., and Yagel, S. K. Effects of dexamethasone in hypoxic-ischemic brain injury in the neonatal rat. Biol. Neonate 46:149–156, 1984.
2. Anderson, D. C., and Cranford, R. E. Corticosteroids in ischemic stroke. Stroke 10:68–71, 1979.
3. Asano, T., Sasaki, T., Koide, K., et al. Experimental evaluation of the beneficial effect of an antioxidant on cerebral vasospasm. Neurol. Res. 6:49–53, 1984.
4. Bauer, R. B., and Tellez, H. Dexamethasone as treatment in cerebrovascular disease. 2. A controlled study in acute cerebral infarction. Stroke 4:547–555, 1973.
5. Betz, A. L., and Coester, H. C. Effect of steroid therapy on ischemic brain edema and blood to brain sodium transport. Acta Neurochir. [Suppl.] (Wien) 51:256–258, 1990.
6. Betz, A. L., Ennis, S. R., Schielke, G. P., and Hoff, J. T. Blood to brain sodium transport in ischemic brain edema. Adv. Neurol. 52:73–80, 1990.
7. Braughler, J. M., and Hall, E. D. Correlation of methylprednisolone levels in cat spinal cord with its effects on Na^+-K^+ ATPase, lipid peroxidation, and alpha motor neuron function. J. Neurosurg. 56:838–844, 1982.
8. Bucci, M. N., Black, K. L., and Hoff, J. T. Arachidonic acid metabolite production following focal cerebral ischemia: time course and effect of meclofenamate. Surg. Neurol. 33:12–14, 1990.
9. Chan, R. C., Durity, F. A., Thompson, G. B., et al. The role of the prostacyclin-thromboxane system in cerebral vasospasm following induced subarachnoid hemorrhage in the rabbit. J. Neurosurg. 61:1120–1128, 1984.
10. Chyatte, D., Fode, N. C., Nichols, D. A., and Sundt, T. M., Jr. Preliminary report: effect of high dose methylprednisolone on delayed cerebral ischemia in patients at high risk for vasospasm after aneurysmal subarachnoid hemorrhage. Neurosurgery 21:157–160, 1987.
11. Chyatte, D., Rusch, N., and Sundt, T. M., Jr. Prevention of chronic experimental cerebral vasospasm with ibuprofen and high dose methylprednisolone. J. Neurosurg. 59:925–932, 1983.
12. Chyatte, D., and Sundt, T. M., Jr. Response of chronic experimental cerebral vasospasm to methylprednisolone and dexamethasone. J. Neurosurg. 60:923–926, 1984.
13. Conley, R. F., and Sundt, T. M., Jr. Effect of

14. Demopoulos, H. B., Flamm, E. S., Pietronigro, D. D., and Seligman, M. L. The free radical pathology and the microcirculation in the major central nervous system disorders. Acta Physiol. Scand. [Suppl.] 492:91–119, 1980.
15. De Reuck, J., Vandekerckhove, T., Bosma, G., et al. Steroid treatment in acute ischemic stroke: a comparative retrospective study of 556 cases. Eur. Neurol. 28:70–72, 1988.
16. Dux, E., Ismail, M., Szerdahelyi, P., et al. Dexamethasone treatment attenuates the development of ischemic brain edema in gerbils. Neuroscience 34:203–207, 1990.
17. Findlay, J. M., MacDonald, R. L., and Weir, B. K. A. Current concepts of pathophysiology and management of cerebral vasospasm following aneurysmal subarachnoid hemorrhage. Cerebrovasc. Brain Metab. Rev. 3:336–361, 1991.
18. Fox, J. L., and Yasargil, M. G. The relief of intracranial vasospasm: an experimental study with methylprednisolone and cortisol. Surg. Neurol. 3:214–218, 1975.
19. French, L. A. The use of steroids in the treatment of cerebral edema. Bull. NY Acad. Med. 42:301–311, 1966.
20. Hall, E. D., and Braughler, J. M. Acute effects of intravenous glucocorticoid pretreatment on the in vitro peroxidation of cat spinal cord tissue. Exp. Neurol. 73:321–324, 1983.
21. Hall, E. D., Pazara, K. E., and Braughler, J. M. 21-Aminosteroid lipid peroxidation inhibitor U74006F protects against cerebral ischemia in gerbils. Stroke 19:997–1002, 1988.
22. Hall, E. D., Pazara, K. E., and Braughler, J. M. Effects of tirilazad mesylate on postischemic brain lipid peroxidation and recovery of extracellular calcium in gerbils. Stroke 22:361–366, 1991.
23. Hall, E. D., and Travis, M. A. Attenuation of progressive brain hypoperfusion following experimental subarachnoid hemorrhage by large intravenous doses of methylprednisolone. Exp. Neurol. 99:594–606, 1988.
24. Hall, E. D., and Travis, M. A. Effects of the nonglucocorticoid 21-aminosteroid U74006F on acute cerebral hypoperfusion following experimental subarachnoid hemorrhage. Exp. Neurol. 102:244–248, 1988.
25. Hall, E. D., and Yonkers, P. A. Attenuation of postischemic cerebral hypoperfusion by the 21-aminosteroid U74006F. Stroke 19:340–344, 1988.
26. Hall, E. D., Yonkers, P. A., McCall, J. M., and Braughler, J. M. Effects of the 21-aminosteroid U74006F on experimental head injury in mice. J. Neurosurg. 68:456–461, 1988.
27. Hammerschmidt, D. E., White, J. G., Craddock, P. R., et al. Corticosteroids inhibit complement-induced granulocyte aggregation: a possible mechanism for their efficacy in shock states. J. Clin. Invest. 63:798–803, 1979.
28. Haraldseth, O., Grönas, T., and Unsgård, G. Quicker metabolic recovery after forebrain is-

chemia in rats treated with the antioxidant U74006F. Stroke *22*:1188–1192, 1991.

29. Hasan, D., Lindsay, K. W., Wijdicks, E. F. M., *et al.* Effect of fludrocortisone acetate in patients with subarachnoid hemorrhage. Stroke *20*:1156–1161, 1989.

30. Hatashita, S., and Hoff, J. T. Brain edema and cerebrovascular permeability during cerebral ischemia in rats. Stroke *21*:582–588, 1990.

31. Hatashita, S., and Hoff, J. T. Role of a hydrostatic pressure gradient in the formation of early ischemic brain edema. J. Cereb. Blood Flow Metab. *6*:546–552, 1986.

32. Hattori, T., Nishimura, Y., Sakai, N., *et al.* Inhibitory effect of pentobarbital on phospholipase C activity in ischemic rat brain. Neurol. Res. *9*:164–168, 1987.

33. Heros, R. C. Intracranial aneurysms: a review. Minn. Med. *73*:27–32, 1990.

34. Heros, R. C. Acute hydrocephalus after subarachnoid hemorrhage. Stroke *20*:715–717, 1989.

35. Heros, R. C., and Korosue, K. Hemodilution for cerebral ischemia. Stroke *20*:423–427, 1989.

36. Heros, R. C., and Zervas, N. T. Subarachnoid hemorrhage. Annu. Rev. Med. *34*:367–375, 1983.

37. Heros, R. C., Zervas, N. T., and Varsos, V. Cerebral vasospasm after subarachnoid hemorrhage: an update. Ann. Neurol. *14*:599–608, 1983.

38. Hirata, F., Schiffman, E., Venkatsubramanian, K., *et al.* A phospholipase A_2 inhibitory protein in rabbit neuropils induced by glucocorticoids. Proc. Natl. Acad. Sci. USA *77*:2533–2536, 1980.

39. Hoff, J. T. Cerebral protection. J. Neurosurg. *65*:579–591, 1986.

40. Ito, U., Ohno, K., Suganuma, Y., *et al.* Effect of steroid in ischemic brain edema. Stroke *1*:166–172, 1980.

41. Jackson, F. E. Optic chiasmatic arachnoiditis: improvement of rapidly failing vision following surgical lysis of chiasmatic adhesions and postoperative steroid therapy. Milit. Med. *139*:127–128, 1974.

42. Jastremski, M., Sutton-Tyrrell, K., Vaagenes, P., *et al.* Glucocorticoid treatment does not improve neurological recovery following cardiac arrest. JAMA *262*:3427–3430, 1989.

43. Julow, J. The influence of dexamethasone on subarachnoid fibrosis after subarachnoid hemorrhage: scanning electron microscopic study in the dog. Acta Neurochir. (Wien) *51*:43–51, 1979.

44. Kanamaru, K., Weir, B. K. A., Findlay, J. M., *et al.* A dosage study of the effect of the 21-aminosteroid U74006F on chronic cerebral vasospasm in a primate model. Neurosurgery *27*:29–38, 1990.

45. Karnik, R., Valentin, A., Prainer, C., *et al.* Zum Problem der Steroidtherapie bei Subarachnoidalblutungen. Wien. Klin. Wochenschr. *102*:1–4, 1990.

46. Klazo, I. Neuropathological aspects of brain edema. J. Neuropathol. Exp. Neurol. *26*:1–14, 1967.

47. Lee, M. C., Mastri, A. R., Waltz, A. G., and Loewenson, R. B. Ineffectiveness of dexamethasone for treatment of experimental cerebral infarction. Stroke *5*:216–218, 1974.

48. Little, J. R. Modification of acute focal ischemia by treatment with mannitol and high-dose dexamethasone. J. Neurosurg. *49*:517–524, 1978.

49. Lo, W. D., Betz, A. L., Schielke, G. P., and Hoff, J. T. Transport of sodium from blood to brain in ischemic brain edema. Stroke *18*:150–157, 1987.

50. Marzatico, F., Gaetani, P., Buratti, E., *et al.* Effects of high-dose methylprednisolone on Na^+-K^+ ATPase and lipid peroxidation after experimental subarachnoid hemorrhage. Acta Neurol. Scand. *82*:263–270, 1990.

51. Marzatico, F., Gaetani, P., Rodriguez, Y., *et al.* Bioenergetics of different brain areas after experimental subarachnoid hemorrhage in rats. Stroke *19*:378–384, 1988.

52. Maxwell, R. E., Long, D. M., and French, L. A. The clinical effects of a synthetic glucocorticoid used for brain edema in the practice of neurosurgery. In: Steroids and Brain Edema, edited by H. J. Reulen and K. Schurmann, pp. 219–232. Springer-Verlag, New York, 1972.

53. McCall, J. M., Braughler, J. M., and Hall, E. D. Lipid peroxidation and the role of oxygen radicals in CNS injury. Acta Anaesthesiol. Belg. *38*:373–379, 1987.

54. Norris, J. W., and Hachinski, V. C. High dose steroid treatment in cerebral infarction. Br. Med. J. *292*:21–23, 1986.

55. Okabe, T., Meyer, J. S., Amano, T., *et al.* Prostaglandin inhibition and cerebrovascular hemodynamics in normal and ischemic human brain. J. Cereb. Blood Flow Metab. *3*:115–121, 1983.

56. Okamatsu, S., Peck, R. C., and Lefer, A. M. Protective actions of dexamethasone in acute cerebral ischemia. Circ. Shock *9*:445–456, 1982.

57. Perkins, W. J., Milde, L. N., Milde, J. H., and Michenfelder, J. D. Pretreatment with U74006F improves neurologic outcome following complete cerebral ischemia in dogs. Stroke *22*:902–909, 1991.

58. Schemm, G. W., Benrley, J. P., and Deoffler, M. Wound healing in the subarachnoid space. Neurology *18*:862–869, 1968.

59. Shubin, R. A., and Fisher, M. Steroid therapy in stroke. In: Medical Therapy of Acute Stroke, edited by M. Fisher, pp. 89–202. Marcel Dekker Inc., New York, 1989.

60. Siegel, B. A., Studer, R. K., and Potchen, E. J. Steroid therapy of brain edema. Arch. Neurol. *27*:209–212, 1972.

61. Siesjö, B. K. Cell damage in the brain: a speculative synthesis. J. Cereb. Blood Flow Metab. *1*:155–185, 1981.

62. Siesjö, B. K. Pathophysiology and treatment of focal cerebral ischemia. I. Pathophysiology. J. Neurosurg. *77*:169–184, 1992.

63. Siesjö, B. K. Pathophysiology and treatment of focal cerebral ischemia. II. Mechanism of damage and treatment. J. Neurosurg. *77*:337–354, 1992.

64. Smith, D. S. Free radical scavengers and protection against ischemic brain damage. In: Cerebral Is-

chemia and Resuscitation, edited by A. Schur and B. M. Rigor, pp. 373–388. CRC Press, Boca Raton, FL, 1990.

65. Spetzler, R. F., and Nehls, D. G. Cerebral protection against ischemia. In: Cerebral Blood Flow: Physiologic and Clinical Aspects, edited by J. H. Wood, pp. 651–676. McGraw-Hill Book Company, New York, 1987.

66. Suzuki, J., Imaizumi, S., Kayama, T., and Yoshimoto, T. Chemiluminescence in hypoxic brain: the second report: cerebral protective effect of mannitol, vitamin E and glucocorticoid. Stroke *16:*695–700, 1985.

67. Umansky, F., Kaspi, T., and Shalit, M. N. Regional cerebral blood flow in the acute stage of experimentally induced subarachnoid hemorrhage. J. Neurosurg. *58:*210–216, 1983.

68. Vollmer, D. G., Kassell, N. F., Hongo, K., *et al.* Effect of the nonglucocorticoid 21-aminosteroid U74006F on experimental cerebral vasospasm. Surg. Neurol. *31:*190–194, 1989.

69. Wijdicks, E. F. M., Vermeulen, M., van Brummelen, P., and van Gijn, J. The effect of fludrocortisone acetate on plasma volume and natriuresis in patients with aneurysmal subarachnoid hemorrhage. Clin. Neurol. Neurosurg. *90:*209–214, 1988.

70. Wijdicks, E. F. M., Vermeulen, M., Ten Haaf, J. A., *et al.* Volume depletion and natriuresis in patients with a ruptured intracranial aneurysm. Ann. Neurol. *18:*211–216, 1985.

71. Young, W., and Flamm, E. S. Effect of high dose corticosteroid therapy on blood flow, evoked potentials, and extracellular calcium in experimental spinal injury. J. Neurosurg. *57:*667–673, 1982.

72. Young, W., Wojak, J. C., and DeCrescito, V. 21-Aminosteroid reduces ion shifts and edema in the rat middle cerebral artery occlusion model of regional ischemia. Stroke *19:*1013–1019, 1988.

73. Ziylan, Y. Z., Lefauconnier, J. M., Bernard, G., and Bourre, J. M. Regional alterations in blood-to-brain transfer of α-aminoisobutyric acid and sucrose, after chronic administration and withdrawal of dexamethasone. J. Neurochem. *52:*684–689, 1989.

Principles of Management of Subarachnoid Hemorrhage: Antifibrinolysis

SEAN MULLAN, M.D.

INTRODUCTION

Before 1953, there was virtually no effective treatment for subarachnoid hemorrhage. Medical management consisted of rest in bed, with occasional intermittent lumbar puncture to relieve headache. Pioneering intracranial surgical attempts produced considerable interest but few disciples. Common carotid ligature was explored, because it was realized that the bursting pressure of an aneurysm is related to the blood pressure within it. Then in 1953, Norlen and Olivecrona (57) dramatically showed that satisfactory occlusion by craniotomy could be achieved with a mortality rate of only 3–4%.

Others attempted to duplicate the results, but without full recognition of the fact that Norlen and Olivecrona had delayed operations until 2–3 weeks after hemorrhage. The success rates of these early operations (mostly unpublished) fell far short of those of Norlen and Olivecrona. After the figures from Magladery (49) became available, there was major disenchantment with the intracranial approach, and common carotid ligature was increasingly employed. New interest was taken in optimizing medical control of blood pressure (73), but control by common carotid artery ligation dominated the surgical scene. That experience made it clear that common carotid artery ligation, in the short term, greatly reduced early bleeding of internal carotid artery aneurysms and, to a lesser extent, of middle cerebral and anterior

cerebral artery aneurysms. It was also apparent that this was accompanied by a distressing incidence of delayed postocclusion hemiplegia (28). In time this was recognized as either the liberation of an embolus from the occluded artery or a manifestation of the newly recognized arterial spasm (12). Then, as the natural history of the condition and especially the role of spasm became better understood and as the problems of intracranial surgery were slowly resolved and its techniques perfected, craniotomy, following an interval of recovery as pioneered by Norlen, slowly displaced ligature as the treatment of choice. A delay of 12 days became more or less accepted (37).

Rationale

From the medical perspective, it was next postulated that, if the hemostatic effect of the regional blood clot could be prolonged by inhibiting its lysis, then the Norlen interval of presurgical improvement in the condition of the patient could be retained with an acceptably low risk of rebleeding during that interval. The delay would then make the final definitive surgery safe. In a series of studies beginning in 1968, it became evident that the use of antifibrinolytic drugs did in fact reduce the rebleeding rate, but from the beginning there was a suspicion that perhaps the drugs incurred enhanced intravascular thrombosis in some instances, (25, 26, 53, 65, 78). By the late 1970s, it had become increasingly clear that these drugs did intensify the morbidity of the spasm phase of subarachnoid hemorrhage, so that what was gained by decreasing rebleeding was lost by an increase in spasm morbidity (19, 35, 40, 83). At this stage, emboldened by 30 years of experience in the evolution of surgical techniques, throughout which early operation was never totally abandoned (33, 52, 53), surgeons became again more interested in early surgery (5, 47, 67, 75, 85). A pilot study of international scope was set up in the early 1980s to explore the possibilities of early surgery. Because of the inherent difficulties, almost impossibilities, of setting up a valid statistical study, this was simply an observational study without formal controls. When concluded, it suggested, to the surprise of some and to the disappointment of others, that early operation was neither as bad as was feared nor as good as was hoped (30, 41, 42). In terms of final outcome, it made little difference whether the operation was planned early or planned late, except that outcome between days 7 and 10 was significantly disappointing on the whole. An attempt to recognize some benefit from early operation was made by extracting the North American figures from the total, but again the results were unconvincing. For drowsy patients, the 6–14-day planned interval still brought disappointing results. For alert patients, perhaps there was a marginal improvement in outcome for those for whom the operation was planned in the 0–3-day interval. The overall management results of the total study, as seen 6 months later, revealed a 27% mortality rate and 58% good recovery rate. For the North American section, the mortality rate was 22% and the good results were 57%. It must be recalled that this was an observational study and not in any way a controlled study. By design, it could only suggest; it could not prove. It emphasized that ruptured aneurysms are a multifactorial problem not easily solved by one single management decision applicable to all patients. The timing of operation was simply one of very many factors which must be considered in relation to others. As in all surgical operations, patient selection and adjuvant medical care must be considered as carefully as timing and technique.

As further experience accumulated and as this International Cooperative Aneurysm Study was compared to previous studies, especially the earlier cooperative studies of the 1960s and 1970s, a change in the rebleeding pattern was observed. In the classical study by Locksley (48), a peak in rebleeding had been recognized at the end of the first week and the beginning of the second week. This recent study (30, 41, 42) did not recognize such a peak period. Instead, one occurred during the first 24 hours, with a 4.1% rebleeding rate. Thereafter, the rate was approximately 1.5%/day. The acute rebleeding rate was 19% in 14 days. There are three possible explanations. Probably earlier referral to neurosurgical centers simply disclosed this earlier peak, which previously had been lost in the transport and referral pattern. Another possibility is that deterioration due to spasm was wrongly diagnosed in those studies as a bleed, before the clinical entity of spasm was fully appreciated (15, 87). The third possibility is the influence of antifibrinolytic medication. Fibrinolysis is not significant on the first day, nor can a proper level of antifibrinolytic drug activity be achieved on the first day, if the drug is given orally or by intravenous injection. Intravenous infusion produces adequate levels more quickly (15). The first and probably the second days are unprotected. These early rebleeds are "blow-out" hemorrhages. In addition, only approximately 25% of patients were given antifibrinolytic drugs on the first day. On the other hand, 75% of patients in whom surgery was planned for the 7–10-day interval did have antifibrinolytic medication, thereby smoothing out the peak of that interval. This first-day peak has been observed by others. Inagawa et al. (34) have reported on 150 patients who were admitted within 6 hours of their initial hemorrhage. Twenty-three bled within 6 hours. Twenty-nine bled within the first 24 hours. Because of an early operation policy, there was no significant figure for later rebleeding. It should be noted that, of 75 patients who underwent angiography within 6 hours of the initial subarachnoid hemorrhage, four developed rebleeding during angiography. This was twice the rate of rebleeding during any other time interval (34).

Vasospasm

The introduction of nimodipine by Allen et al. (2) in 1983 then opened up a new chapter in medical management. This study of 116 good-risk patients, which was multi-institutional, double-blinded, randomized, and placebo-controlled, with surgery interval at will up to 14 days, reported one death among 56 patients given nimodipine and three deaths and five serious outcomes among 60 patients given placebo. The total number of deaths was three in the nimodipine-treated group and seven among the controls (2). Auer (5) also reported a series using early operation and nimodipine, with a mortality rate of 10.8% and a full recovery rate of 60%. Had poor-risk cases been excluded, the mortality rate would have dropped to 1.5%. He, too, commented upon the protective role of nimodipine despite arterial spasm. The series reported by Ljunggren et al. (46), of 60 nimodipine-treated patients of all grades, mostly operated upon within 72 hours, had a mortality rate of 1.5% and a serious morbidity rate of 3%. This was better than previous experience reported by the same authors, utilizing early operation but not nimodipine (47). The former mortality rate for early surgery with good-grade patients was about 10%, with an additional late death rate of 6%. Although the authors expressed the opinion that the good results in the later series were due to early surgery and nimodipine, the dominant factor appears to be nimodipine. The lack of correlation between spasm and cerebral ischemia addressed the possibility that the effect of nimodipine was mediated by a factor other than large-vessel spasm. Öhman and Heiskanen (58), in their study of patients of grades I, II, and III, using nimodipine, noted a significantly lowered mortality rate for the treated patients, compared to the controls (1.6% and 12.3%, respectively), for patients operated upon within 1 week. Petruk et al. (60), in a multicentered, randomized, placebo-controlled, double-blind study, specifically investigated patients of grades III, IV, and V, utilizing nimodipine and mostly early operation (71% operated upon on days 0–3). The mortality rate for the nimodipine-treated group (47.2%) was greater than that for the placebo-treated group (39%), but the good recovery rate was the reverse (29.2% for treatment and 9.8% for control). An advantage was not seen in the grade V category. There was no significant difference in the radiographic evidence of spasm between the treated and the control groups (60). It should be noted that the mortality factor was only marginally better than the spontaneous outcome reported by Alvord et al. (3), which is the base-line against which all treatments must be measured. The study of Mee et al. (50) is of particular interest, in that serial xenon-133 studies revealed not the expected increase but a minimal decrease in cerebral blood flow with the use of nimodipine. Despite this, only one patient of 50 died in the treatment group, compared to six among the controls. The timing of surgery was a matter of individual judgement (50).

Outcome

It might thus be stated that there is good evidence that the introduction of nimodipine has led to a very significant improvement in operative outcome in terms of mortality and morbidity rates, especially in alert patients. It also appears to be of significant benefit in terms of morbidity rates for less alert patients, but not necessarily for those of grade V. The role of operation timing is not so clear. Days 7–10, or possibly days 6–14, have been documented as hazardous, especially for drowsy patients, but the extent to which nimodipine alters or removes this hazard is not clear. In the entire field, decisions must be made based on individual judgement, because statistically valid studies which might provide an answer simply do not exist. Early operation removes the risk of subsequent rebleeding, which is perhaps 1.5%/day, and it has come to dominate neurosurgical thinking, just as delayed intervention once did, but it has not solved the problem by any means (30, 42, 60).

Theoretically there is reason to believe that the arterial spasm problem will be solved relatively soon by use of fibrinolytic drugs (e.g., T.E.P.A.), continuous intra-arterial papaverine, or intraluminal dilatation, or by all three, leaving the way open for a surgically undisputed early operation for most patients (14, 36, 38, 69). However, that time has not yet arrived. None of these three antispasm remedies is universally proven or universally in place, nor will they be universally available outside of research institutions for some years. Neither is the possibility of immediate operative occlusion of the aneurysm. There are logistical considerations relating to diagnosis, transport, availability of facilities, and availability of personnel which have not been universally solved. Moreover, there is a number of medical conditions which may demand attention before operation. Lastly, the patient may not consent to operation. Thus, for some time into the future, the neurosurgeon or responsible physician will be confronted with the need to manage medically patients with a subarachnoid hemorrhage for a period before operation is undertaken.

Early surgical clipping was tried, shown to be effective, and then rejected because of its complications. Hypotension and antifibrinolysis were tried and also shown to be effective. They too were rejected because of their complications. Early clipping is now back in use for properly defined patients, in association with better control of intracranial pressure and the use of nimodipine. The question, therefore, arises as to whether there remains a legitimate role for hypotension and antifibrinolysis in properly selected patients in conjunction with better intracranial pressure control and the use of nimodipine. All of these factors are inter-related. A study designed to measure one of them without recognition of the others would reveal little useful information. By paying strict attention to all of them (except nimodipine, which was not available), we were able to report in 1978 (54) a medical mortality rate of 15% (21%, if those too moribund to have an angiogram were included). The associated surgical mortality rate was zero. These overall figures, which compare favorably with those for the natural outcome (3) and with those of the International Cooperative Study (30, 41, 42), indicate that there is merit in very intensive medical management before surgery. The task is to examine this merit in detail, as it pertains to either the referring or the accepting institu-

tion, and minimize both the preoperative rebleed and complication figures and the overall mortality and morbidity rates.

Mechanism of Action

Antifibrinolysis delays lysis of the original hemostatic clot and thereby should delay or reduce rebleeding (25, 26, 35, 53, 65, 78). A normal blood clot is lysed by the enzyme plasmin. This is derived from plasminogen, a normal constituent of the blood. It is contained in every blood clot. A blood clot in a glass vial will spontaneously lyse. Plasminogen is converted to plasmin by tissue activators which increase in response to disturbances such as trauma, infection, and hemorrhage. If fibrous tissue and endothelial repair of a ruptured aneurysm is completed before lysis of the hemostatic clot takes place, then the patient recovers uneventfully. If repair is not completed, there is another hemorrhage. It has been known since 1948 that this activation can be inhibited by ϵ-aminocaproic acid (EACA). This is a synthetic amino acid (monoaminocarboxylic acid). There are two others with similar properties, tranexamic acid (AMCA) and *para*-aminobenzoic acid (PAMBA). On a molar basis AMCA is 5–10 times more potent than EACA and twice as strong as PAMBA. This much-quoted 5–10-fold figure reflects a major dosage imprecision that has related to these drugs since their introduction (15, 17, 19–22, 25, 26, 35, 53, 59, 65, 77–80, 83).

At the time of their introduction, there was no truly successful monitoring method to determine optimum dosage, and there has been no extensive effort to compare the several drugs that are available (9). Fibrin degradation products are regularly found in the cerebrospinal fluid following subarachnoid hemorrhage. They are reduced by the fibrinolytic drugs, but a level which could be closely related to the risk of rebleeding has not been determined. There are many additional factors which determine this, such as the size of the opening, the direction of its axis in relation to the main flow of the artery, and blood pressure. Measurements of the plasminogen level of the blood have been inconsistent. Perhaps the whole-clot lysis and accelerated clot lysis times were as good as any. Figures of 72 hours and 48 hours, respectively, for these values were aimed at, but these targets were quite arbitrary and reasonable rather than accurately determined by outcome results (51). They had a major drawback, in that they did not provide immediate information to regulate management on an hourly or even daily basis. The euglobulin lysis test, with a 45–60-min normal range, would now provide a better standard.

The dose initially used was based upon laboratory experiments. One week after thrombosis of dog femoral artery by an electric current, the clot had disappeared in six of eight animals. A similar group was given EACA in drinking water at a dose of 350 mg/kg/day. At the end of 1 week, the clot was still present in seven of eight animals, not totally disappearing in all animals until the fifth week. A chromium-tagged blood clot, suspended in the cisternum magnum of a rabbit given EACA, remained largely intact at day 12 as determined by external counting, but was fully dissolved and dispersed by day 25 (51, 52). It therefore appears that clot in the wall of an artery and surrounding an artery in the subarachnoid space begins to dissolve in <1 week and is largely dissolved within 3 weeks. The moment when lysis would make it loose, in relation to arterial pressure, was not determined. It was estimated that the major value of such medication would be seen in the first week (15). There was evidence that lysis did

not begin significantly within 24 hours, nor was antifibrinolysis fully established within 48 hours. Thus, the greatest protection would exist between the second and seventh day, but further protection might be expected for another week or perhaps more.

In the 20-year period following introduction of the concept, there have been 16 EACA, 13 AMCA, eight EACA plus AMCA, and two PAMBA clinical studies, for a total of 39. Some were controlled (1, 9, 24, 29, 31, 51, 53, 62, 63, 65, 68, 71, 76, 78, 81). Others were controlled but not randomized (4, 6, 8, 10, 23, 25, 26, 39, 44, 45, 55, 56, 61, 66, 70, 72). In 26 of these 31, which were uncontrolled or controlled but not randomized, a reduction of bleeding was reported. In one of the earliest, it was recognized that thrombosis of the vessel could occur, so that the method was not without some potential problems (53). In five, there was either no effect or even an apparently negative effect. Cerebral ischemic events were recognized in six patients in the two PAMBA studies (the drugs were given intrathecally). Studies combining antifibrinolytic drugs and Kallikren inhibitors were inadequate for final conclusions. Kallikren inhibitors are antiplasmin drugs extracted from bovine salivary gland. Trasylol is one such drug. The eight randomized and controlled trials are of greater interest because of their intrinsic design (Table 5C.1). Four were not blinded (16, 19, 27, 86). In three of these AMCA was used and in one EACA was employed. In all four which were blinded AMCA was used (7, 43,

TABLE 5C.1
Clinical Trials

Year	Study	Drug	Day	Total		Rebled (%)		Died (%)	
				Drug	Control	Drug	Control	Drug	Control
Not blinded									
1973	Girvin (27)	EACA	24	39	27	36	15	18	15
1978	Fodstad et al. (19)	AMCA	3–6	23	23	4	39	26	43
1978	Williams (86)	AMCA	6	25	25	24	56	12	44
1981	Fodstad (16)	AMCA	4–6	30	29	20	24	43	31
Double-blinded									
1977	Von Rossum et al. (84)	AMCA	4	26	25	19	16	58	44
1978	Chandra (7)	AMCA	6	20	19	5	21	5	26
1979	Kaste and Ramsey (43)	AMCA	6	32	32	22	19	13	13
1984	Vermeulen et al. (83)	AMCA	4–6	241	238	9	24	35	37
Total				436	418	14	34	32	34

83, 84). Thus, it might be said that the definitive studies were done with AMCA and EACA has not had an adequate trial. The total number of treated patients in these eight studies was 436, with a bleeding rate of 14% and a mortality rate of 32%. The total number of controls was 418, with a rebleeding rate of 34% and a mortality rate of 34%. The report of Vermeulen et al. (83) is probably the most definitive, because it enrolled 479 aneurysm patients. It is of interest that, of the total of 904 patients in this study who were admitted to major hospitals in Amsterdam, Glasgow, London, and Rotterdam, 26% were excluded because they were not admitted within 72 hours of bleeding, indicating a substantial problem in initiating treatment and the fact that the total aneurysm population was not studied. This was only a subsection of the total. AMCA was given intravenously initially and, in two of the institutions, orally after 2 weeks. Six grams/day were given during the first week and 4 g/day thereafter. Those receiving the medication orally received 6 g/day. Two hundred and forty-one treated patients had a rebleeding rate of 9% and a mortality rate of 35% in comparison to 238 controls, who had a rebleeding rate of 24% and a mortality rate of 37%. Clearly, rebleeding was prevented in the treatment group, indicating not only a smaller number of hemorrhage but also a delay in those who did have a hemorrhage. This delay confirmed previous studies (25, 53, 76). Clearly the ischemic factor was worse in the treated group, so that the total mortality rate almost equalled that for the controls.

Evaluation

The International Cooperative Study on the Timing of Aneurysm Surgery was not designed to study antifibrinolysis but contained sufficient numbers of patients, 2265, to make an evaluation of interest (39). Despite the total lack of selection, it happened that the groups matched relatively well in terms of risk. This was a pre-nimodipine study. Of the total, 672 patients were arbitrarily chosen to have surgery during the 7–14-day interval. Of these, 467 were given antifibrinolytic medication (69%) and 205

(31%) were not. The proportion given EACA and given AMCA is not reported, but the recommended dose of EACA was 36 g/day and that of AMCA was 6–12 daily, again reflecting the inadequate knowledge of what constituted an optimum dose, particularly of AMCA. The recommended duration of medication was 14 days or until operation, whichever came first. The incidence of bleeding at 14 days was 17.7% within the treatment group and 19% for the controls. The peak time of ischemic events was day 7. The 30-day mortality rate was 22.3% and 20%, respectively. It should be noted that these results refer to a time in the rebleeding cycle (day 7–16 interval) when the theoretical support offered by an antifibrinolytic drug was in decline and spasm was at its peak, making any conclusion somewhat problematic, other than that, as in the study of Vermeulen et al., the drug was given too late.

Microanalysis of all of these studies would probably add little that would guide future care, although some interesting questions could be asked. One might wonder why, for example, the rebleeding rate reported by Fodstad and co-workers (15) was 4% in the early series and 20% in the later series or why was the mortality rate for treated patients was 26% in the early series and 43% in the later series. One might wonder whether the dose of AMCA generally given was unnecessarily high and was in fact toxic. The overall conclusion remains that antifibrinolytic treatment, as used in these studies, significantly delays and reduces the rebleeding rate (perhaps by 50%) but is associated with an increase in infarct morbidity rates that makes the outcome mortality rate of the treated and control groups comparable. These clinical studies have been reviewed by Fodstad and Ljunggren (20) and Ramirez-Lassepas (64).

Complications

Complications with the use of antifibrinolytic drugs have been few. When taken orally, vomiting is not uncommon. Diarrhaea has occurred. There have been a few reports of myopathy, but the incidence of this has been extraordinarily low (20, 82).

The possibility of deep venous thrombosis and pulmonary embolism were alluded to in the earlier publications. One might have expected a higher incidence of pulmonary embolism, but perhaps it could be a lesser incidence, since resolution of the leg clot was delayed rather than enhanced and therefore the clot was afforded more opportunity to fibrose *in situ*. In the first series of Fodstad *et al.* (19) there was one pulmonary embolus in the controls, and in the second series (16) there were three in the treatment group (16, 19). In our own experience there was no pulmonary embolus before day 20. It might be stated that, from a survey of the literatures as a whole, there was no evidence of an enhanced pulmonary embolus problem. Spontaneous occlusion of a ruptured aneurysm has been recognized to be sometimes associated with a thrombosed artery (32, 74). In some there has been a late reappearance of the aneurysm. In others there has been an arterial without an aneurysm thrombosis. Fodstad and co-workers (18, 20) and Davies Howell (11) have discussed the issue in detail.

The role of antifibrinolytic medication in relation to hydrocephalus is a debatable one. Theoretically, it might merely prolong the duration of the moderate hydrocephalus which so often accompanies subarachnoid hemorrhage, because of the slower resolution of the extravasated blood. It is also possible that it might cause a more lasting change by setting up a fibrin-enhanced adhesive process in the subarachnoid space or even in the arachnoid granulations. There is some experimental evidence in dogs, both supporting and contradicting this idea. (13) At the clinical level, there has been evidence both for and against this concept. The Dutch-English study reported an incidence of hydrocephalus that required drainage of 15% in the treated group, compared to 12% in the control group (83). The International Cooperative Study reported an overall incidence of 14% *vs.* 12% (41). In the initial series of Fodstad *et al.* (19), echoencephalography showed ventricular dilatation in 13 treated and 14 control patients. It occurred postoperatively in five treated and seven control patients, and it occurred after repeat hemorrhage in four patients. It developed 2–3 weeks after the hemorrhage and was most marked at 2–3 months. In a second group, computerized tomography scans demonstrated acute ventricular dilatation in seven treated and five control patients. Two treated patients required a shunt, but the post-admission day was not given. After 3–41 months, slight to moderate dilatation was seen in eight treated and 12 control patients (16, 19, 20). On the whole, it might be stated that antifibrinolytic treatment can prolong the duration of hydrocephalus in some patients, but it does not contribute to mortality or morbidity in any significant manner.

Suggested Use

In determining how to separate and retain the good effects and reject the bad, one must recognize that these results apply to the specific drugs, dosage schedules, and time schedules reported. Two general criticisms may be applied. Treatment was frequently started too late and continued too long into the period of spasm. One might wonder if, in the total cascade of events, there might exist a window of therapeutic opportunity. One might consider that in fact EACA, at the dose of 24 g/day originally reported, has not had an adequate trial. It had been noted that many of the earlier nonrandomized, more optimistic reports were based on EACA, although the one controlled EACA trial was certainly unfavorable (27). All of the other controlled studies which were negative employed AMCA. In attempting to select patients who are most likely to benefit, there are, unfortunately, no good guidelines. Those who are most ill on admission seem most likely to rebleed, but unfortunately this is the group that is also most likely to sustain ischemic deficit. Therefore, the course of treatment for these patients and for those other groups prone to spasm and infarction, *e.g.*, the elderly and the diabetic, should be deliberately of short duration. A reasonable program might begin with the realization that antifibrinolysis does not protect patients due for operation during the first 48 hours, and it might recommend concentration on blood pressure control (plus nimodipine, 360 mg/day, to control the late effects of spasm) for this group. For those for whom a later operation is planned, blood pressure control in the early days, together with nimodipine for late spasm, could be supplemented by intravenous EACA infusion at a dose of 24 g/day, since this seemed to be as effective as any other dose selection. It should be started immediately on admission, to be effective 24–48 hours later. It should be continued until there is evidence of angiographic spasm, a decrease in cerebral blood flow, the clinical onset of spasm, or an arbitrary period of about 7 days. For all patients daily, and for those in the special risk group for spasm more frequent, intracranial Doppler examinations would probably give the earliest warning to terminate the drug. For those with least risk of spasm but for whom further delay of surgery (for whatever reason) is required, the medication could be continued on a daily basis beyond 7 days, paying particular attention to a changing blood flow pattern. For patients admitted after the fourth day, as were in fact so many patients in the reported studies, there may be relatively little indication. By the time that the antifibrinolysis becomes effective in this situation, (after the fifth day), the period of spasm risk begins.

Summary

In conclusion, it might be stated that the role for an antifibrinolytic agent is at the moment equivocal. Antifibrinolysis slows the access of plasmin into the clot. It slows but does not prevent clot lysis. It has little or no role for patients who will have their operation during the first day or two, since early hemorrhages are the product of "blowout," not clot lysis. It has been shown repeatedly to reduce the incidence of rebleeding after an aneurysmal rupture, perhaps overall by one half. It has been shown to enhance the ischemic effects of spasm if continued into the spasm phase, thereby offering no overall benefit to the patient. Theoretically it is probable that antifibrinolysis has a role during the early days, perhaps as late as the fifth day in all patients and later in those with minimal spasm. Possibly the ill effects recorded in the past can be reduced by use of nimodipine and the newer spasmolytic methods, just as the ill effects of early clipping have been ameliorated by these means. Possibly, with these methods and with blood flow monitoring, the period of usefulness for antifibrinolysis may be extended. The small window of therapeutic merit which it affords may be of great value to a few patients in a disease that remains greatly in need of every therapeutic window that is available.

REFERENCES

1. Adams, H. P., Nibbenling, D. D. W., Torner, J. C., et al. Antifibrinolytic therapy in patients with aneurysmal subarachnoid haemorrhage. Arch. Neurol. 38:25–29, 1981.
2. Allen, G. S., Ahn, H. S., Preziosi, T. J., et al. Cerebral arterial spasm: a controlled trial of nimodipine in patients with subarachnoid haemorrhage. N. Engl. J. Med. 308:619–624, 1983.
3. Alvord, E., Loeser, J., Bailey, W., and Copass, M. Subarachnoid hemorrhage due to ruptured aneurysms. Arch. Neurol. 27:273–284, 1972.
4. Ameen, A. A., and Illingworth, R. Antifibrinolytic treatment in the preoperative management of subarachnoid haemorrhage caused by ruptured intracranial aneurysm. J. Neurol. Neurosurg. Psychiatry 44:220–226, 1981.
5. Auer, L. M. Acute operation and preventive nimodipine improve outcome in patients with ruptured cerebral aneurysms. Neurosurgery 15:57–66, 1984.
6. Cameron, M. J. Neurol. Neurosurg. Psychiatry 42:963, 1979.
7. Chandra, B. Treatment of subarachnoid haemorrhage from ruptured intracranial aneurysm with tranexamic acid: a double-blind clinical trial. Ann. Neurol. 3:502–504, 1978.
8. Chowdhary, U. M., Carey, P. C., and Hussein, M. M. Prevention of early recurrence of spontaneous subarachnoid hemorrhage by ε-aminocaproic acid. Lancet 2:741–743, 1979.
9. Chowdhary, U. M., and Sayed, K. Comparative clinical trial of epsilon-aminocaproic acid and tranexamic acid in the prevention of early recurrence of subarachnoid haemorrhage. J. Neurol. Neurosurg. Psychiatry 44:810–813, 1981.
10. Corkill, G. Earlier operation and antifibrinolytic therapy in the management of aneurysmal subarachnoid haemorrhage. J. Neurol. Neurosurg. Psychiatry 44:810–813, 1981.
11. Davies, D., and Howell, D. A. Tranexamic acid and arterial thrombosis. Lancet 1:49, 1977.
12. Ecker, A., and Riemenschneider, P. A. Arteriographic demonstration of spasm of the intracranial arteries with special reference to saccular arterial aneurysms. J. Neurosurg. 8:660–667, 1951.
13. Ewald, T., Mahaley, S., Goodrich, J., et al. Experimental epsilon-aminocaproic acid (EACA) administration in the presence of subarachnoid blood. J. Neurosurg. 35:657–663, 1971.

14. Findlay, J. M., Weir, B., Kanamaru, K., *et al.* Intrathecal fibrinolytic therapy after subarachnoid hemorrhage: dosage study in a primate model and review of the literature. Can. J. Neurol. Sci. *16*:28–40, 1989.

15. Fodstad, H. Tranexamic acid as therapeutic agent in aneurysmal subarachnoid haemorrhage: clinical, laboratory and experimental studies. Umea Univ. Med. Dissertations New Ser. *60*:1–74, 1980.

16. Fodstad, H., Forssell, A., Liliequist, B., *et al.* Antifibrinolysis with tranexamic acid in aneurysmal subarachnoid haemorrhage: a consecutive controlled clinical trial. Neurosurgery *8*:158–165, 1981.

17. Fodstad, H., Kok, P., and Algers, G. Fibrinolytic activity of cerebral tissue after experimental subarachnoid haemorrhage: inhibitory effect of tranexamic acid (AMCA). Acta Neurol. Scand. *64*:29–46, 1981.

18. Fodstad, H., and Liliequist, B. Spontaneous thrombosis of ruptured intracranial aneurysms during treatment with tranexamic acid (AMCA): report of three cases. Acta Neurochir. (Wien.) *49*:129–144, 1979.

19. Fodstad, H., Liliequist, B., Schannong, M., *et al.* Tranexamic acid in the preoperative management of ruptured intracranial aneurysms. Surg. Neurol. *10*:9–15, 1978.

20. Fodstad, H., and Ljunggren, B. Antifibrinolytic drugs in subarachnoid hemorrhage. In Fibrinolysis and the Central Nervous System. Edited by R. Sawaya, pp. 257–273. Hanley-Belfus, Inc., Philadelphia, 1990.

21. Fodstad, H., and Nilsson, I. M. Coagulation and fibrinolysis in blood and cerebrospinal fluid after aneurysmal subarachnoid haemorrhage: effect of tranexamic acid (AMCA). Acta Neurochir. (Wien.) *56*:25–38, 1981.

22. Fodstad, H., Pilbrant, A., Schannong, M., *et al.* Determination of tranexamic acid and fibrin/fibrinogen degradation products in cerebrospinal fluid after aneurysmal subarachnoid haemorrhage. Acta Neurochir. (Wien.) *58*:1–13, 1981.

23. Gelmers, H. J. Prevention of recurrence of spontaneous subarachnoid haemorrhage by tranexamic acid. Acta Neurochir. (Wein.) *52*:45–50, 1980.

24. Geronemus, R., Hertz, D. A., and Shulman, K. Streptokinase clot lysis time in patients with ruptured intracranial aneurysms. J. Neurosurg. *40*:499–503, 1974.

25. Gibbs, J. R., and Corkill, A. G. L. Use of an antifibrinolytic agent (tranexamic acid) in the management of ruptured intracranial aneurysms. Postgrad. Med. J. *47*:199–200, 1971.

26. Gibbs, J. R., and O'Gorman, P. Fibrinolysis in subarachnoid haemorrhage. Postgrad. Med. J. *43*:779–784, 1967.

27. Girvin, J. P. The use of antifibrinolytic agents in the preoperative treatment of ruptured intracranial aneurysms. Trans. Am. Neurol. Assoc. *98*:150–152, 1973.

28. Graf, C. J., Torner, J. C., Perret, G. E., *et al.* Long-term Follow-up Evaluation of Randomized

29. Guidetti, B., and Spallone, A. The role of antifibrinolytic therapy in the preoperative management of recently ruptured intracranial aneurysms. Surg. Neurol. *15*:239–248, 1981.

30. Haley, E. C., Kassell, N. F., and Torner, J. C. The International Cooperative Study on the Timing of Aneurysm Surgery. The North American Experience Stroke. *23(2)*:205–214, 1992.

31. Heidrich, R., Mackwardt, F., Endler, S., *et al.* Antifibrinolytic therapy of subarachnoid haemorrhage by intrathecal administration of *p*-amino-methyl-benzoic acid. J. Neurol. *219*:83–85, 1978.

32. Hoffman, E. P., and Koo, A. H. Cerebral thrombosis associated with amicar therapy. Radiology *131*:687–689, 1979.

33. Hunt, W. E., and Hess, R. M. Surgical risk as related to time of intervention in the repair of intracranial aneurysms. J. Neurosurg. *28*:14–19, 1968.

34. Inagawa, T., Kamiya, K., Ogasawara, H., Yano, T. Rebleeding of ruptured intracranial aneurysms in the acute state. Surg. Neurol. *28(2)*:93–99, 1987.

35. Kagstrom, E., and Palma, L. Influence of antifibrinolytic treatment on the morbidity in patients with subarachnoid haemorrhage. Acta Neurol. Scand. *48*:257–258, 1972.

36. Kaku, Y., Yonekawa, Y., Tsukahara, T., and Kazekawa, K. Superselective intra-arterial infusion of papaverine for the treatment of cerebral vasospasm after subarachnoid hemorrhage. J. Neurosurg. *77*:842–847, 1992.

37. Kassell, N. F., and Drake, C. G. Timing of aneurysm surgery. Neurosurgery *10*:514–519, 1982.

38. Kassell, N. F., Helm, G., Simmons, N., *et al.* Treatment of cerebral vasospasm with intra-arterial papaverine. J. Neurosurg. *77*:848–852, 1992.

39. Kassell, N. F., Torner, J. C., and Adams, H. P. Antifibrinolytic therapy in the acute period following aneurysmal subarachnoid hemorrhage. J. Neurosurg. *61*:225–230, 1984.

40. Kassell, N. F., Torner, J. C., and Adams, H. P. Antifibrinolytic therapy in the acute period following aneurysmal subarachnoid hemorrhage. J. Neurosurg. *61*:225–230, 1984.

41. Kassell, N. F., Torner, J. C., Haley, C., *et al.* The International Cooperative Study on the Timing of Aneurysm Surgery. J. Neurosurg. *73*:18–36, 1990.

42. Kassell, N. F., Torner, J. C., Jane, J., *et al.* The International Cooperative Study on the Timing of Aneurysm Surgery. J. Neurosurg. *73*:37–47, 1990.

43. Kaste, M., and Ramsay, M. Tranexamic acid in subarachnoid hemorrhage: a double-blind study. Stroke *10*:519–521, 1979.

44. Knuckey, N. W., and Stokes, B. A. R. Medical management of patients following a ruptured cerebral aneurysm with ε-aminocaproic acid, kanamycin and reserpine. Surg. Neurol. *17*:181–185, 1982.

Study, pp. 203–245. Urban & Schwarzenberg, Baltimore, 1981.

45. Leska, P., Krupka, J., Naktadal, J., *et al.* Intrathecal administration of antifibrinolytics in primary subarachnoid haemorrhage in acute period. Cs. Neurol. Neurochir. *50/83:*17–23, 1987 (Czech).

46. Ljunggren, B., Brandt, L., Saveland, H., *et al.* Outcome in 60 consecutive patients treated with early aneurysm operation and intravenous nimodipine. J. Neurosurg. *61:*964–973, 1984.

47. Ljunggren, B., Brandt, L., Sundbarg, G., *et al.* Early management of aneurysmal subarachnoid hemorrhage. Neurosurgery *11:*412–418, 1982.

48. Locksley, H. Natural history of subarachnoid haemorrhage, intracranial aneurysm and arteriovenous malformations. J. Neurosurg. *25:*321–368, 1966.

49. Magladery, J. W. On subarachnoid bleeding: an appraisal of treatment. J. Neurosurg. *12:*437–449, 1955.

50. Mee, E., Dorrance, D., Lowe, D., and Neil-Dwyer, G. Controlled study of nimodipine in aneurysm patients treated early after subarachnoid hemorrhage. Neurosurgery *22:*484–491, 1988.

51. Mullan, S. Conservative management of the recently ruptured aneurysm. Surg. Neurol. *3:*27–32, 1975.

52. Mullan, S. The Initial Medical Management of Ruptured Intracranial Aneurysms. In: Current Controversies in Neurosurgery, edited by Morley, T. P., W. B. Saunders, Philadelphia, pp. 259–269. 1976.

53. Mullan, S., and Dawley, J. Antifibrinolytic therapy for intracranial aneurysms. J. Neurosurg. *28:*21–23, 1967.

54. Mullan, S., Hanlon, K., and Brown, F. Management of 136 consecutive supratentorial berry aneurysms. J. Neurosurg. *49:*794–804, 1978.

55. Nibbelink, D. W. Cooperative Aneurysm Study: Antihypertensive and antifibrinolytic therapy following subarachnoid haemorrhage from ruptured intracranial aneurysms. In: Cerebral Vascular Disease, edited by J. P. Whisnant and B. A. Sandek, Grune and Stratton, New York, pp. 155–173. 1975.

56. Nibbelink, D. W., Torner, J. C., and Henderson, W. G. Intracranial aneurysms and subarachnoid haemorrhage: a cooperative study: antifibrinolytic therapy in recent onset subarachnoid haemorrhage. Stroke *6:*622–629, 1975.

57. Norlen, G., and Olivecrona, H. The treatment of aneurysms of the circle of Willis. J. Neurosurg. *10:*404–415, 1953.

58. Öhman, J., and Heiskanen, O. Effect of nimodipine on the outcome of patients after aneurysmal subarachnoid hemorrhage and surgery. J. Neurosurg. *69:*683–686, 1988.

59. Pechet, L. Fibrinolysis. N. Engl. J. Med. *273:*1024–1034, 1965.

60. Petruk, K., West, M., Mohr, G., *et al.* Nimodipine treatment in poor-grade aneurysm patients. J. Neurosurg. *68:*505–517, 1988.

61. Pinna, G., Pasqualin, A., Viveza, C., *et al.* Rebleeding, ischaemia, and hydrocephalus following antifibrinolytic treatment for ruptured cerebral aneurysms: a retrospective clinical study. Acta Neurochir., (Wien.) *93:*77–87, 1988.

62. Post, K. D., Flamm, E., Goodgold, A., *et al.* Ruptured intracranial aneurysms: case morbidity and mortality. J. Neurosurg. *46:*290–295, 1977.

63. Profeta, G., Castellano, F., Guarnieri, L., *et al.* Antifibrinolytic therapy in the treatment of subarachnoid haemorrhage caused by arterial aneurysms. J. Neurosurg. Sci. *19:*77–78, 1975.

64. Ramirez-Lassepas, M. Antifibrinolytic therapy in subarachnoid haemorrhage caused by ruptured intracranial aneurysm. Neurology *31:*316–322, 1981.

65. Ransohoff, J., Goodgold, A., and Benjamin, M. V. Preoperative management of patients with ruptured intracranial aneurysm. J. Neurosurg. *36:*525–530, 1989.

66. Rosenorn, J., Eskesen, V., Espersen, J. O., *et al.* Antifibrinolytic therapy in patients with aneurysmal subarachnoid haemorrhage. Br. J. Neurosurg. *2:*447–453, 1988.

67. Saito, I., Ueda, Y., and Sano, K. Significance of vasospasms in the treatment of ruptured intracranial aneurysms. J. Neurosurg. *47:*412–429, 1977.

68. Schisano, G. The use of antifibrinolytic drugs in aneurysmal subarachnoid haemorrhage. Surg. Neurol. *10:*217–222, 1978.

69. Seifert, V., Eisert, W. G., Stolke, D., and Goetz, C. Efficacy of single intracisternal bolus injection of recombinant tissue plasminogen activator to prevent delayed cerebral vasospasm after experimental subarachnoid hemorrhage. Neurosurgery *25:*590–598, 1989.

70. Sengupta, R. P., So, S. C., and Villarejo-Ortega, F. J. Use of *epsilon*-aminocaproic acid (EACA) in the preoperative management of ruptured intracranial aneurysms. J. Neurosurg. *44:*479–484, 1976.

71. Shaw, M. D. M., and Miller, J. D. *Epsilon*-aminocaproic acid and subarachnoid haemorrhage. Lancet *1:*847–848, 1974.

72. Shucart, W. A., Hussain, S. K., and Cooper, P. R. *Epsilon*-aminocaproic acid and recurrent subarachnoid haemorrhage. J. Neurosurg. *53:*28–31, 1980.

73. Slossberg, P. S. Treatment of ruptured aneurysms with induced hypotension. In: Intracranial Aneurysms and Subarachnoid Haemorrhage, edited by W. S. Fields, and A. L. Sahs, Charles C. Thomas, pp. 211–236. Springfield, IL, 1965.

74. Sonntag, V. K. H., and Stein, B. M. Arteriopathic complications during treatment of subarachnoid hemorrhage with *epsilon*-aminocaproic acid. J. Neurosurg. *40:*480–485, 1974.

75. Suzuki, J., Yoshimoto, T., and Onuma, T. Early operation for ruptured intracranial aneurysms: a study of 31 cases operated on within the first four days after ruptured aneurysm. Neurol. Med. Chir. (Tokyo) *18:*82–89, 1978.

76. Tovi, D. The use of antifibrinolytic drugs to prevent early recurrent aneurysmal subarachnoid haemorrhage. Acta Neurol. Scand. *49:*163–175, 1973.

77. Tovi, D., and Nilsson, I. M. Increased fibrinolytic activity and fibrin degradation products after experimental intracerebral haemorrhage. Acta

Neurol. Scand. *48:*403–415, 1972.

78. Tovi, D., Nilsson, I. M., and Thulin, C. A. Fibrinolysis and subarachnoid haemorrhage: inhibitory effect of tranexamic acid: a clinical study. Acta Neurol. Scand. *48:*393–402, 1972.

79. Tovi, D., Nilsson, I. M., and Thulin, C. A. Fibrinolytic activity of the cerebrospinal fluid after subarachnoid haemorrhage. Acta Neurol. Scand. *48:*1–9, 1973.

80. Tovi, D., and Thulin, C. A. Ability of tranexamic acid to cross the blood-brain barrier and its use in patients with ruptured intracranial aneurysms (Abstract). Acta Neurol. Scand. *49:*163–175, 1973.

81. Uttley, D., and Richardson, A. E. ε-Aminocaproic acid and subarachnoid haemorrhage. Lancet *2:*1080–1081, 1974.

82. Vanneste, J. A., and van Wijngaarden, G. K. *Epsilon*-aminocaproic acid myopathy: report of a case and literature review. Eur. Neurol. *21:*242–248, 1982.

83. Vermeulen, M., Lindsay, K. W., Murray, G. D., *et al.* Antifibrinolytic treatment in subarachnoid haemorrhage. N. Engl. J. Med. *311:*432–437, 1984.

84. Von Rossum, J., Wintzen, A. Z. R., Endtz, L. J., *et al.* Effect of tranexamic acid on rebleeding after subarachnoid haemorrhage: a double-blind controlled clinical trial. Ann. Neurol. *2:*238–242, 1977.

85. Weir, B., and Aronyk, K. Management mortality and the timing of surgery for supratentorial aneurysms. J. Neurosurg. *54:*146–150, 1981.

86. Williams, M. Prolonged antifibrinolysis: an effective nonsurgical treatment for ruptured intracranial aneurysms. Br. Med. J. Clin. Res. *1:*945–947, 1978.

87. Williams, M. Ruptured intracranial aneurysms: has the incidence of early rebleeding been over-estimated? J. Neurol. Neurosurg. Psychiatry *45:*774–779, 1982.

Principles of Management of Subarachnoid Hemorrhage: Induced Hypotension

SEAN MULLAN, M.D.

INTRODUCTION

A review of the recent literature on ruptured cerebral aneurysms reveals a problem hitherto not recognized and not yet adequately addressed. It is the high incidence of rebleeding during the first 24 hours, perhaps especially during the first 6 hours (5, 9). Another fact of interest is that "early operation" is not really early (9, 10, 16). It commonly refers to surgery within the first 3 days, rather than within the first 3 hours. There is a general acknowledgement that truly early operation is not logistically possible. In patients who are significantly drowsy or in coma, it may not be advisable. It remains to be seen whether the newer forms of treatment of spasm, namely nimodipine, fibrinolysis, intra-arterial paperverine, and arterial balloon dilatation, will make truly early operation theoretically advisable for all (2, 7, 8, 14, 19, 21). Until these problems are all resolved, and this may not be soon, the surgeon or responsible physician must manage patients preoperatively by medical means in a manner that minimizes the still formidable mortality and morbidity rates of both the preoperative and postoperative periods.

Reduction of the blood pressure (BP), to reduce the incidence of rebleeding, is an obvious method (20). Perhaps one should think rather in terms of bursting pressure, *i.e.*, recognizing the fact that BP and intracranial pressure (ICP) should be considered together. Reduction can be done systematically or regionally by constricting the parent artery mechanically; it has been demonstrated by direct measurement that pressure within a carotid or middle cerebral artery aneurysm mirrors that within the common carotid artery (1). Both methods have been tried extensively in the past. The clinical results on common carotid ligature as a definitive treatment for subarachnoid hemorrhage are included in the experience of the earlier Cooperative Aneurysm Study. In that report (18), the cumulative mortality rate for subarachnoid hemorrhage, based upon 6368 protocols collected between 1957 and 1965, was 46%, not much different from that with the completely conservative management of an earlier decade (15). A very definitive rebleeding peak was recognized at the end of the first week. A subsequent series of 972 patients with anterior circle of Willis aneurysms, collected between 1963 and 1970, was randomly assigned to bed rest, drug-induced hypotension, carotid ligature, or intracranial clipping. The 5-year mortality rates were 56.5%, 48.3%, 36.5%, and 45.3%, respectively. Apparently carotid ligature had some merit, and drug-induced hypotension had little (4). Adequate effort was not made to separate the good effect of hypotension prior to spasm from the bad effect of hypotension during spasm, the result being that all hypotension was rejected. In our own experience, we have learned to separate these and to recognize a small but definite role for hypotension in the prespasm phase (12, 13). This niche would include the peak rebleeding time on the first day which, until now, has not been dealt with adequately.

In attempting to identify the current role, if any, for hypotension, it is perhaps best to take a detailed look at the natural history. Enough aneurysms have been observed to bleed during surgery and enough experimental bleeding and blood clotting have been observed in animals to give the experienced surgeon a very good idea of what happens in the natural state. There is a sudden spurt of blood, not an ooze. The ICP rises. A platelet plug commences at the site of hemorrhage and a perianeurysmal blood clot forms. In the majority of instances, bleeding ceases. If it continues beyond a few minutes, the ICP mounts and the patient dies then, or soon after, as brain swelling or cerebrospinal fluid obstruction, or both, add to the progressive rise in ICP and progressive herniation. Since the bursting pressure reflects the difference between the intra-aneurysmal BP and the intracranial "capping" pressure, a modest rise in ICP could be regarded as a protective factor. Once rising ICP triggers an increase in systemic BP, the danger of a clot blow-out increases. This mechanism probably contributes to the recently recognized peak of rebleeding during the first 24 hours (7), and perhaps especially during the first 6 hours, or during angiography (5). It enhances risk up until clipping of the aneurysm. It has been repeatedly documented that patients with more severe initial hemorrhage are more prone to repeated hemorrhage (5, 11, 17). Their steady or progressive rise in ICP may be one explanation. A larger weak blister, and therefore a larger initial opening, could be another. Over the first week, the ICP problem is expected to stabilize spontaneously in most patients. A connective tissue cellular response commences about the third day, leading to a fibrous and endothelial closure of the site of aneurysmal rupture (3). This proceeds concomitantly with dissolution of the fibrin content of the hemostatic clot. Depending upon the size of the opening, the size of the clot, the efficacy of connective tissue repair, and the rapidity of dissolution of the fibrin, the aneurysm proceeds to an uneventful repair or is subject to repeated hemorrhage. Whether the tradi-

tional peak at the end of the first week or the beginning of the second week occurs (5, 9, 11) probably relates to whether antifibrinolytic treatment is used. With increasing numbers of early operations, it is becoming more difficult to recognize.

As the days progress, rising BP continues to suggest the possibility of rising ICP, but it could also be produced by an increasing degree of spasm-induced ischemia. As the clot breaks down and the cells are lysed, the spasm-inducing oxyhemoglobin molecule comes into free contact with the cerebrospinal fluid and with the blood vessels in the subarachnoid space (2). Angiographic spasm can be detected by the third day, but clinical spasm is more commonly a problem by the end of the first week. If it appears early, by the fourth or fifth day, it will become severe. If not manifest until the end of the first week or the beginning of the second week, it may be mild. It tends to decrease by the 12th day, or in more severe instances by the 17th. It should be clearly understood that there are wide variations and that multiple individual exceptions to these stated time intervals are encountered. Blood flow determinations with either the xenon-133 washout method or the transcranial Doppler method can monitor the course of spasm. The exact values determined are of less importance than the graph or trend in events, namely the time of onset of a detectable decrease in flow and the time when a progressive fall in flow begins to reverse. It is always dangerous to operate on the downslope, even if a patient shows no adverse clinical signs. It may be permissible to operate on the upslope in the presence of minimal clinical change. The clinical condition may improve considerably in advance of improvements in the angiographic pattern but not in advance of improvements in blood flow.

It is postulated that hypotension induced to reduce rebleeding appears to be safe, effective, and desirable in noncomatose patients up until surgery is undertaken or until the onset of spasm, as determined either radiologically or by cerebral blood flow (CBF) measurements. It may be further pursued guardedly until the onset of clinical spasm. It should not be used in a patient in whom CBF is compromised by an elevated

ICP, as occurs in the more severe grade of hydrocephalus, or, especially, by the presence of a large blood clot. Hypotension is usually monitored by clinical judgement and by serial CBF examinations. The latter permits more liberal and safer utilization. After spasm has passed and CBF begins to increase, if surgery is not undertaken, hypotension may again be used judiciously. There are several rules for reduction of BP in the alert patient. 1) The systolic BP can always be reduced by 25%. 2) The systolic BP can always be reduced to the diastolic level. 3) The pressure may be reduced until some symptom is experienced by the patient, more often as a subjective feeling of mild distress rather than an objective symptom such as a weak limb. At that point the systolic pressure is raised 20 mm Hg. Reduction of pressure is best done with the head and trunk elevated, so that advantage can be taken of the totally flat position if the target is over-reached. It has been our experience that few patients who clinically tolerated such a systemic reduction rebled while hypotensive, although as a rule the systolic level was rarely sustained at better than the prereduction mean. Bleeding did recur when, with the onset of spasm, it was necessary to stop the hypotensive regimen.

There are some problems and exceptions.

1. Normal BP. On admission the patient's normal BP is not always known. The presenting BP may be a reaction to stress induced by the hemorrhage. It is best to make reductions based upon the actual BP observed until the previous medical history becomes available.
2. It must be recognized that it may be much more difficult to reduce a patient's normal BP to subnormal levels than to reduce a hypertensive BP to normal.
3. Sedation. Rather than paralyzing and intubating the patient to perform a computerized axial tomography (CAT) scan, it is best to use a sedative of choice. Chlorpromazine (25 mg, intramuscularly) is an old favorite which tends to reduce BP slightly. Valium can ease the patient's anxiety but has a specific adverse effect upon breathing and should be avoided. There is a wide choice.
4. Localized neurological defect. If a blood clot is present and is removed, and if the CBF is normal, then hypotension may proceed. A localized clinical defect in the absence of a blood clot denotes ischemia, in which case hypotension may not be used.
5. General medical condition. Use of hypotensive medication could be a serious problem in a patient with atherosclerosis who has marginal coronary flow, carotid flow, or even renal or femoral flow. In older patients especially, a medical history should be sought. A preliminary electrocardiograph (EKG) and auscultation of the carotid arteries are minimal requirements. An EKG may be difficult to interpret, since subarachnoid hemorrhage notoriously produces EKG abnormalities.

In managing hypotension, mannitol has proven to be an invaluable drug, both in controlling ICP, and therefore reactive BP, and in promoting CBF. We have made extensive observations on its use in experimental animals and in patients with subarachnoid hemorrhage. Any hypertonic solution increases the diameter of small blood vessels. Hemodilution with saline to a hematocrit value of 25% in normal monkeys increased CBF by 15% but with a rise in ICP, presumably as blood vessels dilated. Mannitol (1.5 g/kg), with added saline to keep the central venous pressure from falling, has produced a similar increase in blood flow but without any increase in ICP. Jafar *et al.* (6) observed the effect of mannitol upon 21 patients with unruptured aneurysms. Seven, given a bolus injection of 1.5 g/kg, had an average increase in CBF of 15% (xenon-133) by 12 hours, reaching 19% by 24 hours. Seven given 1.5 g over an 8-hour period had an increase of 25% at 3 hours and 20% at 6 hours, with a return to base-line at 18 hours. Seven given 4.5 g/kg over a 24-hour period had an increase of 16% by 3 hours and 20% by 12 hours, remaining at 22% throughout the next 12 hours. This slow infusion did not result in any decrease in ICP. ICP was not measured in those given a bolus injection, but it was known from other studies that bolus injections produced a decrease. Cardiac output measured in the 8-hour and bolus studies showed 12-hour peaks of 24% and 16%, respectively. Sixteen patients of grades I and II, 4–10 days after a subarachnoid hemorrhage, were studied, using 4.5 g/kg administered continuously over 24 hours. Base-line flows were 19% below controls, indicating that the patients had already entered into the period of potential spasm although they were clinically intact. By 6 hours, flows had increased to 28% above that base level. The figure was 50% at 12 hours but then decreased and remained at 33% throughout the period of study. ICP, initially 220 mm H_2O, dropped to 130 mm H_2O by 6 hours and rose to 180 mm H_2O by 24 hours. This steady infusion of mannitol, which can be carried on for hours or, if necessary, for days, requires large fluid replacement (usually 5% glucose, 0.45% NaCl) and electrolyte monitoring.

Immediate Management of Alert Patients

The clinical diagnosis usually takes only a few minutes. At that moment, it should be recognized that the patient's instant danger is that of rebleeding. In this emergency, hypotension is immediately instituted.

There are three intravenous methods for reducing blood pressure:

1. Trimethaphan camsylate (Arphonad) at an initial rate of 1–15 μg/kg/m.
2. Nitroprusside at the rate of 1–10 μg/kg/m/min.
3. Esmalol at 50–300 μg/kg/m.

Perhaps one can arrive at the desired level more rapidly with nitroprusside than with Arphonad. Esmalol, a β-blocker, is probably more effective for those with a rapid pulse and has not been our initial drug of choice. Once the BP has been reduced, the patient receives a CAT scan to confirm the diagnosis, estimate the severity of the hemorrhage, and scan for intracranial clot or obstructed ventricular system. When this is completed, with good hypotensive control, the patient

receives an angiogram. This may be done before or after admission to an intensive care facility. It should be noted that there is some evidence that angiography has been associated with a 100% increase in rebleeding for the time spent during that procedure (5). This may be related to restlessness, stress, and reactively raised BP. It is desirable that an anesthesiologist, using suitable medication (perhaps Propofol and fentanyl) be available.

Immediate Management of Obtunded Patients

For these patients the immediate goal is to prevent reactive surges of BP, rather than to produce marked hypotension. A goal of 10% reduction in BP should secure this, provided the patient remains stable or improves. If he or she deteriorates under constant supervision, hypotension should be abandoned until CAT scan and blood flow measurements are complete. With the use of rapid CAT scanning machines, it is rarely necessary to intubate these obtunded but conscious patients at an early stage merely to obtain the scan. Once the CAT scan has eliminated the possibility of major intracranial mass lesions, it is appropriate to introduce hypotension, under blood flow and clinical supervision. If it is believed that there is elevated ICP, then a slow infusion of mannitol may be appropriate.

Immediate Management of Comatose or Semicomatose Patients

These patients present a major dilemma, in terms of bursting pressure control. There may be a large hematoma present, with a potentially poorly perfused brain due to intracranial hypertension. This ischemia could be worsened by hypotension. The early use of mannitol to control ICP and thereby prevent a reactionary climb in BP is more appropriate than deliberate hypotension. Nevertheless, hypotensive medication should be available to suppress dangerous surges in BP should they occur. An emergency CAT scan is mandatory and, for this, careful intubation is generally required. If, however, skilled intubation service is not immediately available it might be better to delay a short time until it is, rather than risk the surges in BP that unskilled intubation may induce. If intubation is required for respiratory indications, delay is not permissible. One should also avoid rapid infusion of mannitol, lest a sudden decrease in ICP remove the "cap," thus raising the bursting pressure and thereby risking a hemorrhage.

It might be noted that there are two types of grade IV or grade V patients, those with a clot or a blocked ventricle and those with a diffusely swollen brain. The good results from operations for these grades come largely from evacuation of the hematoma or correction of the hydrocephalus, not from immediate clipping of an aneurysm in a swollen brain. Thus, if the CAT scan reveals a surgically correctable lesion such as a clot or hydrocephalus that needs draining, these procedures should be instituted immediately. This improves the cerebral perfusion pressure and eliminates both the risk of herniation and the surges of BP. In these patients, Doppler blood flow measurements should be instituted in the postsurgical period to assess the safety of any planned hypotension, although it is unusual to use it in these seriously ill patients. If a pressure-relieving operation is not indicated, angiography may not be urgent.

Postadmission Management Up to the Fifth Day

The main problems of these early days remain rebleeding and the control of ICP. If the patient is already receiving BP medication, this should be initially maintained, except that calcium channel blockers may be reduced or withdrawn as nimodipine is introduced. Long-acting drugs such as Aldomet are best avoided. When indicated, hypotension is effected by intravenous infusion. Tachyphylaxis may be established with Arphonad by 24 hours, and by that time a switch is made to nitroprusside. After 24 hours with this drug, some risk of toxicity from cyanide accumulation develops. To prevent this, it is best to switch back routinely to Arphonad within 24 hours. Cyanide intoxication is associated with a falling PCO_2, respiratory difficulty, and increasing confusion. In the alert patient, it is expected

that the high ICP initiated by the hemorrhage will decrease in the early days, although it will not necessarily reach normal values. As this proceeds, the patient's alertness improves, giving confirmatory evidence. If the initial intensity and duration of the hemorrhage were sufficient, they created some degree of ischemia at that time and perhaps some herniation. Consequent to these, the brain may undergo some significant swelling and, thus, the ICP remains high or increases. Later, the adverse effects of spasm may appear. Resistance to medication control may indicate a rising BP due to a rising ICP or ischemia, rather than tachyphylaxis. If there is a concomitant increase in obtundation or the appearance of a neurological defect, this is confirmatory of an alternative explanation. Management consists of increasing or initiating ICP control and CBF enhancement and stopping the hypotensive effort. Even without deterioration, in the case of hypertensive patients a progressive switch might be made from oral to intravenous infusion control as the period of spasm approaches, to regulate the perfusion and bursting pressure more precisely. For those patients who show continuing or even increasing drowsiness during the early days, and in whom a diagnosis of brain swelling is made, an infusion of mannitol at the rate of 1.5 g/kg, over 8 hours, may help control an increase in ICP and, at the same time, lay the basis for better cerebral perfusion as the time for spasm approaches. The frequency of such infusions or the need for a bolus injection to control a more desperate pressure problem are within the realm of individual management.

If at this stage signs of deterioration continue, one might be prepared to initiate respiratory control early electively, rather than later in an emergency situation, with attendant risks of surges in BP. A decrease or loss of the respiratory pause, a rate greater than 22/min, or any periodicity might be taken as signs to intubate. The central venous pressure should be maintained between 8 and 10 mm H_2O. Blood osmolality should not exceed 320 mOsm/kg (normal, 289–310 mOsm/kg). Serum creatinine determinations are necessary to recognize early renal impairment (normal, 0.5–1.4 mg/dl). In the control of BP, a ventricular catheter may be a useful monitor of I.C.P., since increases may trigger mechanisms which cause elevations in BP. In addition, knowledge of the existing ICP permits calculations of the perfusing and bursting pressures at all times. A disadvantage of a catheter is the risk of infection. Its use is a matter of judgment for which there are no established rules. In general, it is most useful for patients in coma for whom prolonged medical management is necessary. A ventricular peritoneal shunt prevents the rise of ICP but does not continue to give information regarding ICP and might, in fact, reduce cap pressure below that which is ideal from the aneurysm-bursting point of view. If it ceases to drain, this fact might not be recognized clinically. One option is to use an external drain for a few days to verify functioning and then convert the drain to a shunt.

Management of Vasospasm

Not all patients have clinical manifestations of spasm, probably not more than one of three. A larger number may have radiographic evidence of spasm or, as in Jafar's experience (6), of reduction in CBF. Nimodipine, which should be started shortly after admission, may reduce potential damage from spasm. Mannitol is recommended to prevent a reactive rise in BP in patients with an increased ICP and may also enhance CBF. Hemodilution is another mechanism of augmenting blood flow. It demands increased cardiac output and should not be used in patients with impaired cardiac reserve. An added benefit is that the incidence of pulmonary embolism is reduced as the hematocrit falls. Hemodilution is induced by withdrawing one or more units of blood until the hematocrit falls to 30%, with storage of the blood for possible replacement at the time of surgery. Blood volume is maintained by fluid replacement concomitant with withdrawal. Hypotension can be continued into the spasm time period only with those patients who are alert and for whom CBF measurements show only minimal decreases, in other words, those who demonstrably do not have spasm or impending spasm.

Preoperative Evaluation

Once the patient has entered the period of spasm, CBF determinations will help establish the time for operation. If, for example, on the fifth day the CBF shows a 20% reduction in a grade II or III patient, operation on the sixth day could be hazardous, because further reduction might be anticipated. On the other hand, if the same patient deteriorates to a lower level but returns to the 20% figure on the ninth day, then operation of the 10th day could be quite safe since flow is improving. In the absence of facilities to monitor blood flow, a trial reduction of BP might clinically demonstrate whether the patient has a margin of safety which would make operative intervention safe. A tolerated 20 mm Hg reduction in systolic pressure in a patient recovering from spasm would be such a figure.

Since opening the dura with increased ICP decreases the capping pressure to zero, the bursting pressure on the aneurysm increases correspondingly. On the day before or on the morning of the operation, a trial reduction of BP might be made to determine a permissible intraoperative decrease to control this risk. In the author's 40-year experience of aneurysm surgery, hemorrhage occurred upon opening of the dura on two occasions and before opening on one occasion, all in good-risk patients. Had hypotension been employed, the statistics would not have changed significantly, but one death and two serious disabilities might have been averted. Good management requires attention to a myriad of details. Again, knowing in advance the exact level of safe tolerance of hypotension in the waking state, one might allow the entire operation to be carried out at this level without risk of impairment. The operator must be especially careful of retractor pressure during the use of hypotension. Once the proximal artery is reached so that effective control of the risk of aneurysmal hemorrhage may be secured, hypotension is no longer necessary. It is not recommended that both methods be used simultaneously. Once the aneurysm is clipped, all hypotension medication is discontinued and, if necessary, a switch is made to hypertensive medications. Even in patients with known hypertension, it is probably better to accept the perils of moderate spontaneous hypertension than to risk postoperative ischemia until the period of spasm is completely over.

Alternative Hypotensive Method

Total common carotid artery occlusion greatly reduces the incidence of rebleeding (4) in carotid and middle cerebral artery aneurysms but carries a significant complication rate from ischemia either due to propagated clot or in association with the later development of spasm. Subtotal occlusion, resulting in almost as great a reduction of intra-aneurysmal pressure, provides virtually identical protection and eliminates the risk of clot propagation. A subtotally occluding clamp may be opened fully with the advent of spasm. Repeated experiences with the subtotal common carotid artery clamp, together with distal pressure measurements in the superficial temporal artery, have shown that a distal mean pressure of approximately 60–80 mm Hg can be well tolerated for days or weeks. It has also been our experience that no such patients rebled during such regional hypotension (13), although some bled subsequent to its release during the period of spasm.

Subtotal occlusion can be effected by applying a Selverstone clamp to the common carotid artery between the two heads of the sterno-mastoid muscle. The artery is totally occluded, at which point superficial temporal pulsation disappears. The clamp is then opened until a pulsation reappears (usually 5–10 mm Hg higher). A mean pressure of 75–80 mm Hg may be obtained by this mechanism. The clamp is opened and removed after the aneurysm is clipped. Application can be made under local anesthesia with Propofol or other suitable sedation or under general anesthesia. The clamp may be adjusted from time to time in relation to the monitored pressure. This method has limited indication at present but could be used in a patient whose hypertension is particularly difficult to control medically. It may be particularly well suited to some patients with hypertension who may tolerate this regional reduction but not a systemic reduction. It is possible that the reduced pulsation is an important element, in addition to the absolute level achieved.

In conclusion, it is postulated that the main indication for hypotension is to reduce the rebleeding rate between admission and surgery, an interval measured as a rule by many hours or several days. This can be done quite safely in the pre-spasm phase in alert patients and even in patients who are slightly obtunded under adequate CBF and clinical control. It is believed that close attention to this and similar details of medical management will continue to erode the still distressing mortality and morbidity rates for subarachnoid hemorrhage.

REFERENCES

1. Bakay, L., and Sweet, W. Intra-arterial pressures in the neck and brain. J. Neurosurg. *10:*353–359, 1953.
2. Findlay, J. M., Weir, B., Kanamaru, K., et al. Intrathecal fibrinolytic therapy after subarachnoid hemorrhage: dosage study in a primate model and review of the literature. Can. J. Neurol. Sci. *16:*28–40, 1989.
3. Fodstad, H. Tranexamic acid as therapeutic agent in aneurysmal subarachnoid haemorrhage: clinical, laboratory and experimental studies. Umea Univ. Med. Dissertations New Ser. *60:*1–74, 1980.
4. Graf, C. J., Nishioka, H., Torner, J. C., et al. *Cooperative Aneurysm Study: Long-Term Follow-up Evaluation of Randomized Study*, pp. 203–248. Urban & Schwarzenberg, Baltimore, 1981.
5. Inagawa, T., Ogasawara, H., et al. Rebleeding of ruptured intracranial aneurysms in the acute state. Surg. Neurol. *27:*93–99, 1987.
6. Jafar, J. J., Johns, L. M., and Mullan, S. F. The effect of mannitol on cerebral blood flow. J. Neurosurg. *64:*754–759, 1986.
7. Kaku, Y., Yonekawa, Y., Tsukahara, T., and Kazekawa, K. Superselective intra-arterial infusion of papaverine for the treatment of cerebral vasospasm after subarachnoid hemorrhage. J. Neurosurg. *77:*842–867, 1992.
8. Kassell, N. F., Helm, G., Simmons, N., et al. Treatment of cerebral vasospasm with intra-arterial papaverine. J. Neurosurg. *77:*848–852, 1992.
9. Kassell, N. F., Torner, J. C., Haley, C., et al. The international cooperative study on the timing of aneurysm surgery. J. Neurosurg. *73:*18–36, 1990.
10. Ljunggren, B., Fodstad, H., von Essen, C., et al. Aneurysmal subarachnoid haemorrhage: overall outcome and incidence of early recurrent haemorrhage despite a policy of acute stage operation. Br. J. Neurosurg. *2:*589–593, 1988.

11. Maurice-Williams, R. S. Ruptured intracranial aneurysm: has the incidence of early rebleeding been overestimated? J. Neurol. Neurosurg. Psychiatry 45:774–779, 1982.

12. Mullan, S. *The Initial Medical Management of Ruptured Intracranial Aneurysms.* Current Controversies in Neurosurgery, edited by Morley, T. P. pp. 259–269. W. B. Saunders Co., New York, 1976.

13. Mullan, S., Hanlon, K., and Brown, F. Management of 136 consecutive supratentorial berry aneurysms. J. Neurosurg. 49:794–804, 1978.

14. Newell, D. W., Eskridge, J. M., Mayberg, M. R., et al. Angioplasty for the treatment of symptomatic vasospasm following subarachnoid hemorrhage. J. Neurosurg. 71:654–660, 1989.

15. Pakarinen, S. Incidence, aetiology, and progress of primary subarachnoid haemorrhage: a study based on 589 cases diagnosed in a defined urban population during a defined period. Acta Neurol. Scand. 43(suppl. 29):8–128, 1967.

16. Pickard, D., Murray, G. D., Illingworth, R., et al. Effect of oral nimodipine on cerebral infarction and outcome after subarachnoid haemorrhage: British Aneurysm Nimodipine Trial (B.R.A.N.T.). Br. Med. J. 298:636–642, 1989.

17. Rosenorn, J., Eskesen, V., Espersen, J. O., et al. Anti-fibrinolytic therapy in patients with aneurysmal subarachnoid haemorrhage. Br. J. Neurosurg. 2:447–453, 1988.

18. Sahs, A. L. *History of the Cooperative Aneurysm Study and Central Registry,* pp. 3–13. Urban & Schwarzenberg, Baltimore, 1981.

19. Seifert, V., Eisert, W. G., Stolke, D., and Goetz, C. Efficacy of single intracisternal bolus injection of recombinant tissue plasminogen activator to prevent delayed cerebral vasospasm after experimental subarachnoid hemorrhage. Neurosurgery 25:590–598, 1989.

20. Slosberg, P. S. Medical treatment of intracranial aneurysm: an analysis of 15 cases. Neurology 10:1085–1089, 1960.

21. Zubkov, Y. N., Nikiforov, B. M., and Shustin, V. A. Balloon catheter technique for dilatation of constricted cerebral arteries after aneurysmal SAH. Acta Neurochir. (Wein) 70:65–79, 1984.

Principles of Management of Subarachnoid Hemorrhage: Monitoring

HOWARD YONAS, M.D.

Aneurysm rupture sets in motion a series of processes that often lead to infarction or death. Management of the patient after subarachnoid hemorrhage (SAH) is further complicated by the need to intervene to eliminate an aneurysm, a process which may cause additional temporary or permanent ischemia. The ability to monitor cerebral blood flow (CBF) and the metabolic function and neuronal activity that are normally linked to CBF is proving to be important for guiding clinical management.

Basic Physiology

The approaches to monitoring patients after SAH are based on the underlying physiology. CBF is a logical initial focus because compromise of cerebral perfusion is a common pathway for most injuries after SAH (7). CBF is normally coupled to metabolic activity, with local variations of 20% occurring with normal activity. Following SAH a moderate reduction of CBF and metabolism occurs irrespective of neurological grade, with an additional reduction of both variables occurring inversely with increasing neurological grade (2, 15).

Uncoupling of CBF and metabolism can occur in two ways during the acute phase of ischemia (20, 25). When perfusion pressure is compromised, CBF falls and metabolism remains unaltered until all reserves for flow and oxygen supply are exhausted. If reperfusion occurs following an ischemic challenge, flow may exceed metabolic demand (luxury perfusion). To utilize physiological monitoring, it is important to understand in greater detail the relationships between CBF, cerebral blood volume (CBV), the oxygen extraction fraction, the metabolic rate of oxygen or glucose, and neuronal activity (Fig. 5E.1). When perfusion pressure decreases, resistance vessels relax, resulting in an increase of CBV. If perfusion pressure continues to fall, CBF falls from a normal level of about 50 ml/100 g/min, and metabolism is not altered until all reserves for oxygen delivery are exhausted. At this level of perfusion (about 20 ml/100 g/min) neuronal function becomes impaired, and alterations of voltage and slowing of conduction become evident upon neurophysiological monitoring (24). A further decrease of perfusion pressure can cause reversible or irreversible ischemic injury, depending on the depth and the duration of the ischemic challenge (9). These facts explain why increasing the perfusion pressure can reverse neurological deficits due to vasospasm and why it is important to reverse such deficits without delay. This time/depth relation can, however, be altered by interventions that reduce metabolic demand. The combination of hypothermia and barbiturate coma can theoretically prolong the window of reversibility for a "no-flow" state from about 15 min to 60 min (22).

While a CBF study should be valuable for monitoring patients after SAH, a single study is limited in its diagnostic value unless flow is near zero or far in excess of normal

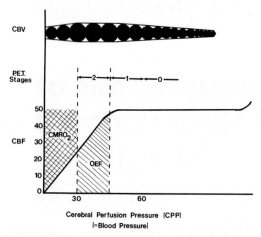

Cerebral Perfusion Pressure [CPP]
[≈Blood Pressure]

Figure 5E.1. With a reduction of perfusion pressure, vasodilatation occurs and CBF is maintained (stage 1) (21). CBF falls after maximal CBV, with compensation for an increase of oxygen extraction fraction (OEF) (stage 2). Alteration of metabolic activity with the reduction of the cerebral metabolic rate for oxygen ($CMRO_2$) occurs with flow values below 20 ml/100 g/min.

(28). High flow levels indicate an acute reperfusion of tissue which has undergone prior severe ischemic injury. Only with a more demanding assessment of hemodynamics (10) or a CBF study coupled with a measure of metabolism can the diagnosis of active ischemia be made (21). Because the latter type of information is not widely available, approaches using more accessible technologies appear more reasonable. Assuming that a region of the brain either at high risk for ischemia or already acutely ischemic is maximally vasodilated, double-CBF studies that examine the response to vasodilatory challenge or the integrity of autoregulation provide an alternate means of identifying a territory at increased ischemic risk (11, 27).

Approaches to Monitoring

Clinical and Anatomical Imaging

While the bedside examination remains the basis for most clinical judgement, the clinical exam offers little help for managing the care of a patient who is unresponsive or in whom ischemia is limited to less eloquent areas of the brain. Also, the purpose of monitoring technologies is to provide warning that a region is at increased ischemic risk.

With this kind of insight strategies can be developed for reversing and preventing infarction.

Angiography, computerized tomography (CT), and magnetic resonance imaging (MRI) primarily provide information concerning the anatomy of the brain and its vasculature. While angiography is the gold standard for the assessment of the structure of the aneurysm and the quality and quantity of collateral vessels, intraoperative verification of aneurysm clipping, and assessment of the degree of narrowing during or after surgery, it cannot determine the adequacy of perfusion. Perfusion is determined by the summation of the blood supply from all collateral channels, which angiography cannot assess (19). For this reason, while angiographically evident vasospasm remains common, symptomatic vasospasm, *i.e.*, symptoms due to ischemia, is far less common. While CT provides valuable information about the location of a hemorrhage in and/or about the brain and the presence of low-density areas consistent with infarction, it does not provide information about the quality of perfusion. At least 5–6 hours of severely low flow and more often 12–24 hours of more moderate ischemia are required for the appearance of lower CT densities in areas of infarction (28). Moreover, regions with low density may have no elevated or normal levels of perfusion; this depends on the patency of the microcirculation and whether reperfusion has occurred. MRI is expected to provide an assessment of vascular and brain anatomy as well as an assessment of perfusion and metabolism. While the potential applications of MRI following SAH appear significant, the fact that this technology cannot identify acute hemorrhage limits its usefulness.

Intracranial pressure (ICP) monitoring is used to provide information concerning perfusion pressure (mean arterial pressure minus ICP), which serves as an indirect monitor of CBF. In a focal disorder such as ischemia due to vasospasm, global ICP monitoring is not sensitive enough to identify an ischemic problem until it is large, and when it is often too late, in the course of the injury, for significant prevention (18). While ICP measurements can be useful in guiding the timing of surgery, CT is better for distinguishing raised ICP due to hydrocephalus, intracerebral clot, or diffuse edema, each of which has very different therapeutic implications. Intermittent ICP recordings are still useful for assessing the status of cerebrospinal fluid absorption following SAH, with the elevation of ICP due to hydrocephalus directly lowering CBF due to a reduction of perfusion pressure.

CBF Measurement

A number of approaches to the clinical study of CBF are currently available, due to the important role of CBF alterations and the limitations of the current methodologies. The initial work in this field involved efforts toward quantitative CBF measurements using diffusible tracers. More recent approaches provide a qualitative assessment using either "microsphere-like" radionucleotides, MRI-based diffusion imaging, or transcranial Doppler (TCD) studies of velocities within proximal intracranial vessels.

While global quantitative CBF measurements can be obtained by the concurrent arterial and venous analysis of N_2O delivery and washout, the focal nature of ischemia after SAH demands more regional information if the measurements are to be clinically useful. External scintillation counting of gamma emissions from xenon-133 provides either regional or local CBF information, depending on whether 4–32 independent counters or a fixed and integrated ring of counters are utilized (23). Because xenon is highly diffusible, CBF studies can be repeated at 20-min intervals, providing the ability to study physiological responses in one session (13). Although xenon-133 studies can be performed at the bedside, their clinical utility is limited by a lack of high resolution, poor quantitation especially within the depths of the brain, and no direct anatomic reference (26). The combination of stable xenon (which is radio-dense, like iodine) with CT imaging has overcome many of these limitations (8). Xe/CT CBF monitoring provides high-resolution, quantitative CBF measurements with equal sensitivity at the center and the surface of the brain. Xe/CT measurements are accurate to the extremes of high and low flow (28), as

well as providing sensitivity to the threshold for ischemia (29). Xenon-based CBF studies permit the examination of the vasodilatory status of the cerebral vasculature with paired studies that examine the local response of CBF either to a vasodilatory challenge or to a pharmacological manipulation of blood pressure. The effectiveness of Xe/CT CBF studies is limited by the need to bring the patient to a CT scanner, as well as by the intolerance of the study to patient motion during the 6–7 min of data acquisition.

Qualitative imaging of flow is provided by the combination of single-photon emission computerized tomography (SPECT) and tracers such as Tc-99m hexamethylpropylene amineoxime that are bound within brain tissue in proportion to CBF. The ability to inject the tracer and capture a picture of flow at a later time has proved useful for studying transient processes. The inadequacy of this technology for recording absolute flow values limits its capacity for diagnosing ischemia and identifying a global disturbance of flow (26). Because these isotopes have relatively long half-lives, most repeat studies require a delay of 24 hours, although partial dosing can be done with different tracers to obtain studies within a shorter interval. The ability to record blood volume and CBF information with SPECT has, however, proven useful for the study of ischemia (12), but this is a more costly and demanding analysis than CBF measurement alone.

Continuous focal cortical CBF monitoring is available in the operating room as well as in the intensive care unit, with thermal dilution (3) or laser Doppler flow probes (1) that must be placed directly on the cortical surface. Both systems provide a continuous, highly focal, cortical flow assessment that can examine the response to clinical intervention. A major limitation of this technology is the inability to maintain a probe-cortex relationship, so that one cannot be certain whether a reduction of signal is due to a reduction of flow or a loss of cortical contact.

TCD provides an increasingly popular, noninvasive, bedside assessment of the velocity of blood flow in the proximal vessels of the circle of Willis. Because vasospasm is often most severe within these vessels, elevated velocity is used to signify narrowing. While individual high-velocity readings have not proven to be predictive or diagnostic of ischemia due to vasospasm, a significant daily rise in velocity of one or more vascular territories can be more predictive (4, 6). Potentially, more information can be obtained by measuring ratios of rates in internal carotid artery and middle cerebral artery or by carefully analyzing the waveform for restrictions of distal run-off. The fact that high velocity may also be due to high bulk flow, elevated blood pressures, and reduced blood viscosity, and may be reduced by elevated ICP, introduces unmeasured variables that restrict the ability to extract CBF values directly from a TCD analysis. TCD is also limited by its inability to identify spasm within more distal vessels. In 15–20% of patients measurements cannot be made because of the absence of a "window" for TCD recording.

Neurophysiological Monitoring

Based on known physiological relationships, neurophysiological monitoring provides a noninvasive and continuous means of identifying when metabolism is altered and presumably when CBF has fallen below 20 ml/100 g/min (5). The diminution and loss of electrical activity tell us that perfusion has fallen below the threshold for reversible ischemia, whether electroencephalography (EEG), somatosensory evoked potential (SSEP) brainstem evoked response (BSER), or central conduction time is monitored. Although a more abrupt and complete loss of electrical activity implies a more severe ischemic challenge, the loss of electrical activity does not supply essential information concerning the depth of ischemic challenge.

Metabolic Monitoring

Studies that assess metabolism and flow should be most useful for the assessment of patients after SAH. Although it is comparatively simple to acquire rates of oxygen and glucose delivery and extraction from the concurrent measurement of arterial and venous jugular bulb sampling, these measurements provide only global information, which may be insensitive to important focal

disorders. While positron emission tomography can measure all of the relevant variables, its relative in accessibility and its high acquisition and operation costs make it an unlikely choice for the routine monitoring of patients after SAH. Positron emission tomography has, however, provided the foundation on which less expensive and more widely available technologies are being developed.

In summary, although there are many technologies available for monitoring hemodynamics and/or metabolism in patients after SAH, each has its own limitations. Thus, patient care is best guided by an analysis of data obtained from several sources.

Integration of Information For Clinical Guidance

Preoperative Monitoring

It is essential to be able to make rapid decisions after SAH concerning surgical intervention to prevent re-rupture of an aneurysm. While brain death can be established by neuroimaging techniques that define the absence of cerebral perfusion, a more difficult problem is encountered with patients of Hunt and Hess grade 4 or 5 who have no anatomically defined injury. While a bad outcome is suspected, the measurement of low flow (<20 ml/100 g/min) in spite of normal pCO_2 level is a useful indicator that the prior ischemic injury was severe. The persistence of flow values below normal but above the ischemic threshold has also been used to militate against early aneurysm surgery (5).

Intraoperative Monitoring

Neurophysiological monitoring is ideally suited for intraoperative use, because it provides continuous regional information directly related to flow and metabolism. The type of monitoring chosen for clinical use depends on the specific problem being addressed and the physical constraints inherent in the surgical exposure. While EEG data provide regionally specific information, the placement of a full cortical array of electrodes is not possible during aneurysm surgery, and focal cortical information is usually not required. EEG information is, however, essential for guiding the safe and effective loading of barbiturates if deemed necessary during surgery.

Evoked potential monitoring has gained general acceptance for intraoperative use at our center because it permits the acquisition of vital information despite limited electrode placements. The value of evoked potential monitoring is enhanced by its ability to provide systematic continuous analysis of neuronal activity. Usually SSEPs are recorded from peroneal and median nerve stimulation during aneurysm surgery of the anterior circulation, while BSERs are added if surgery involves the vertebral or basilar arteries. SSEP alterations are more predictive of postoperative deficits than are BSERs (14). While some centers prefer, routinely, to maintain drug-induced metabolic suppression of all aneurysm patients for prolonged periods, it has been our preference to use these agents selectively and only when neurophysiological monitoring indicates that temporary vessel occlusion causes physiological changes. SSEP monitoring has also increased our ability to detect potential intraoperative complications that may occur from the accidental retractor compression of a major vessel, excessive cortical retraction, or even moderate unintended hypotension.

Postoperative Monitoring

When planned or inadvertent large-vessel occlusion occurs during aneurysm surgery, immediate postsurgical evaluation of CBF and vascular reserve capacity can assess whether a vascular territory has been placed at increased ischemic risk. The identification and persistence of low CBF and compromised vascular reserves provide guidance to aggressively maintain perfusion pressures and may support the decision to perform a vascularization procedure if medical therapies prove sufficient to correct the hemodynamic disorder.

The identification of ischemia as a cause for delayed onset of new deficits after SAH remains a major area of concern (Fig. 5E.2). Objective means of diagnosing symptomatic vasospasm are needed because clinical assessment is often inaccurate and aggressive therapies carry a risk of morbidity. While TCD studies have won wide clinical accept-

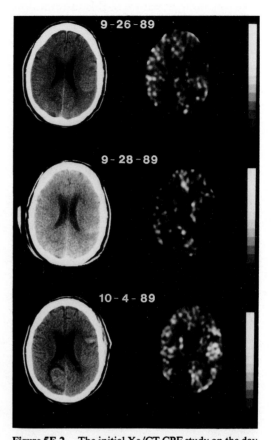

Figure 5E.2. The initial Xe/CT CBF study on the day of referral, 8 days after SAH from a left anterior choroidal artery aneurysm, confirmed inadvertent embolization of the right PCA territory during angiography and disclosed an unsuspected severe reduction of left hemispheric flow. TCD recordings were within normal limits but angiography disclosed distal spasm of the M2 and M3 vessels (left > right), despite blood pressure remaining in the 170–180 mm Hg range. This 58-year-old man developed a right hemiplegia and aphasia on September 28, at which time CBF measurements confirmed further deterioration of flow values primarily within the left hemisphere but also within the right hemisphere. Surgery was delayed until October 4, when CBF showed recovery to nonischemic levels of flow. In this case the first CBF study identified right occipital infarction and unsuspected ischemia, providing insight that the patient probably would not tolerate intraoperative maneuvers needed for exposure and clipping of a large aneurysm. CBF data also provided guidance to maintain elevated pressures despite an unclipped aneurysm. The patient later regained normal flow, indicating a better time for surgical intervention. The scale for CBF is in ml/100 g/min.

ance, the indirect nature of this information restricts its application as the single parameter guiding clinical decisions. The combination of TCD data with a qualitative CBF study appears to increase the sensitivity to symptomatic vasospasm (16). Combining two qualitative CBF studies still has limited specificity because, in addition to the limitations of TCD, CBF is often asymmetrically low after SAH and surgical intervention. We have utilized daily rises of TCD measurements as a highly sensitive indicator that large-vessel narrowing may be occurring and that studies with higher specificity are indicted.

Double-CBF studies that examine the

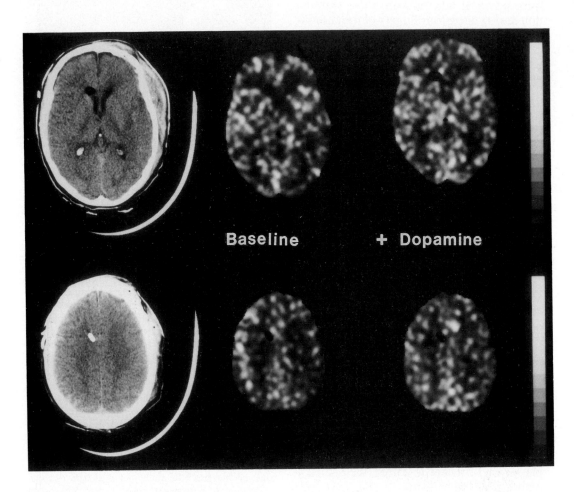

Baseline   **+ Dopamine**

Figure 5E.3. Seven days after SAH and 5 days after surgery for a right internal carotid artery aneurysm, this 42-year-old woman developed a more severe left hemiparesis. Blood pressure was immediately raised with dopamine from 130/90 to 185/100 mm Hg and the patient was brought to the CT scanner. The CT scan revealed low density within the right middle cerebral artery territory. The Xe/CT CBF study done at the higher blood pressure showed a slight reduction of mixed cortical flow on the right side but values well within normal range. The second study was obtained 20 min later, within 5 min of the reduction of dopamine infusion. At the lower perfusion pressure the right cortical flows as well as flow within the white matter on the left side fell into the level of <10 ml/100 g/min. The study confirms the need for hypertensive therapy to minimize further ischemic injury. The color scale is a quantitative CBF scale in ml/100 g/min.

quantitative CBF response to tests of auto-regulation or to a vasodilatory challenge have made these studies more effective as a diagnostic test for active ischemia. The lack of CBF elevation, despite a drug-induced >20-torr elevation of pressure, confirms the integrity of autoregulation, and indicates that hypertensive therapy is not necessary. Conversely, the appropriate elevation of ischemic to nonischemic levels of flow with hypertensive therapy validates the need for such intervention (Fig. 5E.3). Because of the inherent difficulties in maintaining medically induced hypertension, we utilize this test as an objective indicator of whether alternative therapies such as angioplasty are indicated. Waiting until ischemic symptoms recur despite hypertension or until hyperten-sion can no longer be maintained often means that infarction has already occurred and that angioplasty is less likely to be of benefit.

The capacity to augment flow in response to vasodilatory challenge with CO_2 elevation or Diamox confirms that CBV is not maximally increased, and that low flow values are not a result of compromise of perfusion (29). The absence of CBF elevation, especially a paradoxical reduction of CBF with CO_2 elevation, suggests that CBV is maximal and that CBF is critically dependent on perfusion pressure (Fig. 5E.4). The CBF response to CO_2 lowering must, however, be distinguished from a vasodilatory challenge because the former is a local chemical response which remains intact until infarction has occurred.

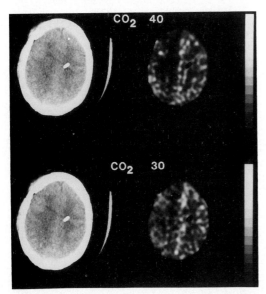

Figure 5E.4. This 24-year-old woman presented with an intraventricular and temporal lobe hemorrhage from a right middle cerebral artery aneurysm 7 days earlier. After aneurysm clipping on day 1, she remained intubated and on ventilation support. On day 8 a CBF study was obtained at a pCO₂ of 30 mm Hg and then with elevation, with normalization, to a level of 40 mm Hg. The study disclosed a paradoxical lowering of right anterior cerebral artery and middle cerebral artery flow values and a clear intolerance to the withdrawal of ventilation support. The patient had severely elevated right middle cerebral artery velocities on TCD. Moderate hyperventilation was continued in addition to hemodilution/hypertension/hypervolemia therapy, resulting in a resolution of hemodynamic compromise without additional middle cerebral artery infarction.

REFERENCES

1. Arbit, E., DiResta, G. R., Bedford, R. F., et al. Intraoperative measurement of cerebral and tumor blood flow with laser Doppler flowmetry. Neurosurgery 24:166–170, 1989.
2. Carpenter, D. A., Grubb, R. L., Jr., Tempel, L. W., and Powers, W. J. Cerebral oxygen metabolism after aneurysmal subarachnoid hemorrhage. J. Cereb. Blood Flow Metab. 11:837–844, 1991.
3. Carter, L. P., White, W. L., and Atkinson, J. R. Regional cortical blood flow at craniotomy. Neurosurgery 2:223–229, 1978.
4. Davis, S. M., Andrews, J. T., Lichtenstein, M., et al. Correlations between cerebral arterial velocities, blood flow and delayed ischemia after subarachnoid hemorrhage. Stroke 23:492–497, 1992.
5. Ferguson, G. C., Farrar, J. K., Meguro, K., et al. Serial measurements of CBF as a guide to surgery in patients with ruptured intracranial aneurysms. J. Cereb. Blood Flow Metab. (suppl. 1):S518, 1981.
6. Grossett, D. G., Straiton, J., Trevou, M., and Bullock, R. Prediction of symptomatic vasospasm after subarachnoid hemorrhage by rapidly increasing Transcranial doppler velocity and cerebral blood flow changes. Stroke 23:674–679, 1992.
7. Grubb, R. L., Jr., Raichle, M. E., Eichling, J. O., and Gado, M. H. Effects of subarachnoid hemorrhage on cerebral blood volume, blood flow and oxygen utilization. J. Neurosurg. 46:446–453, 1977.
8. Johnson, D. W., Stringer, W. A., Marks, M. P., et al. Stable xenon CT cerebral blood flow imaging: rationale for and role in clinical decision making. AJNR 12:201–213, 1991.
9. Jones, T. H., Morowitz, R. B., Crowell, R. M., et al. Thresholds of focal cerebral ischemia in awake monkeys. J. Neurosurg. 54:773–782,

1981.

10. Kanno, I., Uemera, K., Higano, S., *et al.* Oxygen extraction fraction at maximally vasodilated tissue in the ischemic brain estimated from the regional CO_2 responsiveness measured by positron emission tomography. J. Cereb. Blood Flow Metab. *8:*227–235, 1988.

11. Kleiser, B., and Widder, B. Course of carotid artery occlusions with impaired cerebrovascular reactivity. Stroke *23:*171–174, 1992.

12. Knapp, W. H., Kummer, R., and Kbuler, W. Imaging of cerebral blood flow-to-volume distribution using SPECT. J. Nucl. Med. *27:*465–470, 1986.

13. Leinsinger, G., Furst, H., Schmiedek, K., *et al.* Cerebrovascular reserve capacity measured with 133-xenon dynamic SPECT before and after carotid endarterectomy. In: Stimulated Cerebral Blood Flow, edited by K. Schmiedek, K. Einhaupt, and C. M. Kirsch, pp. 250–260. Springer Verlag, Berlin, 1992.

14. Little, J. R., Lesser, R. P., and Luders, H. Electrophysiological monitoring during basilar aneurysm operation. Neurosurgery *20:*421–427, 1987.

15. Matsuda, M., Shiino, A., and Handa, J. Sequential changes of cerebral blood flow after aneurysmal subarachnoid hemorrhage. Acta Neurochir. (Wien.) *105:*98–106, 1990.

16. Mizuno, M., Asakura, K., Hadeishi, H., *et al.* Combination of serial transcranial Doppler examinations and cerebral blood flow studies in the management of cerebral vasospasm after subarachnoid hemorrhage. No Shinkei Geka *18:*905–913, 1990.

17. Mourier, K. L., George, B., Raggueneau, J. L., *et al.* Value of the measurement of cerebral blood flow before and after diamox injection in predicting clinical vasospasm and final outcome in aneurysmal subarachnoid hemorrhage. Neurochirurgie *37:*318–322, 1991.

18. Noterman, J., Berre, J., Vandesteene, A., and Brotchi, J. Monitoring of intracranial pressure during the postoperative period of aneurysms. Neurochirurgie *34:*161–163, 1988.

19. Powers, W. J. Cerebral hemodynamics in ischemic cerebrovascular disease. Ann. Neurol. *29:*231–240, 1991.

20. Powers, W. J., Grubb, R. L., Jr., Baker, R. P., *et al.* Regional cerebral blood flow and metabolism in reversible ischemia due to vasospasm. J. Neurosurg. *62:*539–546, 1985.

21. Powers, W. J., Press, G. A., Grubb, R. L., Jr., *et al.* The effect of hemodynamically significant carotid artery disease on the hemodynamic status of the cerebral circulation. Ann. Intern. Med. *106:*27–35, 1987.

22. Spetzler, R. F., Hadley, M. H., Rigomonti, D., *et al.* Aneurysms of the basilar artery treated with circulatory arrest, hypothermia, and barbiturate cerebral protection. J. Neurosurg. *68:*868–879, 1988.

23. Sugiyama, H., Christianson, J., Olsen, T. S., and Lassen, N. A. Monitoring CBF in clinical routine by dynamic single photon emission tomography (SPECT) of inhaled xenon[133]. Stroke *17:*1179–1182, 1986.

24. Sundt, T. M., Sharbrough, F. W., Anderson, R. E., *et al.* Cerebral blood flow measurements and electroencephalograms during carotid endarterectomy. J. Neurosurg. *41:*310–320, 1974.

25. Voldby, B. Pathophysiology of subarachnoid hemorrhage: experimental and clinical data. Acta Neurochir. [Suppl.] (Wien.) *45:*1–6, 1988.

26. Welch, K. M., Levine, S. R., and Ewing, J. R. Viewing stroke pathophysiology: an analysis of contemporary methods. Stroke *17:*1071–1077, 1986.

27. Yonas, H., Durham, S. R., Smith, H. A., *et al.* Stroke risk assessment using a vasodilatory challenge. J. Cereb. Blood Flow Metab. *11:*S658, 1991.

28. Yonas, H., Gur, D., Classen, D., *et al.* Stable Xe-enhanced CT measurement of cerebral blood flow in reversible focal ischemia in baboons. J. Neurosurg. *73:*266–273, 1990.

29. Yonas, H., Sekhar, L., Johnson, D. W., and Gur, D. Determination of irreversible ischemia by xenon-enhanced computed tomographic monitoring of cerebral blood flow in patients with symptomatic vasospasm. Neurosurgery *24:*368–372, 1989.

CHAPTER 5F

Principles of Management of Subarachnoid Hemorrhage: Ultrasound

JIMMY D. MILLER, M.D., ROBERT R. SMITH, M.D.

INTRODUCTION

Ultrasound has been a part of the neurosurgical armamentarium for more than 40 years. French *et al.* (16, 17) used sonography to document intracerebral tumors following postmortem brain removal. They also evaluated the brains of animals subjected to transcranial pulsed ultrasound with frequencies of 15 MHz and found no evidence of cerebral damage (17). Insonation through the temporal bone using low-frequency ultrasound of 2–4 MHz was used by Leksell (27, 28), and he noticed that "arterio-venous aneurysms" may cause recording of abnormal pulsating echoes. Ford and Ambrose (18), using operating frequencies of 2.5 MHz and 1.5 MHz, performed ultrasound examinations through the intact skull in the temporo-parietal area just above the tip of the ear (5). They discovered four cases of "angiomas" and demonstrated pulsating echoes from a suprasellar aneurysm that were used to measure the width of the aneurysm. The temporal region was also advocated for insonation of the midline to determine shift (7, 41). On the basis of the thinness of the bone. Although use of ultrasound to evaluate midline shift was thought to have been made obsolete by computerized tomography (CT) and magnetic resonance imaging scanning, real-time sonography has recently been shown to be useful in the evaluation of basal cisterns and ventricular size (8). The most useful neurosurgical application of ultrasound is the transcranial Doppler (TCD) to evaluate blood flow velocity in the basal arteries, which was introduced by Aaslid *et al.* (5) in 1982. They believed that this would be particularly helpful in the evaluation of vasospasm following subarachnoid hemorrhage (SAH) (9).

During the past decade, TCD has found widespread application as both a clinical and research tool due to the ease of use and repeatability. However, blood flow velocity differs from volume blood flow, and TCD is an adjunctive measurement that adds to but does not replace radiographic or clinical examinations or direct flow measurements. Its usefulness relates to the ability to evaluate the physiological situation repeatedly, allowing dynamic correlation with the course of the patient. This is particularly important following SAH, when patients may demonstrate rapid clinical change. If the CT scan does not demonstrate further bleeding or acute hydrocephalus, vasospasm is often inferred. In this situation, TCD may be particularly useful, in that serial studies may demonstrate changes in velocities related to decreasing vessel lumen size.

Physics of the Doppler Effect

The Doppler effect was first described by Christian Doppler in 1842 (12). He theorized that sound can be used to measure the velocity of moving objects by calculating the difference in frequency between the reflected signal (echo) and the transmitted frequency if the objects are moving parallel with the direction of insonation. If the object under study is moving away from the transducer and receiver the time for the echo to return is longer, and if the study object is moving toward the receiver the echo time is shortened. The angle of insonation is of critical importance, in that the true object velocity can be accurately determined if the movement is directly toward or away from the transducer/receiver but the calculated velocity decreases as the insonation angle increases. Insonation at an angle of 90° to the moving objects results in no recordable velocity. Thus, the calculated velocity may accurately reflect the actual velocity if the angle of insonation is sufficiently low, but if the angle is between 0° and 180° the calculated velocity is less than the actual velocity. A 60° angle results in a value of 50% of the actual velocity, and a 30° insonation angle results in the calculated velocity being 87% of the true velocity. When the temporal window is used, the angles of insonation can usually be assumed to be less than 30°. Therefore the calculated velocity will likely be lower than the actual velocity, and the most valid calculated velocity will be the highest recorded.

The speed of sound propagation through various tissues is known, allowing the depth of the study to be controlled by computerized range gating. This is performed by having the receiver accept only signals that return in a specified time interval, with other echoes being rejected. Sequential evaluations of regions of vessels at various depths can be calculated. However, even with recording restricted to specified echoes, a range of velocities are detected, because a certain range of time is allowed and the reflected echoes are generated from flowing red blood cells that are traveling at varying rates. A velocity spectrum from different depths along the vessel being studied, rather than a single value, is therefore recorded. The usual sample length is about 5–10 mm. The velocity reported may be the maximum velocity (V_{max}), reflecting the velocity from the so-called spectral envelope, or the mean velocity. With laminar flow these two parameters should have a linear relationship. Even with changing clinical conditions, the two parameters have been shown to reflect changes accurately; therefore the use of one or the other should be based on the type of instrument used to obtain the measurement.

Color-flow instruments have been developed to allow rapid evaluation of flow directions and velocity. Red colors are typically used to identify flow toward the transducer, and blue colors flow away from the transducer. Flow direction change, such as with collateral flow across the anterior communicating artery in internal carotid artery (ICA) occlusion, is easily detected using color-flow techniques. These techniques can be combined with mapping by including a headpiece aligned with reference points on the patient's head (1). The *x*-reference is the distance from the transducer at the temporal window-to the area of study, the *y*-reference is from the forehead in the supraorbital region, and the *z*-reference is from the top of the head near the bregma. A computer generated map of the circulation, can be obtained using the data from the range-gated insonation in two or three orientations to assist in assessment. This technique is commonly used in the anterior circulation; but may prove useful in evaluation of the vertebrobasilar circulation. Combining mapping and color-flow greatly enhances the examiner's ability to rapidly and accurately identify various vessels under study.

Methods of Monitoring Hemorrhage Patients with SAH by Using TCD

The TCD evaluation is readily learned, but requires methodical technique to achieve reliable and reproducible results. Each laboratory should develop its own protocol for consistency in the examination and results. Ideally, the examination is performed in the sonography laboratory with the patient in the supine position. Frequently, however patients with SAH cannot be safely transported if they are seriously ill or have not received surgical clipping and the test must then be performed at the patient's bedside. Modifications may be required to meet the individual patients' requirements. The examination begins with use of the temporal window just above the zygomatic arch. Insonation is usually first attempted at a depth of 55–60 mm, to insonate the ICA bifurcation. A bidirectional signal can usually be seen, but on occasion flow toward or away from the probe may be observed. By insonating at progressively shallower depths, the middle cerebral artery (MCA) can be mapped out, providing velocities along the MCA in the basal cistern. Once the MCA is followed as far as possible, insonation depth is increased to the region of the ICA bifurcation and the anterior cerebral artery (ACA) is followed distally. In the ACA, the flow direction is away from the transducer unless this vessel is providing collateral flow. The insonation depth for the ACA is about 60–80 mm and the transducer requires slightly anterior angulation to keep the vessel in the field of study. As the midline is crossed, the contralateral ACA may be insonated, in which case flow changes and is toward the probe. The velocity of the ACA is 49–60 cm/sec, which is usually slightly less than the MCA velocity. The posterior cerebral artery (PCA) can be insonated by directing the probe slightly posteriorly and inferiorly from the ICA bifurcation and increasing the depth of insonation about 5 mm deeper than the ICA bifurcation. The PCA can be insonated as it curves around the brainstem to its origin from the basilar artery, and sometimes the contralateral vessel can be insonated. The ipsilateral PCA flow direction is toward the probe at the usual location of insonation and the velocity is 30–50 cm/sec. If the flow direction is away from the probe, the location of insonation may be from the P_2 segment after the PCA has circled around the brainstem. The posterior communicating artery is rarely insonated, but flow may be detected in this vessel if it is providing collateral flow. The ophthalmic artery can be insonated via an orbital window at depths of 40–60 mm. The flow direction is toward the probe unless this vessel is providing collateral flow and the mean velocity is around 20 cm/sec. With deeper insonation through the transorbital window, the carotid artery can be insonated. Flow direction can be either toward or away from the probe. With practice, the carotid siphon can be insonated to document flow toward the probe inferiorly and away from the probe superiorly at the carotid siphon level. The normal velocity is 30–60 cm/sec. The vertebral and basilar arteries can be insonated via the foramen magnum. Insonation of these vessels is more difficult, but with practice they can be insonated with some consistency. The velocities of these vessels are 28–51 cm/sec and the flow is away from the transducer.

The technique requires that the person performing the study have some knowledge of the anatomy of the intracranial arteries as well as a working knowledge of the flow directions and velocities. In general, handheld probes are used, necessitating careful manipulation of the transducer to follow the course of the vessel and to adjust for the maximum velocity at each particular depth. With practice, the technique requires minimal time for a complete examination. Detailed instruction regarding the technique has been well outlined in several good texts (2, 19).

Results of the TCD Examination and Timing of Vasospasm

Following SAH, patients often have no evidence vasospasm seen in early angiography. Likewise, have TCD velocities measured within 72–96 hours following SAH have revealed normal values (20, 22, 34). Seiler et al. (35) found that 10 of 24 patients had normal values within the first 3 days following SAH, but 14 patients had velocities increasing above 80 cm/sec in the second and third days, with all patients achieving velocities greater than 80 cm/sec between days 4 and 10, 24 (24) reported that all of their patients demonstrated velocities in the MCA above 100 cm/sec by day 8. The greatest elevations occur in the MCA ipsilateral to the blood side with only slight changes in the ACA and PCA (Fig. 5F.1) (22). Romner et al. (34) have shown that there are no differences in velocities in 14 patients surgically treated within 48 hours, compared to those treated between 49 and 96 hours, when comparing TCDs performed within 72 hours of bleed. The velocities in both groups increased by days 5–7, with the patients undergoing later surgery having significantly higher velocities ($p < 0.01$) and with the difference remaining at days 10–12. The two groups were similar with regard to aneurysm location, clinical grade, and CT

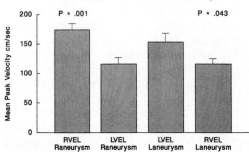

Figure 5F.1. Peak velocities are higher in the MCA ipsilateral to the side of the aneurysm which resulted in the SAH. RVEL = right velocities, LVEL = left velocities.

appearance. The highest velocity in this study was only 176 cm/sec, which the authors attributed to testing only up to day 12.

The day of maximum velocity increase is of obvious clinical importance for monitoring treatment options and advising families and patients. In two studies the maximum velocity was reached on days 8–14 (20, 24). Patients who develop clinically symptomatic vasospasm tend to reach maximum TCD velocity on day 8 or 9, while those without clinical vasospasm attain maximum TCD velocity on days 10–14 (20, 24). Sekhar *et al.* (37) commented that in eight patients developing delayed ischemic deficits (DIDs), the highest average daily velocity occurred just before or during the clinical vasospasm (see Fig. 5F.2). The critical velocity for clin-

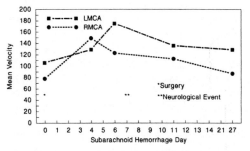

Figure 5F.2. This patient had a left ICA aneurysm, with multiple TCD evaluations. As can be seen, the left MCA (LMCA) achieved a higher velocity than the right MCA (RMCA), and the left MCA velocity increased prior to the neurological deterioration.

ical vasospasm is 200 cm/sec (see Fig. 5F.3). At this level, the risk of infarction is great, yet some patients still remain asymptomatic (36). Velocities in the 120–140 cm/sec range usually are not associated with infarction, and with velocities less than 100 cm/sec the chance of clinical vasospasm is minimal (24, 36). Seiler *et al.* (36) reported a series of 118 patients with repeated TCD measurements between days 3 and 10 following SAH. They found only six (5%) patients with velocities below 80 cm/sec, and all of these were more than 65 years of age. Forty-three percent had velocities up to 140 cm/sec, 32% had velocities of 140–200 cm/sec, and 20% had velocities over 200 cm/sec. All of these patients were being treated with nimodipine. Eleven patients had transient problems, five had delayed ischemic deficit (infarction), and three others died from large infarctions (36). The velocity differences between asymptomatic patients and those who died reached significance ($p = 0.008$); however, there was a middle group in which it was difficult or impossible to separate the clinical profile from the TCD velocities. The authors also noted that patients who developed infarctions had early and steep increases in velocities. Grosset *et al.* (21) also stressed the steep or rapid rise in TCD velocities as being ominous for significant clinical vasospasm, and they defined a velocity rise of greater than 50 cm/sec/24 hours as the critical level (21).

With decreasing consciousness level, as in SAH of grades III–V, cerebral blood flow may decrease significantly, and this may result in a decrease in the expected elevated velocities. Lindegaard *et al.* (24) used the hemispheric velocity of the MCA divided by the hemispheric velocity of the ICA (V_{MCA}/V_{ICA} index) to avoid this problem. A change in volume flow should alter flow velocities proportionately in both the ICA and the MCAs. A ratio above 3 indicates vasospasm. The authors also indicated that the index corrected for differences related to age and gender.

Transluminal angioplasty has shown considerable promise in alleviating the clinical as well as the radiographic features of cerebral vasospasm that follows SAH from an intracranial aneurysm. The method seems most effective when applied to the treatment of patients who have significant angiographic vasospasm without cerebral infarction. Because the timing of intervention is critical, we sought to identify patients who would develop these events prior to the onset of irreversible ischemic changes (14). Twenty-five patients were included in this study, in which at least three serial TCD examinations were carried out following SAH from an intracranial aneurysm. Fifteen patients (60%) became symptomatic. In symptomatic patients, mean peak MCA velocities occurred between days 8 and 11, and a second peak occurred after day 20. The latter event may have been associated with

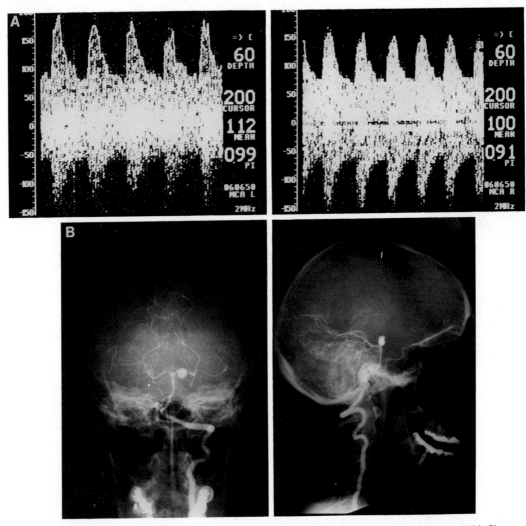

Figure 5F.3. This case involved a 49-year-old white woman who sustained a SAH on January 30, 1992. She was initially very lethargic but improved over 48 hours and was referred for neurosurgical evaluation. (*A*) TCD revealed mildly elevated MCA velocities on February 3, 1992 (*left*, left side; *right*, right side). (*B*) Angiography revealed a PCA aneurysm. There was no evidence of vasospasm. Shown are views of the basilar artery (*left*, anterior-posterior; *right*, lateral). The patient subsequently underwent clipping of her aneurysm. Postoperatively, she developed a right hemiparesis. (*C*) TCD velocities were markedly elevated on February 5, 1992, and the patient was treated with hypertension/hypervolemia but failed to improve (*left*, left side; *right*, right side). (*D*) Angiography performed at the time of angioplasty documented severe vasospasm, as shown in the left MCA.

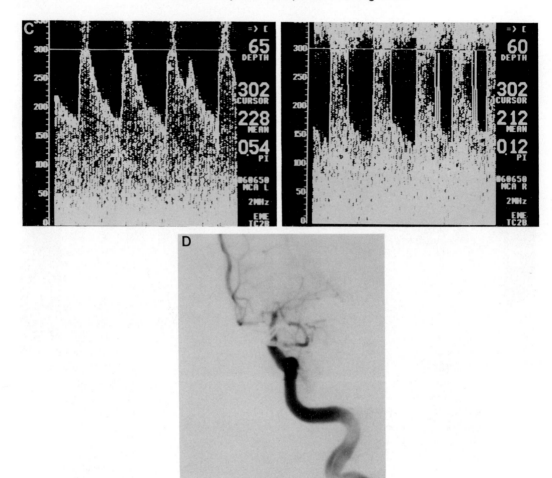

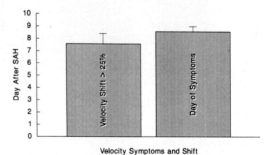

Figure 3—continued.

infarction. There was no velocity that was a reliable indicator of which patients would become symptomatic. However, in every patient who became symptomatic, velocity increased >25%/day during the 2 days preceding the onset of symptoms (see Fig. 5F.4). One patient in the asymptomatic group also showed a 25% velocity shift (specificity, 100%; sensitivity, 90%).

We found that MCA velocity usually showed two peaks (Fig. 5F.5). The first peak occurred on day 13 after SAH. The second peak appeared between days 21 and 23. If only the ipsilateral MCA velocity is considered, two earlier peaks can be identified. The first one occurs between days 8 and 11 and the second peak between days 15 and 17

(see Fig. 5F.5). Based upon these findings, we suggest that following SAH from an aneurysm, if the velocity increases 25%/day,

Figure 5F.4. Velocity shift of >25% is associated with neurological deterioration and occurs prior to the onset of symptoms.

Peak Mean Velocity Each Day After SAH

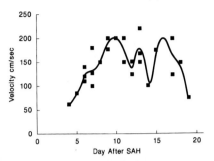

Figure 5F.5. The peak mean velocity has two major peaks; one occurs early, at days 8–10, and the other later, at days 15–17. Patients whose profile fits the early peak are more likely to develop symptomatic vasospasm.

repeat angiography should be performed in preparation for endovascular intervention. The TCD must be carried out serially, starting before the fourth day of hemorrhage.

Comparison with Other Parameters

Attempts at correlating TCD velocity changes with arteriographic vessel narrowing have yielded mixed results. Some authors have reported a positive correlation between the velocity and the diameter of the MCA on the angiogram ($r = 0.75$) (4). Musical murmurs may be associated with high velocity and severe vasospasm on angiography probably related to configuration of the vessels or wall changes (6). Others have found a poor correlation ($r = 0.25$) between vessel radius to the fourth power and TCD MCA velocities, but those authors stated that their data must be interpreted with caution because the diameter of the vessels prior to SAH was not known, thus possibly leading to flawed evaluation (37). Both of the aforementioned studies found poor correlation between the TCD velocity of the ACA and the angiographic appearance of vasospasm. Aaslid *et al.* (4) compared patients with SAH to patients with no known cerebrovascular disease and found that those tested within 4 days of SAH had velocities that were 40% elevated and those tested between days 5 and 12 had 81% velocity elevation, compared to controls. Of those with SAH, the

MCA diameter was 2.7 ± 0.3 mm in the group tested early and 2.1 ± 0.6 mm in the group, tested later.

Cerebral blood flow (CBF) decreases usually follows the elevation of TCD velocities and correlate with the clinical condition of the patients (37). Patients with CBF below 20 ml/100 g/min had very high TCD velocities in the vessels supplying the ischemic territory. In patients with rapid rises in TCD velocity, single photon emission computed tomography findings have revealed regional abnormal patterns consistent with ischemia (21). In the majority of patients, the abnormality consisted of focal hypoperfusion that usually correlated with the site of the aneurysm, but the evidence was stronger for the MCA than the ACA data. There were a few patients with mixed zones of hypoperfusion and hyperperfusion that the authors attributed to reperfusion of ischemic tissue. Some patients were found to have increased TCD velocities and single photon emission computed tomography perfusion defects but remained clinically asymptomatic, presumably because the flow remained above threshold levels for cellular function or infarction.

The amount of blood on the CT scan correlates with the likelihood of clinical vasospasm (15, 25, 30). Comparison of CT results with TCD has shown that velocity increase is related to the amount of cisternal blood. In one study, patients with normal CT scans following SAH had velocities up to about 140 cm/sec, patients with diffuse or thin layers of cisternal-blood had a slow increase of velocity up to about 150 cm/sec, and 15 patients with localized cisternal clots or diffuse thick layers of blood had a steep increase in velocity to about 190 cm/sec (17). In addition, patients with thick or localized clots reached maximum velocity by day 7, while those with normal scans attained peak velocities on days 11–15. In this study, the velocities in patients with normal scans or only diffuse or thin layers of blood were significantly different from those in patients with thick clots. However, Hutchison and Weir (24) were unable to find a difference between patients with CT scans revealing thick rather than thin clots, but those with blood evident on CT scans had higher velocities, compared to those with no blood evident on CT scan.

TCD Velocity Changes with Treatment of Vasospasm

TCD velocity elevation occurs prior to clinical evidence of ischemia and potentially could be used to indicate treatment for asymptomatic patients, as suggested by Sekhar *et al.* (37). Conversely, a decrease in TCD velocity may guide a rational withdrawal of therapy. Seiler *et al.* (36) have reported on the use of TCD to determine the change of nimodipine from an intravenous preparation to an oral form. Most reported studies have utilized nimodipine prophylactically. Harders and Gilsbach (22) found that velocities increased after discontinuation of intravenous nimodipine and start of the oral medication.

The most dramatic effects of TCD velocity changes have been associated with angioplasty. To date, the number of reported cases remains small, but angioplasty appears promising in decreasing the velocity without recurrence (10, 32). Newell *et al.* (32) reported one case in which the velocity initially decreased, only to increase again on the second day following angioplasty. The cause of this recurrence is unknown. The decrease in velocity following dilatation is particularly well illustrated by the case of Konishi *et al.* (26). Their patient had SAH from a ruptured left anterior cerebral artery. Clipping was performed on the second day after SAH. On the fifth day the patient's neurological condition deteriorated, with an associated right MCA velocity of 200 cm/sec and pulsating index (PI) of 0.32 and a left MCA velocity of 158 cm/sec and PI of 0.46. Angiography documented vasospasm, and bilateral MCA angioplasty was performed. Immediately following the procedure, the right MCA had a velocity of 62 cm/sec and PI of 0.74 and the left MCA had a velocity of 72 cm/sec and PI of 0.85. Carotid angiography and TCD were performed on day 18 and 6 months following SAH, and these tests showed continued vessel dilatation and normal TCD values.

At the present time there are few, if any, data on the effect of volume loading and hypertension therapy with regards to TCD monitoring in patients with vasospasm. It is difficult to predict changes that might occur, but increasing blood pressure and hemodilution effects would be expected to increase recorded velocity despite an improvement in cerebral perfusion and the clinical condition. This might be detected through use of the hemispheric V_{MCA}/V_{ICA} index, as proposed by Lindegaard *et al.* (29). If autoregulation remains intact, in at least some of the microvasculature, there may be additional vasoconstriction in some arteriolar fields, which may counteract the effects of the increased blood flow from hemodilution (31). This complex issue remains open for evaluation.

Advantages and Disadvantages of TCD

Many of the advantages and disadvantages have been covered above. Certainly, a major advantage is the ease of use at the patient's bedside. Because the test is painless, it has met with patient acceptance even in the pediatric population. TCD testing can also be repeated, thus defining the dynamic course of each patient. Grosset *et al.* (21) have proposed that rapidly increasing velocity (>50 cm/sec/24 hours) may be a useful finding to help predict impending vasospasm, especially if combined with the ratio of the MCA or ACA to the extracranial ICA by the submandibular approach. Others have stressed that TCD testing may reduce costs and morbidity associated with repeated angiography (35). Because velocity elevation may be detected prior to clinical evidence of ischemia, TCD may be used to guide angiography and surgical or medical treatment (37). Some patients may present for treatment 3 or 4 days following SAH, and TCD may be of value in the timing of surgery (34). Alert patients admitted after day 3 without a steep increase in velocity over 24 hours were operated on as soon as possible, thereby avoiding angiography and surgery during the critical phase of vasospasm, according to two reports (35, 36). TCD evaluation may assist in determining the side of bleeding in patients with bilateral aneurysms. Lateralized aneurysms tend to show higher velocities on the side of the aneurysm by the fourth day following SAH, but the difference has not consistently been shown to reach statistical significance (24, 35). From a research standpoint, another major advantage of TCD is the fact that changes occur rapidly. Velocity changes have been recorded within 2.3–8 sec following a stimulus (3, 13).

Physiological testing may prove useful to evaluate cerebrovascular reserve and more precisely select patients who are at danger of delayed ischemia. This can be performed relatively easily using CO_2 reactivity. Normally there is a 4.7% increase in flow velocity for each rise in pCO_2 of 1 mm Hg, while the increase is lessened in patients with vasospasm (23). With mild vasospasm (velocity, 80–120 cm/sec) the increased flow velocity was 2.3% mmHg pCO_2 rise, with moderate vasospasm (velocity, 120–160 cm/sec) reactivity was 1.9%, and with severe vasospasm (velocity, >160 cm/sec) rising pCO_2 caused only a 0.9% change/mm Hg pCO_2. Presumably these changes were related to distal vasodilation to compensate for proximal vasoconstriction in the basal vessels. As shown by Hassler and Chioffi (23), the PI also decreased with progressive severity of vasospasm, and the change in the PI with alteration of pCO_2 was less as the severity of vasospasm increased. Romner et al. (33) found a poor correlation between absolute cerebral blood flow and TCD, but there was a linear relationship between CBF and pCO_2 (r = 0.70) and a positive but less marked relationship between pCO_2 and TCD (r = 0.52). The correlation between responses in CBF and TCD to pCO_2 changes was poor (r = 0.33). The disparity between the two methods was pronounced with CBF values above 30 ml/100 g/min, where there were large variations in TCD values. The authors stressed that the two methods have differences, in that TCD measures velocity in major basal vessels, whereas CBF is a mean flow value for many vessels of different size and the area covered is not known. In addition, vasoreactivity and autoregulation may not be uniformly altered in single patients or in several patients. It should be noted that TCD changes in response to pCO_2 alterations occur within seconds, while CBF

methods use summed data accrued over many minutes. Which method is more appropriate remains to be determined.

There are several problems with TCD that must be recognized, to most effectively use this tool for the treatment of patients. First, the velocity increase depends on the vessel diameter change and on the available collateral blood supply. Marked spasm in the A_1 segment of the ACA may cause only modest flow velocity changes, because flow can bypass this region via the contralateral A_1 segment if the anterior communicating artery is present. Second, vasospasm in distal branches may not be detected by insonation of the basilar vessels. This occurred in one patient of eight in the series reported by Sekhar et al. (37). In addition to the aforementioned problems, DeWitt and Wechsler (11) outlined several other pitfalls in their review of TCD, including the observations that vasospasm involving the ICA may result in lower MCA velocities and that the reliability of determining vasospasm in the vertebrobasilar circulation is uncertain. Velocity increases may potentially occur with hemodilution during treatment of vasospasm with volume loading, despite improved supply of cerebral tissue needs.

Future Possibilities

The use of sonography may allow visualization of aneurysm anatomy. One case of intraoperative color-flow Doppler imaging has been reported, involving an aneurysm of the MCA (9). After clipping there was obliteration of flow in the aneurysm and patency of the MCA could be verified. Becker et al. (8) have reported on the use of transcranial color-coded real-time sonography that could be combined with Doppler evaluation. Using real-time sonography, they were able to visualize ventricular hemorrhage except when there was only a small amount of blood in the occipital horns. Parenchymal hemorrhage was characterized by increased echo density, although the polar regions could not be scanned. In 76% of aneurysm patients, the aneurysm could be identified, thus allowing noninvasive evaluation suitable for presumptive diagnosis. Hydrocephalus could be evaluated, and increased echo density in the basal cisterns could be seen in 75%. Repeated evaluation could potentially document impending or present uncal herniation. Although embolism from an aneurysm is probably uncommon, TCD may prove useful in detecting emboli from large aneurysms with thrombi, as it is following cardiopulmonary bypass and carotid endarterectomy (39, 40). It may be possible to utilize TCD in the functional evaluation of specific cerebral arterial territories. For example, an increase in PCA velocity following visual stimuli has been reported. Such evaluations may prove useful in the evaluation of patients with SAH (3, 38). Other potential tests would include tests of mental activities, as reported by Droste *et al.* (13).

Conclusion

The use of TCD has proven to be a valuable adjunct to the care of patients with aneurysmal SAH. The test is noninvasive, repeatable, safe, and accepted readily by patients. The dynamic course of velocity elevation can be elucidated by serial testing prior to clinical symptomatology. This allows the clinician to make rational decisions regarding the timing of angiography and surgical clipping and the optimal time of treatment withdrawal as vasospasm improves. Real-time sonography will enhance the use of ultrasound by combining visualization of intracranial structures with the Doppler examination.

Acknowledgments

The authors thank Robin French for secretarial assistance and Lucia Griffin for editorial assistance in preparing this manuscript.

REFERENCES

1. Aaslid, R. The Doppler principle applied to measurement of blood flow velocity in cerebral arteries. In: Transcranial Doppler Sonography, edited by R. Aaslid, pp. 22–38. Springer-Verlag, Wien, 1986.
2. Aaslid, R. Transcranial Doppler examination techniques. In: Transcranial Doppler Sonography, edited by R. Aaslid, pp. 39–59. Springer-Verlag, Wien, 1986.
3. Aaslid, R. Visually evoked dynamic blood flow response of the human cerebral circulation. Stroke *18*:771–775, 1987.
4. Aaslid, R., Huber, P., and Nornes, H. Evaluation of cerebrovascular spasm with transcranial Doppler ultrasound. J. Neurosurg. *60*:37–41, 1984.
5. Aaslid, R., Markwalder, T.-M., and Nornes, H. Noninvasive transcranial Doppler ultrasound recording of flow velocity in basal cerebral arteries. J. Neurosurg. *57*:769–774, 1982.
6. Aaslid, R., and Nornes, H. Musical murmurs in human cerebral arteries after subarachnoid hemorrhage. J. Neurosurg. *60*:32–36, 1984.
7. Barrows, H. S., Dyck, P., and Kurze, T. The diagnostic applications of ultrasound in neurological disease: the intracerebral midline. Neurology *15*:361–365, 1965.
8. Becker, G., Greiner, K., Kaune, B., *et al.* Diagnosis and monitoring of subarachnoid hemorrhage by transcranial color-coded real-time sonography. Neurosurgery *28*:814–820, 1991.
9. Black, K. L., Rubin, J. M., Chandler, W. F., and McGillicuddy, J. E. Intraoperative color-flow Doppler imaging of AVM's and aneurysms. J. Neuorosurg. *68*:635–639, 1988.
10. Bracard, S., Picard, L., Marchal, J. C., *et al.* Role of angioplasty in the treatment of symptomatic vascular spasm occurring in the post-operative course of intracranial ruptured aneurysms. J. Neuroradiol. *17*:6–19, 1990.
11. DeWitt, L. D., and Wechsler, L. R. Transcranial Doppler. Stroke *19*:915–921, 1988.
12. Doppler, C. A. Uber das farbige Licht der Doppelsterne und einiger anderer Gestirne des Himmels. Proceedings of the Royal Bohemian Society of Sciences Vth Ed., Vol 2, pp 1–12. In communion with Barrosch & Andre, Prague, 1842.
13. Droste D. K., Karders, N.C., Rastogi, E. A transcranial Doppler study of blood flow velocity in the middle cerebral arteries performed at rest and during mental activities. Stroke *20:*1005–1011, 1989.
14. Fahmy, M. A., and Smith, R. R. Identification of presymptomatic cerebral vasospasm by transcranial Doppler sonography. (Abstract). Stroke *23:*84, 1992.
15. Fisher, C. M., Kistler, J. P., and Davis, J. M. Relation of cerebral vasospasm to subarachnoid hemorrhage visualized by computerized tomographic scanning. Neurosurgery *6:*1–9, 1980.
16. French, L. A., Wild, J. J., and Neal, D. Detection of cerebral tumors by ultrasonic pulses. Cancer *3:*705–708, 1950.
17. French, I. A., Wild, J. J., and Neal, D. The experimental application of ultrasonics to the localization of brain tumors. J. Neurosurg. *8:*198–203, 1951.
18. Ford, R., and Ambrose, J. Echoencephalography: the measurement of the position of mid-line structures in the skull with high frequency pulsed ultrasound. Brain *86:*189–196, 1963.
19. Fujioka, K. A., and Douville, C. M. Anatomy and freehand examination techniques. In: Transcranial Doppler, edited by D. D.W., Newell, and R. Aaslid, pp. 9–36. Raven Press, New York, 1992.

20. Gilsbach, J. M., and Harders, A. Early aneurysm operation and vasospasm: intracranial Doppler findings. Neurochirurgia (Stuttg.) *28:*100–102, 1985.

21. Grosset, D. G., Straiton, J. du Trevou, M., and Bullock, R. Prediction of symptomatic vasospasm after subarachnoid hemorrhage by rapidly increasing transcranial Doppler velocity and cerebral blood flow changes. Stroke *23:*674–679, 1992.

22. Harders, A. G., and Gilsbach, J. M. Time course of blood velocity changes related to vasospasm in the circle of Willis measured by transcranial Doppler ultrasound. J. Neurosurg. *66:*718–728, 1987.

23. Hassler, W., and Chioffi, F. CO_2 reactivity of cerebral vasospasm after aneurysmal subarachnoid hemorrhage. Acta Neurochir. (Wien.) *98:*167–175, 1989.

24. Hutchison, K., and Weir, B. Transcranial Doppler studies in aneurysm patients. Can. J. Neurol. Sci. *16:*411–416, 1989.

25. Kistler, J. R., Crowell, P. M., Davis, K. R., et al. The relation of cerebral vasospasm to the extent and location of subarachnoid blood visualized by CT scan: a prospective study. Neurology *33:*424–436, 1983.

26. Konishi, Y., Maemura, R., Sato, F., et al. A therapy against vasospasm after subarachnoid haemorrhage: clinical experience of balloon angioplasty. Neurol. Res. *12:*103–105, 1990.

27. Leksell, L. Echoencephalography. I. Detection of intracranial complications following head injury. Acta Chir. Scand. *110:*301–315, 1955.

28. Leksell, L. Echoencephalography. II. Midline echo from the pineal body as an index of pineal displacement. Acta Chir. Scand. *115:*255–259, 1958.

29. Lindegaard, K.-F., Nornes, H., Bakke, S. J., et al. Cerebral vasospasm diagnosis by means of angiography and blood velocity measurement. Acta Neurochir. (Wien.) *100:*12–24, 1989.

30. Mizukami, M., Takemae, T., Tazawa, T., et al. Value of computed tomography in the prediction of cerebral vasospasm after aneurysm rupture. Neurosurgery *7:*583–586, 1980.

31. Muizelaar, J. R., Wei, F. R., Kontos, H. A., and Becker, D. P. Mannitol causes compensatory cerebral vasoconstriction and vasodilation in response to blood viscosity changes. J. Neurosurg. *59:*822–828, 1983.

32. Newell, D. W., Eskridge, J. M., Mayberg, M. R., et al. Angioplasty for the treatment of symptomatic vasospasm following subarachnoid hemorrhage. J. Neurosurg. *71:*654–660, 1989.

33. Romner, B., Brandt, L., Berntman, L., et al. Simultaneous transcranial Doppler sonography and cerebral blood flow measurements of cerebrovascular CO_2-reactivity in patients with aneurysmal subarachnoid haemorrhage. Br. J. Neurosurg. *5:*31–37, 1991.

34. Romner, B., Ljunggren, B., Brandt, L., and Saveland, H. Correlation of transcranial Doppler sonography findings with timing of aneurysm surgery. J. Neurosurg. *73:*72–76, 1990.

35. Seiler, R. W., Grolimund, P., Aaslid, R., et al. Cerebral vasospasm evaluated by transcranial ultrasound correlated with clinical grade and CT-visualized subarachnoid hemorrhage. J. Neurosurg. *64:*594–600, 1986.

36. Seiler, R. W., Reulen, H. J., Huber, P., et al. Outcome of aneurysmal subarachnoid hemorrhage in a hospital population: a prospective study including early operation, intravenous nimodipine, and transcranial Doppler ultrasound. Neurosurgery *23:*598–604, 1988.

37. Sekhar, L. N., Wechsler, L. R., Yonas, H., et al. Value of transcranial Doppler examination in the diagnosis of cerebral vasospasm after subarachnoid hemorrhage. Neurosurgery *22:*813–821, 1988.

38. Sitzer, M., Diehl, R. R., and Hennerici, M. Visually evoked cerebral blood flow responses: normal and pathological conditions. J. Neurouimaging *2:*65–70, 1992.

39. Spencer, M. P., Thomas, G. I., Nicholls, S. C., and Sauvage, I. R. Detection of middle cerebral artery emboli during carotid endarterectomy using transcranial Doppler ultrasonography. Stroke *21:*415–423, 1990.

40. Stump, D. A., Stein, C. S., Tegeler, C. H., et al. Validity and reliability of an ultrasound device for detecting carotid emboli. J. Neuroimaging *1:*18–22, 1991.

41. Tanaka, K., Ito, K., and Wagai, T. The localization of brain tumors by ultrasonic techniques: a clinical review of 111 cases. J. Neurosurg. *23:*135–147, 1965.

Principles of Management of Subarachnoid Hemorrhage: Pathophysiology and Management of Hydrocephalus after Subarachnoid Hemorrhage

PATRICIA A. MANCUSO, M.D., PHILIP R. WEINSTEIN, M.D.

INTRODUCTION

Hydrocephalus is a condition marked by dilatation of the cerebral ventricles and accumulation of cerebrospinal fluid (CSF) within the skull. It is characterized by ataxia, mental deterioration, and urinary incontinence and may result in brain atrophy. Although it is often congenital, hydrocephalus may be acquired after hemorrhage, trauma, infection, or neoplastic infiltration; its onset may be acute or slowly progressive. Obstructive hydrocephalus is caused by blockage of CSF pathways. Communicating hydrocephalus arises when the ventricular system is unobstructed and CSF passes into the subarachnoid space but is not absorbed.

Hydrocephalus is a significant complication of subarachnoid hemorrhage (SAH). This challenging and complex problem occurs in 6–67% of patients after SAH and is associated with increased morbidity and mortality rates (5, 13, 31, 39, 54, 59, 60). Most authors agree that about 20% of patients admitted to a hospital within 24 hours after aneurysmal SAH develop hydrocephalus (39, 59). Acute hydrocephalus can cause ventricular dilation, increased intracranial pressure (ICP), and a decreased level of consciousness, resulting in a substantial increase in clinical grade. With prompt diagnosis and careful management, however, it is possible to avoid potentially disastrous complications and maximize the potential for recovery.

Pathophysiology

CSF is a clear colorless liquid containing high concentrations of sodium chloride and small amounts of protein, glucose, and potassium. It fills the subarachnoid space, surrounds the brain and spinal cord, and normally contains no cells. When blood enters the subarachnoid space, whether after trauma or aneurysm rupture, it can spread freely like a film throughout the subarachnoid space and cisterns, over the convexities, and around the spinal cord. In most cases, the blood remains in the subarachnoid space; however, if there is enough pressure (e.g., after rupture of a saccular aneurysm), the blood can break out of the subarachnoid space and form a subdural, intracerebral, or intraventricular hematoma.

The effects of subarachnoid blood on the meninges and on the flow and reabsorption of CSF have been studied extensively, both experimentally and clinically. In a series of experiments published in 1928, repeated injections of blood into the subarachnoid space of dogs caused chronic meningeal fibrosis and in some cases led to marked ventricular dilatation (4). These observations supported the hypothesis of Winkelman and Fay (63), first proposed in 1930, that communicating hydrocephalus is caused by obstruction of the arachnoid villi (pacchionian granulations). In 1932, an autopsy study revealed hydrocephalus in 31% of 13 patients who died of SAH (55). An example of the clinical correlation between SAH and the development of communicating hydrocephalus was reported in 1939, when the autopsy of a 5-week-old child who had died after SAH due to rupture of an angioma showed hydrocephalus; adhesions and thickening of the arachnoid overtying the convexity due to accumulation of blood from the hemorrhage were observed adjacent to the usual sites of CSF absorption (36).

In 1949, Russell (50) described the spontaneous development of communicating hydrocephalus as a chronic, slowly progressive condition and postulated that it was caused by retarded absorption of CSF into venous blood. Subsequent observations further supported the notion that blockage of the arachnoid villi could cause hydrocephalus. At autopsy in fatal cases of SAH, blood components were identified in arachnoid villi (58). In one study, 12 of 50 adults with hydrocephalus had a history of SAH (24). Histological studies in other autopsy series after recent SAH of traumatic, operative, or spontaneous origin showed structural blockage of the villi (10, 29). The extent of obstruction varied; one villus might be distended and packed with red cells, while an adjacent villus contained only a few cells.

Early experimental studies in dogs showed that intact isotope-labeled red blood cells can cross from the subarachnoid space into the systemic circulation, presumably by passing across normal arachnoid villi (7). In a subsequent study, however, electron microscopic examination of the arachnoid villi 3–5 days after injection of blood into the subarachnoid space of dogs showed that erythrocytes degenerated in the villi, leaving behind a fine debris that was eventually removed by phagocytosis; the endothelium of the villi remained intact (2).

Autopsy studies after SAH have shown that clots in the subarachnoid space form and resorb in much the same fashion as they do elsewhere in the body, albeit more slowly (3). During the first 12 hours after SAH, the pathological changes were minimal, consisting of mild fibrin deposition and scattered phagocytes and hemosiderin granules. Observations during the next 12 hours demonstrated little change. By the third day, however, proliferation of connective tissue was observed. Delicate strands of collagenous tissue extended into the subarachnoid space from the arachnoid and pia, but fibrosis did not envelop the adventitia and blood vessels. It has been inferred from the time course of clot formation and resorption in the subarachnoid space that CSF inhibits fibrin formation (41). The demonstration of normal CSF outflow resistance after intracisternal infusion of heparinized blood, but not after injection of nonheparinized blood, in monkeys has suggested that fibrin deposition contributes to a reduction of CSF flow and absorption, leading to the development of hydrocephalus (6).

Radioisotope cisternography in 42 patients within 4 days after SAH showed that CSF circulation delay correlated well with deterioration in neurological status (8). However, assays of the erythrocyte and hemoglobin content of CSF in these cases indicated that the number of erythrocytes in the CSF did not correlate with the development of CSF circulation disturbances. These results are consistent with the hypothesis that CSF flow disturbances may be due to obstruction of the arachnoid granulations by fibrin deposition rather than by red blood cells.

CSF circulation and outflow resistance have been measured and ICP has been monitored to elucidate the pathophysiology of post-SAH hydrocephalus. Joakimsen *et al.* (25) studied CSF hydrodynamics with isotope cisternography and a CSF infusion test in 47 patients recovering from surgery for aneurysmal SAH. Five patients who required ventricular shunting had arrest of tracer circulation and radiological manifestations of normal-pressure hydrocephalus. However, 12 patients had abnormal CSF hydrodynamics without clinical or radiographic evidence of hydrocephalus. Kosteljanetz (32) studied ICP and outflow resistance of CSF in 17 patients with SAH and/ or intraventricular hemorrhage. Although CSF resistance was found to be increased in all patients, only four of the eight surviving patients required a permanent shunt. The presence of both hydrocephalus and ICP elevation at admission correlated with an increase in CSF resistance, but neither CSF resistance nor the level of ICP predicted the need for permanent CSF diversion.

Clinical Presentation

The observation that obstructive hydrocephalus could evolve within hours and cause acute neurological deterioration was not published until 1970, when Milhorat (37) produced acute hydrocephalus experimentally in rhesus monkeys during balloon obstruction of the fourth ventricle. In the same year, the first description of the clinical syndrome of acute hydrocephalus was published (38). Chronic and acute forms of hydrocephalus as complications of SAH were definitively described in the early 1970s (46, 65).

Patients with posthemorrhagic hydrocephalus may be divided into three groups (20, 21). The first group consists of patients with acute hydrocephalus, usually obstructive rather than communicating, who present in poor neurological condition immediately after SAH and have significant ventriculomegaly on computed tomography (CT) scans. These patients are the most difficult to treat, have high morbidity and mortality rates, and usually have additional complications that contribute to their poor clinical condition (65). However, not all patients with ventricular dilatation after acute SAH are symptomatic (23).

The second group consists of patients with subacute hydrocephalus who develop slowly deteriorating mental status, increasing headache, and mild to moderate ventricular enlargement usually during the first few days after SAH.

The third group consists of patients with delayed-onset hydrocephalus, occurring

days or weeks after SAH. These patients fail to improve as expected or slowly deteriorate after an initial improvement with or without aneurysm surgery. The symptoms and signs mimic the syndrome of normal-pressure hydrocephalus, including dementia, lethargy or somnolence, gait ataxia, and urinary incontinence. The opening pressure at lumbar puncture in such patients is usually in the high-normal range (15–25 mm Hg).

Diagnosis

Hydrocephalus is diagnosed from CT scans or magnetic resonance images showing ventricular enlargement and dilatation of the frontal horns of the lateral ventricles (Fig. 5G.1). Magnetic resonance images can show the aneurysm and the size of the ventricles but may not demonstrate the presence of blood due to acute SAH. Although scan measurements are usually not necessary to establish the diagnosis, equivocal cases may be assessed semiquantitatively with the bicaudate index. This index is defined as the width of the frontal horns at the level of the caudate nuclei divided by the corresponding diameter of the brain (9, 34). In patients without neurological deficit, the upper limit of normal is 0.16 at 30 years of age and under, 0.18 at 50 years, 0.19 at 60 years, and 0.21 at 80 years (9, 34).

CT scans may also demonstrate the development of later signs of acute hydrocephalus, as characterized in experimental and clinical studies (5, 37–39). Further evolution of ventriculomegaly that develops in a rostro-caudal direction can be observed on serial scans. Subsequent dilatation of the remaining lateral ventricle and the third or fourth ventricle occurs unless the obstruction is in the foramen of Monro (39) or the aqueduct. Periventricular hypodensity, representing extracellular periventricular edema due to leakage of intraventricular CSF through tears in the ependymal lining (39, 40), may then evolve in association with ventricular enlargement.

Risk Factors and Outcome

Acute hydrocephalus is a poor prognostic factor in patients with SAH (42). Neurological deterioration or failure to improve after SAH may also occur as a result of systemic

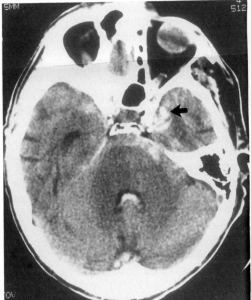

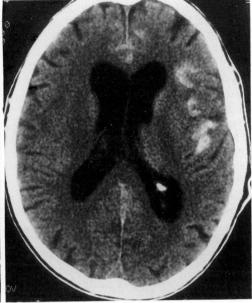

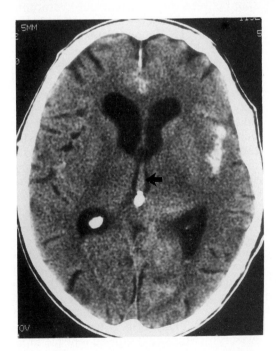

Figure 5G.1. CT brain scans from a 95-year-old man brought to the emergency room, semicomatose with unreactive dilated pupils, after the acute onset of headache followed by loss of consciousness. Blood is present in the fourth ventricle and cisterna magna (*A*), presumably from a large aneurysm (*arrow*) of the left middle cerebral artery. Ventriculomegaly due to obstructive hydrocephalus is obviously demonstrated, despite the presence of cerebral atrophy (*B* and *C*). An isodense blood clot (*arrow*) is present in the third ventricle (*B*) just below the foramen of Munro; subarachnoid blood is present in the left insula. The patient died after therapy was withheld at the family's request.

and central nervous system factors other than hydrocephalus. Systemic complications, such as hyponatremia, dehydration, alcohol withdrawal, cardiac arrhythmias, liver failure, hypoxia, and hypertension, can often be effectively treated to improve neurological function. Other central nervous system complications of SAH, such as he-

matoma, vasospasm, brain edema or infarction, aneurysmal rebleeding, and seizures, aggravate brain injury after SAH and are not always treatable. As a result, it is difficult to determine the contribution of hydrocephalus to outcome after SAH.

Risk factors for the development of hydrocephalus after SAH include the location of the aneurysm, the extent and location of hemorrhage, the occurrence of multiples episodes of SAH, age, hypertension, and vasospasm. Aneurysm location is perhaps the most important of these factors (14). Aneurysms of the anterior communicating artery and of the basilar artery bifurcation have been specifically cited, because they are more often associated with hydrocephalus (29) as well as with an increase in systemic blood pressure. Rupture of anterior communicating artery aneurysms is thought to affect the hypothalamus and to stimulate sympathetic output, elevating blood pressure. Blood or hematoma in the basal cisterns, which is also more common with these aneurysms, is related to the development of communicating hydrocephalus (Fig. 5G.2). Blood within the anterior third ventricle after rupture of posteriorly directed midline lesions is commonly associated with obstructive hydrocephalus.

The relationship between outcome and the extent and location of hemorrhage has been examined in several large series. A prospective study of 174 patients admitted within 72 hours after SAH showed that the occurrence of symptomatic acute hydrocephalus was related to the presence of intraventricular blood and not to the extent of cisternal hemorrhage (59). Intraventricular hemorrhage was more likely to be present in the 34 patients (20%) with acute hydrocephalus, most of whom (88%) were obtunded. However, CT scans showed no evidence of intraventricular blood in seven of these 34 patients. Cisternographic studies in this series showed that blockage of CSF flow in the subarachnoid space, usually at the level of the basal cisterns, was common and was present in all patients who had no CT scan evidence of ventricular obstruction. A correlation was also noted between the occurrence of acute hydrocephalus and subsequent death from cerebral infarction due to vasospasm (57). Furthermore, patients with both hydrocephalus and cerebral infarction were often hyponatremic. These observations suggested that third ventricular dilation contributed to the loss of sodium, perhaps by stimulating inappropriate secretion of antidiuretic hormone (62).

Multiple episodes of SAH also increase the risk of hydrocephalus. In one series, 62% of patients with communicating hydrocephalus after SAH had had previous episodes of SAH (29).

Older patients with SAH are more likely to develop hydrocephalus (5, 14). Possibly as a result of cerebral atrophy, a more diffuse and extensive collection of subarachnoid blood develops, as demonstrated on CT scans. Furthermore, absorption of CSF normally decreases with age (15). Thus, CSF circulation in elderly patients subjected to the added insult of SAH may be more likely to decompensate. Finally, older patients are more likely to have hypertension, which increases the risk of hydrocephalus, regardless of whether it is present before or develops after SAH (14).

Vasospasm and hydrocephalus are complications of SAH that share a common mechanism. Black (5) observed a relationship between the occurrence of hydrocephalus and vasospasm in a retrospective review of 87 patients. He postulated that hydrocephalus diminishes the clearance of vasoactive substances from the CSF, which contributes to the occurrence of vasospasm and subsequent cerebral ischemia. However, only 71% of these patients were symptomatic. Shigeno et al. (51) studied 208 patients with ruptured aneurysms and also found that patients with vasospasm had a higher incidence of hydrocephalus requiring shunt insertion.

Antifibrinolytic agents have been shown to increase the incidence of posthemorrhagic hydocephalus (14, 27, 30, 45). In one study, hydrocephalus was twice as common in patients who received antifibrinolytic agents as it was in those who did not (45). Prolonging the time the blood clot remains in the subarachnoid space may increase the exposure of the arachnoid villi to obstruction by red blood cells and fibrin. The Cooperative Aneurysm Study (27) showed that the mortality rate among patients treated with antifibrinolytic agents appears to be the same as that among patients not treated with these agents, even though treatment reduces the incidence of rebleeding. Thus, the reduction in mortality rates from rebleeding achieved with antifibrinolytic agents is probably counterbalanced by the increase in mortality

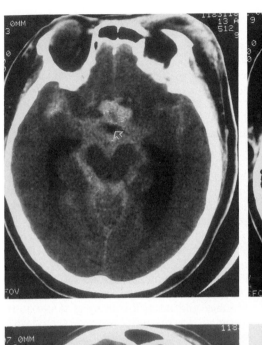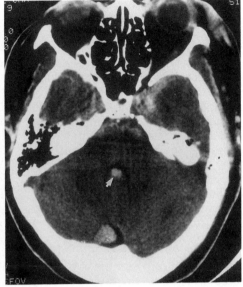

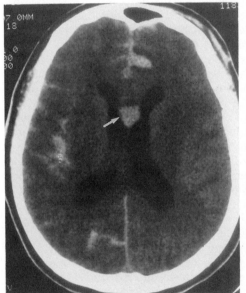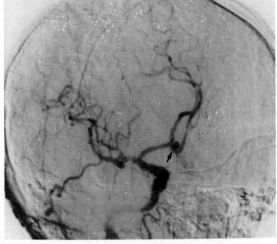

Figure 5G.2. (*A*) CT scan from a 78-year-old woman diagnosed with grade IV SAH, who collapsed while working in her garden, shows subarachnoid blood filling the basal cisterns and outlining an anterior communicating artery aneurysm (*arrow*). CT scans also show enlarged ventricles (*A* and *C*) due to blood (*arrow*) obstructing the fourth ventricle and cisterna magna. Extension of subarachnoid blood into the genu of the corpus callosum is shown (*C*). (*D*) Oblique right internal carotid artery angiogram demonstrates the aneurysm (*arrow*). Hypertension developed that was difficult to control. Ventriculostomy drainage normalized the initially elevated ICP, but the patient deteriorated neurologically and died 7 days after the SAH.

rates due to the more frequent development of hydrocephalus and ischemic neurological complications. Other studies, however, have not demonstrated adverse effects of antifibrinolytic therapy (11).

Management

Clinical Course

Once acute hydrocephalus has been diagnosed, it is necessary to determine whether the ventriculomegaly observed will remain clinically significant. Using the bicaudate index and clinical examination, Hasan *et al.* (18) showed that in approximately one third of patients with CT-proven acute posthemorrhagic hydrocephalus the symptoms of hydrocephalus resolved within 72 hours after the onset of SAH. For example, half of the patients initially diagnosed with hydrocephalus who had a depressed level of consciousness improved spontaneously within 24 hours after presentation. This report confirms the results of some previous studies (59, 60); however, in one study (33) only one of nine patients with symptomatic acute hydrocephalus improved spontaneously.

Ventricular Drainage and CSF Shunting

Although a significant number of patients with acute or chronic hydrocephalus of either the obstructive or communicating type improve spontaneously without surgical intervention, it may be difficult to justify managing a patient with an acutely enlarged ventricular system and depressed mental status without establishing ventricular drainage. Delay in relieving elevated ICP in such patients could lead to cerebral herniation. Dramatic neurological improvement has occurred much more often in patients treated with ventriculostomy than in untreated patients (73% *vs.* 11%) (33). Furthermore, studies in animals (64) have demonstrated a correlation between reduced cerebral blood flow and ventricular enlargement. Similar results were also reported in clinical xenon-inhalation cerebral blood flow studies (35). In another series, cerebral blood flow increased by 19% after ICP was reduced from >35 mm Hg to a mean of 14 mm Hg by lumbar CSF drainage (16).

Drainage or shunting of ventricular fluid can lead to an increase in cerebral vasospasm and infarction as well as a marked increase in the incidence of aneurysmal rebleeding. Kasuya *et al.* (28) evaluated 108 patients with SAH and recorded the volume of CSF removed by continuous ventricular drainage. The incidence of cerebral infarction after SAH without ventricular drainage was 27%. Drainage at a rate of 1–100 ml/day was not associated with a change in the incidence of cerebral infarction. Drainage of 101–200 ml/day was associated with a 39% increase in the incidence of infarction, while drainage of >200 ml/day increased the rate of infarction to 57%. The differences between groups were statistically significant. Moreover, if the total amount of CSF drained during treatment exceeded 1000 ml, the incidence of shunt-dependent hydrocephalus was 44%, compared with only 10% if <1000 ml of CSF was drained. It was concluded from this study that CSF drainage should not be performed too vigorously in patients with SAH because of the increased risk of vasospasm and shunt-dependent hydrocephalus.

The reported association of rebleeding with ventriculostomy or ventricular shunting is variable (18, 22, 33, 43, 47, 49, 59, 60). In a series of 20 patients studied after SAH, abrupt decreases in ICP after CSF drainage and administration of therapeutic agents such as mannitol were associated with rebleeding (43, 49). While the overall incidence of recurrent hemorrhage after SAH in patients without hydrocephalus was reported to be 19% (18), a similar 17% rebleed rate was observed (61) among patients undergoing ventriculostomy in whom drainage was instituted only when ICP was >25 mm Hg. In another study (18), the rebleed rate was 43% for patients with hydrocephalus undergoing ventriculostomy; however, it was only 15% for patients not requiring ventricular drainage. This difference, which was statistically significant, was attributed to the effects of placing the ventricular catheter. However, since patients of poor neurological grade have a greater risk of recurrent hemorrhage (1, 48) and only patients with a Glasgow coma score ≤8 were selected for ventriculostomy in that study, the association between ventriculostomy and rebleeding could be coincidental.

Rapid reduction in ICP can result in aneurysmal rebleeding, with devastating neurological consequences (43). Controlling the rate of continuous ventricular fluid removal has been proposed to avoid complications from ventricular drainage (56, 61). Serial lumbar puncture is a traditional treatment that has been used in cases of subacute communicating hydrocephalus (12, 17, 47). In one series, there was no significant increase in the rebleeding rate among patients with posthemorrhagic communicating hydrocephalus who underwent serial lumbar puncture before surgery (17). Lumbar puncture reduces CSF pressure more gradually than does insertion of a ventricular catheter, and it avoids potential complications of catheter placement, including meningitis, ventriculitis, and hemorrhage along the catheter tract. However, acute hydrocephalus due to ventricular obstruction cannot be treated by lumbar puncture, and ICP cannot be monitored.

Third ventriculostomy to relieve obstructive hydrocephalus has been performed by fenestrating the membrane of Lillequist at the time of surgery for aneurysm clipping (23). However, data from another series of 28 patients did not show reduction of the shunt rate for patients at high risk for persistent hydrocephalus (52).

Placement of a ventriculoperitoneal shunt is required in 9–15% of SAH cases when ICP elevation follows interruption of external ventricular drainage and when delayed onset of communicating hydrocephalus develops (19, 26, 44, 53). Shunting routinely provides good results (57).

Guidelines for Treatment of Posthemorrhagic Hydrocephalus

As described above, patients with hydrocephalus after SAH fall into three groups, based on the clinical presentation. The approach to treatment varies depending on the the severity of the hydrocephalus and the timing of aneurysm surgery.

Group 1. Acute obstructive or severe communicating hydrocephalus in patients with grade II-V SAH should be treated immediately with ventricular drainage, either before or after surgery.

Group 2. Subacute hydrocephalus after SAH usually presents gradually, beginning 3–4 days after the initial hemorrhage or surgery. Ventriculostomy is indicated in symptomatic patients. If the ventriculostomy cannot be removed because of persistent elevation of ICP sufficient to require drainage for relief of symptoms, a shunt must be placed.

Group 3. When a patient has not done well after aneurysm clipping and has never required a ventricular catheter, or if the ventricular catheter has been removed because there was no persistent postoperative ICP elevation, late-onset normal-pressure hydrocephalus must be considered; shunting is required in patients who have delayed neurological deterioration or who fail to improve. Although only 3–4% of patients with subacute or late-onset hydrocephalus required permanent shunting in some series (5, 17, 56), a slightly higher incidence of 10–14% has also been reported (39, 65).

Overall Management Protocol

Patients who present with grade I–III SAH usually receive early surgery. If hydrocephalus develops before or after surgery, ventricular drainage should be established and maintained. If rapid acute neurological deterioration occurs at any time before surgery, a ventricular drain should be inserted immediately. Care should be taken to avoid rapid drainage; the ICP should be maintained between 15 and 25 mg Hg.

Patients who present with grade IV or V SAH, or who have a basilar aneurysm and do not undergo early surgery but have clinical and radiographic signs of hydrocephalus, should also be treated with ventricular drainage. Again, precautions against excessive drainage should be taken. If the clinical status improves rapidly to grade I, II, or III, early surgery is indicated. If there is no clinical change, surgery may be performed late or may be deferred. If delayed surgery is planned, subacute nonobstructive hydrocephalus associated with clinical deterioration should be treated with ventricular drainage. Patients who fail to improve after aneurysm clipping or who later deteriorate clinically may have chronic hydrocephalus. If spontaneous improvement is not observed, a permanent lumbar-peritoneal or a ventriculoperitoneal shunt should be inserted. We advocate placing a lumbar-peritoneal shunt so as to avoid another intracranial procedure, especially in patients with multiple intracranial aneurysms who will require future craniotomy.

Acknowledgment

The authors thank Stephen Ordway for editorial assistance.

REFERENCES

1. Adams, H. P., Jr., Kassell, N. F., and Torner, J. C., et al. Early management of aneurysmal subarachnoid hemorrhage: a report of the Cooperative Aneurysm Study. J. Neurosurg. 54:141–145, 1981.
2. Alksne, J. F., and Lovings, E. T. The role of the arachnoid villus in the removal of red blood cells from the subarachnoid space: an electron microscope study in the dog. J. Neurosurg. 36:192–200, 1972.
3. Alpers, B. J., and Forster, F. M. The reparative processes in subarachnoid hemorrhage. J. Neuropathol. Exp. Neurol. 4:262–268, 1945.
4. Bagley, C., Jr. Blood in the cerebrospinal fluid: resultant functional and organic alterations in the central nervous system. A. Experimental data. Arch. Surg. 17:18–38, 1928.
5. Black, P. M. Hydrocephalus and vasospasm after subarachnoid hemorrhage from ruptured intracranial aneurysms. Neurosurgery 18:12–16, 1986.
6. Blasberg, R., Johnson, D., and Fenstermacher, J. Absorption resistance of cerebrospinal fluid after subarachnoid hemorrhage in the monkey: effects of heparin. Neurosurgery 9:686–690, 1981.
7. Bradford, F. K., and Johnson, P. C., Jr. Passage of intact iron-labeled erythrocytes from subarachnoid space to systemic circulation in dogs. J. Neurosurg. 19:332–346, 1962.
8. Doczi, T., Nemessanyi, Z., Szegvary, Z., and Huszka, E. Disturbances of cerebrospinal fluid circulation during the acute stage of subarachnoid hemorrhage. Neurosurgery 12:435–438, 1983.
9. Earnest, M. P., Heaton, R. K., Wilkinson, W. E., and Manke, W. F. Cortical atrophy, ventricular enlargement and intellectual impairment in the aged. Neurology 29:1138–1143, 1979.
10. Ellington, E., and Margolis, G. Block of arachnoid villus by subarachnoid hemorrhage. J. Neurosurg. 30:651–657, 1969.
11. Fodstad, H., Forssell, A., Lillequist, B., and Schannong, M. Antifibrinolysis with tranexamic acid in aneurysmal subarachnoid hemorrhage: a consecutive controlled clinical trial. Neurosurgery 8:158–165, 1981.
12. Foltz, E. L., and Ward, A. A., Jr. Communicating hydrocephalus from subarachnoid hemorrhage. J. Neurosurg. 13:546–566, 1956.
13. Galera, R., and Greitz, T. Hydrocephalus in the adult secondary to the rupture of intracranial arterial aneurysms. J. Neurosurg. 32:634–641, 1970.
14. Graff-Radford, N. R., Torner, J., Adams, H. P., Jr., and Kassell, N. F. Factors associated with hydrocephalus after subarachnoid hemorrhage: a report of the Cooperative Aneurysm Study. Arch. Neurol. 46:744–752, 1989.
15. Hammes, E. M., Jr. Reaction of the meninges to blood. Arch. Neurol. Psychiatry 52:505–514, 1944.
16. Hartmann, A., Alberti, E., and Lange, D. Effects of CSF drainage of CBF and CBV in subarachnoid hemorrhage and communicating hydrocephalus. Acta Neurol. Scand. 56:336–337, 1977.
17. Hasan, D., Lindsay, K. W., and Vermeulen, M. Treatment of acute hydrocephalus after subarachnoid hemorrhage with serial lumbar puncture. Stroke 22:190–194, 1991.
18. Hasan, D., Vermeulen, M., Wijdicks, E. F. M., et al. Management problems in acute hydrocephalus after subarachnoid hemorrhage. Stroke 20:747–753, 1989.
19. Hayashi, M., Kobayashi, H., Munemoto, S., et al. An analysis of time course of intracranial pressure in patients with communicating hydrocephalus following subarachnoid hemorrhage due to ruptured intracranial aneurysms. Brain Nerve 34:653–660, 1982.
20. Heros, R. C. Preoperative management of the patient with a ruptured intracranial aneurysm. Semin. Neurol. 4:430–438, 1984.
21. Heros, R. C. Acute hydrocephalus after subarachnoid hemorrhage. Stroke 20:715–717, 1989.
22. Heros, R. C., and Kistler, J. P. Intracranial arterial aneurysm: an update. Stroke 14:628–631, 1983.
23. Higashi, K., Hatano, M., and Okamura, T. Cerebral ventricular dilation and disturbance of cerebrospinal fluid circulation following subarachnoid hemorrhage. Neurol. Surg. (Tokyo) 7:1145–1154, 1979.
24. Hogan, P. A., and Woolsey, R. M. Hydrocephalus in the adult. JAMA 198: 1966.
25. Joakimsen, O., Mathiesen, E. B., Monstad, P., and Selseth, B. CSF hydrodynamics after subarachnoid hemorrhage. Acta Neurol. Scand. 75:319–327, 1987.
26. Kassell, N. F., and Boarini, D. J. Perioperative care of the aneurysm patient. Contemp. Neurosurg. 6:1–6, 1984.
27. Kassell, N. F., Torner, J. C., and Adams, H. P., Jr. Antifibrinolytic therapy in the acute period following aneurysmal subarachnoid hemorrhage: preliminary observations from the Cooperative Aneurysm Study. J. Neurosurg. 61:225–230, 1984.
28. Kasuya, H., Shimizu, T., and Kagawa, M. The effect of continuous drainage of cerebrospinal fluid in patients with subarachnoid hemorrhage: a retrospective analysis of 108 patients. Neurosurgery 28:56–59, 1991.
29. Kibler, R. F., Couch, R. S. C., and Crompton, M. R. Hydrocephalus in the adult following spontaneous subarachnoid hemorrhage. Brain 84:45–61, 1961.
30. Knibestol, M., Karadayi, A., and Tovi, D. Echoencephalographic study of ventricular dilatation after subarachnoid hemorrhage, with special reference to the effect of antifibrinolytic treatment. Acta Neurol. Scand. 54:57–70, 1976.
31. Kolluri, V. R. S., and Sengupta, R. P. Symptomatic hydrocephalus following aneurysmal subarachnoid hemorrhage. Surg. Neurol. 21:402–404, 1984.
32. Kosteljanetz, M. CSF dynamics in patients with subarachnoid and/or intraventricular hemorrhage. Neurosurgery 60:940–946, 1984.
33. Kusske, J. A., Turner, P. T., Ojemann, G. A., and Harris, A. B. Ventriculostomy for the treatment

of acute hydrocephalus following subarachnoid hemorrhage. J. Neurosurg. *38:*591–595, 1973.

34. Meese, W., Kluge, W., Grumme, T., and Hopfenmüller, W. CT evaluation of the CSF spaces of healthy persons. Neuroradiology *19:*131–136, 1980.

35. Menon, D., Weir, B., and Overton, T. Ventricular size and cerebral blood flow following subarachnoid hemorrhage. J. Comput. Assist. Tomogr. *5:*328–333, 1981.

36. Merwarth, H. R., and Freiman, I. S. Hydrocephalus following subarachnoid hemorrhage: report of a case with pathologic study. Brooklyn Hosp. J. *1:*149–157, 1939.

37. Milhorat, T. H. Experimental hydrocephalus. 1. A technique for producing obstructive hydrocephalus in the monkey. J. Neurosurg. *32:*385–389, 1970.

38. Milhorat, T. H. Acute hydrocephalus. N. Engl. J. Med. *283:*857–859, 1970.

39. Milhorat, T. H. Acute hydrocephalus after aneurysmal subarachnoid hemorrhage. Neurosurgery 15–20.

40. Milhorat, T. H., Clark, R. G., and Hammock, M. K. Experimental hydrocephalus. 2. Gross pathological findings in acute and subacute obstructive hydrocephalus in the dog and monkey. J. Neurosurg. *32:*390–399, 1970.

41. Minckler, J. Neonatal injury and malformation. In: *Pathology of the Nervous System*, edited by O. T. Bailey, I. Feigin, G. Jervis, *et al.* McGraw-Hill, New York, 1876–1884, 1972.

42. Mohr, G., Ferguson, G., Khan, M., *et al.* Intraventricular hemorrhage from ruptured aneurysm: retrospective analysis of 91 cases. J. Neurosurg. *58:*482–487, 1983.

43. Nornes, H. The role of intracranial pressure in the arrest of hemorrhage in patients with ruptured intracranial aneurysm. J. Neurosurg. *39:*226–234, 1973.

44. Papo, I., Bodosi, M., Merei, T. F., and Luongo, A. L'hydrocephalie après hémorragie sous-arachnoïdienne. Neurochirurgie *30:*159–164, 1984.

45. Park, B. E. Spontaneous subarachnoid hemorrhage complicated by communicating hydrocephalus: ε-aminocaproic acid as a possible predisposing factor. Surg. Neurol. *11:*73–80, 1979.

46. Pertuiset, B., Houtteville, J. P., George, B., and Margent, P. Early ventricular dilatation and hydrocephalus following rupture of supratentorial arterial aneurysms. Neurochirurgia (Stuttg.) *15:*113–126, 1972.

47. Raimondi, A. J., and Torres, H. Acute hydrocephalus as a complication of subarachnoid hemorrhage. Surg. Neurol. *1:*23–26, 1973.

48. Richardson, A. E., Jane, J. A., and Payne, P. M. Assessment of the natural history of the anterior communicating aneurysm. J. Neurosurg. *21:*266–274, 1964.

49. Rosenørn, J., Westergaard, L., and Hansen, P. H. Mannitol-induced rebleeding from intracranial aneurysm: case report. J. Neurosurg. *59:*529–530, 1983.

50. Russell, D. S. *Observations of the Pathology of Hydrocephalus*, p. 138. HM Stationery Office, London, 1949.

51. Shigeno, T., Saito, I., Aritake, K., *et al.* Hydrocephalus following early operation on ruptured cerebral aneurysms: significance of long-term monitoring of intracranial pressure. Neurol. Med. Chir. (Tokyo) *19:*529–535, 1979.

52. Shiobara, R., Toya, S., Iisaka, Y., *et al.* An evaluation of the continuous ventricular drainage for ruptured cerebral aneurysms: treatment of postoperative increased ventricular fluid pressure. Neurol. Med. Chir. (Tokyo) *17:*145–152, 1977.

53. Spallone, A., and Gagliardi, F. M. Hydrocephalus following aneurysmal SAH. Zentralbl. Neurochir. *44:*141–150, 1983.

54. Steinke, D., Weir, B., and Disney, L. Hydrocephalus following aneurysmal subarachnoid haemorrhage. Neurol. Res. *9:*3–9, 1987.

55. Strauss, I., Globus, J. H., and Ginsburg, S. W. Spontaneous subarachnoid hemorrhage: its relation to aneurysms of cerebral blood vessels. Arch. Neurol. Psychiatry *27:*1080–1132, 1932.

56. Sunbbarg, G., and Pontén, U. ICP and CSF absorption impairment after subarachnoid hemorrhage. In: *Intracranial Pressure III*, edited by J. W. F. Beks, D. A. Bosch, and M. Brock. Springer-Verlag, Berlin, 139–146, 1976.

57. Torner, J. C., Jane, J. A., and Kassell, N. F. The relationship of age to outcome following subarachnoid hemorrhage: a report of the Cooperative Aneurysm Study. Presented at the Neurotrauma Conference, September 1986, Charlottesville, VA.

58. Turner, L. The structure of arachnoid granulations with observations on their physiological and pathological significance. Ann. R. Coll. Surg. Engl. *29:*237–264, 1961.

59. van Gijn, J., Hijdra, A., Wijdicks, E. F. M., *et al.* Acute hydrocephalus after aneurysmal subarachnoid hemorrhage. J. Neurosurg. *63:*355–362, 1985.

60. Vassilouthis, J., and Richardson, A. E. Ventricular dilatation and communicating hydrocephalus following spontaneous subarachnoid hemorrhage. J. Neurosurg. *51:*341–351, 1979.

61. Voldby, B., and Enevoldsen, E. M. Intracranial pressure changes following aneurysm rupture. 3. Recurrent hemorrhage. J. Neurosurg. *56:*784–789, 1982.

62. Wijdicks, E. F. M., Vandongen, K. J. H., Vangijn, J., *et al.* Enlargement of the third ventricle and hyponatraemia in aneurysmal subarachnoid haemorrhage. J. Neurol. Neurosurg. Psychiatry *51:*516–520, 1988.

63. Winkelman, N. W., and Fay, T. Pacchionian system: histologic and pathologic changes with particular reference to idiopathic and symptomatic convulsive states. Arch. Neurol. Psychiatry *23:*44–64, 1930.

64. Wozniak, M., McLone, D. G., and Raimondi, A. J. Micro- and macrovascular changes as the direct cause of parenchymal destruction in congenital murine hydrocephalus. J. Neurosurg. *43:*535–545, 1975.

65. Yasargil, M. G., Yonekawa, Y., Zumstein, B., and Stahl, H.-J. Hydrocephalus following spontaneous subarachnoid hemorrhage: clinical features and treatment. J. Neurosurg. *39:*474–479, 1973.

Management of Vasospasm: Hemodynamic Augmentation

MICHAEL L. LEVY, M.D., STEVEN L. GIANNOTTA, M.D.

INTRODUCTION

Cerebral arterial spasm following subarachnoid hemorrhage (*i.e.*, vasospasm) can be defined as an ischemic neurological/deficit in association with narrowing of cerebral vessels. This perhaps overly restrictive definition does not imply correlation between the deficit and angiographically demonstrated narrowing. It does imply that the clinical syndrome is associated with demonstrable ischemia in the microcirculation, regardless of whether large vessels or other factors are responsible for producing it. The definition further avoids discussion of epiphenomena, such as transient mechanically or chemically induced vascular narrowing in certain animal models, that have little relevance to patients with an aneurysmal subarachnoid hemorrhage. Despite >20 years of investigation on possible mechanisms and treatment of vasospasm after subarachnoid hemorrhage, the Second International Workshop on Cerebral Arterial Spasm concluded "...the most effective method of treating cerebral vasospasm in the clinical setting involves restoring, maintaining, and perhaps increasing blood volume and blood pressure, while simultaneously improving the rheological aspects of the cerebral circulation..." (55). Augmentation of rheology and cardiac performance indices have remained an integral part of the management program not only for aneurysmal subarachnoid hemorrhage but also, more recently, for ischemia from acute stroke (1, 7, 20, 21, 28, 45, 54).

Intravascular volume expansion has become an accepted modality in the prevention and subsequent treatment of cerebral ischemia from vasospasm and, with increasing frequency, acute stroke. Complications related to volume expansion include cardiac, hematological, and pulmonary sequelae. To minimize these complications and to maximize cardiac performance during therapy for cerebral vasospasm, we have used a flow-directed balloon-tipped catheter with cardiac output and hemodynamic monitoring. Over the past 5 years the Department of Neurological Surgery at the University of Southern California has developed guidelines with regard to improving cardiac output and the ideal cardiac indices required to potentially improve or maximize cerebral blood flow (CBF) in patients with ruptured intracranial aneurysms. Here we review our guidelines for hypervolemic therapy in terms of the volume and timing of intravenous fluid administration and the target cardiac performance parameters.

We have analyzed the effect of hypervolemic preload enhancement on cardiac performance in patients following aneurysmal subarachnoid hemorrhage. All patients had the placement of a flow-directed balloon-tipped catheter and had measurements of their cardiac parameters made during hypervolemic therapy. We demonstrated that cardiac function was optimal at a pulmonary artery wedge pressure of 14 mm Hg in patients with normal cardiac function. More recently, we described the use of the β-agonist dobutamine in combination with hypervolemic preload enhancement in 23 patients who failed to respond to traditional preload enhancement following aneurysmal subarachnoid hemorrhage. Hyperdynamic therapy with dobutamine in the presence of volume loading resulted in clinical reversal of ischemic symptoms from subarachnoid hemorrhage in 78% of patients. In this chapter we report upon our experience and outline our treatment protocol. We also review the pertinent literature and how it has led to our current understanding of the treatment of vasospasm.

Management Protocol

Initial Medical Management
Patients with suspected subarachnoid hemorrhage are immediately admitted to the neurosurgical intensive care unit. Steps are immediately taken to document the cause of the subarachnoid hemorrhage with computerized tomography (CT) scanning and cerebral angiography. Patients with ruptured intracranial aneurysms are maintained on bed rest with the head elevated to 30 degrees unless significant hypotension intervenes. Vital signs and neurological evaluations are carried out and recorded on an hourly basis. Arterial blood pressure is monitored with automated cuffs or arterial catheters. Young patients or those with no pre-existing cardiac history are given 5% dextrose in lactated Ringer solution at rates approximating 125 ml/hour. Fluid boluses of up to 300 ml are given preparatory to and following cerebral angiography, because of the significant osmotic diuresis related to the contrast load. A short course of high-dose dexamethasone (10 mg every 3 hours, intravenously) is given to patients in poor neurological grades or those awaiting surgery.

An attempt is made to determine the preexisting blood pressure. No effort is made to reduce the blood pressure below 15–20 mm Hg above the pre-morbid level. For those patients with post-subarachnoid hemorrhage blood pressure levels of >20 mm Hg above their normal levels or >185 mm Hg systolic pressure, sedative medications including analgesic agents and phenobarbital are initiated. Refractory elevations in blood pressure are managed using sodium nitroprusside administered intravenously, because of its ability to be easily and rapidly titrated. Hypertensive patients with pre-existing coronary vascular disease are managed on intravenous nitroglycerine. All patients who require antihypertensive intravenous agents are managed also with the use of Swan-Ganz catheterization.

Management of Vasospasm

The majority of the patients in the better grades (grades 1–3) undergo early operative management with clip ligation of the ruptured aneurysm. Thus, the majority of cases of ischemic complications that we experience are in the postoperative period. The new onset of lethargy with or without a focal neurological deficit is presumed evidence of the onset of cerebral vasospasm until proven otherwise. In rapid succession, a CT scan is obtained to rule out other forms of intracranial pathology, intravenous fluid volumes are increased, all patients undergo pulmonary arterial catheterization, and a 7-French, 110-cm, flow-directed, thermodilution pulmonary artery catheter (American-Edward Laboratories) is positioned using a subclavian approach. Complications of Swan-Ganz catheterization, including infection, pneumothorax, hemothorax, pulmonary infarct, and arrythmias, can all be avoided with meticulous technique and sterility in conjunction with catheter changes every 3 days. All catheter tips are cultured when removed. An initial bolus of 300 ml of Albumisol is given and the measurement and recording of cardiac parameters are begun. The administration of copious amounts of Hespan is avoided, given the potential for coagulopathy.

Base-line cardiac index (CI), stroke volume index (SVI), left ventricular stroke work index (LVSWI), and right ventricular stroke work index (RVSWI) are calculated as follows. Central venous pressures (CVP) may also be monitored but are not used as indices of cardiac function.

$$CI \text{ (liter/min} \cdot \text{meters squared } (M^2))$$
$$= \text{cardiac output} \div \text{body surface area}$$

$$SVI \, (ml/M^2) = CI \div \text{heart rate}$$

$$LVSWI \, (g \cdot m/M^2) = SVI$$
$$\times \text{ mean arterial pressure}$$
$$\div \text{ wedge pressure} \, (MAP \div WP)$$
$$\times \, 0.0136$$

$$RVSWI\ (g \cdot m/M^2) = SVI \times mean$$
pulmonary artery pressure (MPAP ÷ CVP)
$$\times\ 0.0136$$

Following base-line measurements, fluid resuscitation is instituted with 5% albumin at 300 ml/hr if the pulmonary capillary wedge pressure (PCWP) is ⋯10 mm Hg. If the PCWP is >16 mm Hg, mannitol (0.25–0.50 g/kg) or Lasix (40 mg) is administered. In patients with cardiac compromise, PCWP values are recorded every 15 min until elevations to 18 mm Hg are documented. Cardiac performance curves are then generated for each patient, and their PCWP is subsequently maintained at a level where CI and LVSWI are maximized.

PCWP

Recently, in our institution, to determine the optimum fluid therapy for enhancement of cardiac performance 10 patients had placement of flow-directed balloon-tipped catheters and measurement of the above-enumerated indices of cardiac function. Following base-line measurements, Albumisol was infused intravenously at 300 ml/hour. There was poor correlation between cardiac output and central venous pressure in the ranges recorded in our study. However, pulmonary artery wedge pressure increases did correlate in a statistically significant manner with increases in CI, stroke volume index, and left ventricular stroke work index. There was no statistical correlation between increases in pulmonary wedge pressure above 14 mm Hg and improvement in cardiac performance, as evidenced by CI, stroke volume index, and left ventricular stroke work index (Fig. 6A.1). Thus, in previously

healthy individuals, we enhance fluid volume status until a pulmonary artery wedge pressure of approximately 14 mm Hg is maintained. Additional checks on CI reduce complications such as cerebral edema, congestive heart failure, and pulmonary edema to a minimum (27).

Protocol for Dobutamine Treatment

Failure of response to classical hypervolemia is defined as no improvement or a decline in neurological status (using the Hunt and Hess grading system) perioperatively, despite hypervolemic management.

Patients who fail to respond to volume expansion alone are then given dobutamine (5–15 µg/kg/min) by intravenous infusion. Infusion rates of dobutamine are predicated upon the maintenance of cardiac performance above the patient's physiological baseline level, as established upon admission to the intensive care unit. Despite the effect of dobutamine in reducing PCWP, fluid resuscitation is continued as before, with 5% albumin at 300 ml/hr, if the PCWP is <8 mm Hg. If the PCWP is >16 mm Hg, mannitol (0.25–0.50 mg/kg) or Lasix (40 mg) is administered.

Dobutamine treatment is continued based upon clinical neurological response. In patients who respond to dobutamine treatment, infusions are weaned 3–4 days following the initial response. Infusions are reinstated with recurrence of ischemic neurological compromise. In patients who fail to respond to dobutamine treatment, infusions are weaned following a 10-day course.

In patients who become refractory to hyperdynamic therapy, cardiac output can be further enhanced with the simultaneous use of sodium nitroprusside (up to 8.5 µg/min). With this regimen, pulmonary artery wedge pressures are no longer reliable for assessing cardiac function directly. This is due to the fact that pulmonary artery wedge pressure is reduced up to 56% with initiation of dobutamine and Nipride. Thus, we rely solely on CI and stroke volume index, which can increase up to 120% following initiation of dobutamine and nipride. This regimen is particularly valuable in patients with ruptured but unsecured aneurysms in the preoperative state.

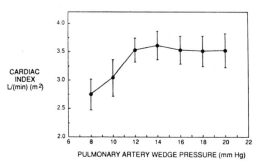

Figure 6A.1. Relationship of CI to pulmonary artery wedge pressure during volume expansion in patients with subarachnoid hemorrhage.

Success of the regimens described above is predicated on prompt institution of therapy at the earliest sign of neurological decline. For the most part, this begins as a reduction in the level of consciousness, which is soon followed by focal neurological deficits. Cardiovascular destabilizing incidents such as orthostatic hypotension, electrolyte fluid balance abnormalities, or contrast loads from cerebral angiography are not infrequently precursors to neurological decline. In that regard, prompt support of intravascular volume soon after admission to the hospital may alleviate more mild cases of cerebral ischemia from cerebral vasospasm. Replacement of all measured and insensible losses plus an extra 1000–1500 ml/day in the early post-subarachnoid hemorrhage period is strongly recommended.

Additional Management Options

In healthy individuals, it may be difficult to maintain a pulmonary wedge pressure in the desired range. As long as the clinical condition is satisfactory, no further measures are taken. If the desired clinical effect is not obtained, hypertensive therapy is instituted. We have had no experience with the use of vasopressin or mineralocorticoids in attempting to maximize fluid retention. Kassell *et al.* (20) have recommended this as an effective measure.

In the past, with a few patients who had high hematocrit values following maximization of hypervolemia and hypertensive therapy and who failed to respond clinically, we resorted to reducing the hematocrit value by therapeutic venesection and removal of 1–2 units of packed cells with replacement of plasma. This has been necessary for two patients in the past 5 years.

Hypervolemic and hypertensive therapy is continued until tapering of the vasopressor and/or volume load is not met with a decrease in neurological function. This has been known to take up to 2 weeks in a few instances. In general, following the critical period for vasospasm, namely, day 5 to day 12 after subarachnoid hemorrhage, most therapeutic maneuvers can be reduced.

When further neurological deterioration occurs in the presence of maximal volume expansion and critical increase in mean arterial blood pressure, ventricular catheterization with subsequent intraventricular pressure monitoring and reduction of intracranial pressure to maximize cerebral perfusion pressure is carried out. Brief periods of hyperventilation are used to acutely reduce intracranial pressure spikes. Removal of cerebral spinal fluid for cerebral perfusion pressures that fall below 70 mm Hg is the next preferred maneuver. Intravenous mannitol administration, which also improves on a temporary basis the hemorrheology in the microcirculation, is used for refractory elevations in intracranial pressure or reduction in cerebral perfusion pressure. With such a comprehensive program, the majority of episodes of cerebral vasospasm can be modified or for the most part ameliorated. There are, however, ischemic sequelae of cerebral vasospasm that are refractory to all forms of treatment. This generally occurs with massive subarachnoid hemorrhage, as documented by early CT scanning, and the inability to operatively remove large amounts of this hemorrhage in a timely fashion. Multiple subarachnoid hemorrhages in our experience have also been responsible for the most malignant forms of cerebrovasospasm.

With the recent institution of the use of dihydropyridine analogues such as nimodipine and nicardipine, a comprehensive program utilizing these preparations prophylactically in concert with hypertensive and hypervolemic therapy should have a dramatic impact on the incidence and severity of pre- and postoperative cerebrovasospasm.

DISCUSSION

Initial Studies of Induced Hypertension

The reversal of ischemic deficits through the concomitant use of induced arterial hypertension via volume expansion and vasopressors was initially described by Brown (5) in 1951. It was noted that neurological deterioration was related to suboptimal blood pressure in cases with presumed altered cerebral hemodynamics. He proposed that it was therefore logical to artificially elevate systemic blood pressure in conditions of circulatory insufficiency. Farhat and Schneider (10) reported reversal of acute ischemic deficits in two patients with cerebral aneurysms with metaraminol-induced hypertension. They theorized that elevations in the mean arterial pressure resulted in increased regional CBF.

Kosnick and Hunt (24) documented reversal of postoperative ischemic deficits from vasospasm in six of seven patients, using vasopressor-induced hypertension and volume expansion. They logically concluded that cerebrovascular autoregulation was disrupted in ischemic areas of the brain and perfusion to these regions could be enhanced with increases in mean arterial pressure (23, 44, 53).

Giannotta *et al.* (5) reported a series of 17 patients with postoperative neurological compromise secondary to cerebral vasospasm. Central venous pressure was augmented and maintained between 8 and 10 cm of water with the infusion of either whole blood or colloid. Pressor agents were employed if clinical improvement could not be reached by hypervolemia alone. They noted the success of low molecular weight dextran in inducing hypervolemia and improving neurological function, based upon its putative ability to improve flow through the microcirculation by reducing both cellular aggregation and arteriovenous shunting.

Associated Hypovolemia

Relative hypovolemia concomitant with subarachnoid hemorrhage was first suggested by Kosnick and Hunt (24) in 1976. Maroon and Nelson (28) documented this phenomenon with further laboratory evaluations of blood volume and red cell mass in 15 patients. Both circulating blood volume and red blood cell mass were found to be diminished in these nonselected subarachnoid hemorrhage patients. Kudo *et al.* (25) further documented a decrease in blood volume following subarachnoid hemorrhage. Putative mechanisms for this phenomenon included rest, supine diuresis, negative nitrogen balance, decrease in erythropoeisis, and iatrogenic blood loss. Such studies suggested that hypovolemia following subarachnoid hemorrhage may play a critical role in delayed ischemia, and they thus explained why hypervolemic therapy may be an appropriate treatment modality.

Solomon *et al.* (45) undertook a blood volume study of 11 patients following subarachnoid hemorrhage. The authors reported that six of seven patients with symptomatic vasospasm had reduced red blood cell volumes or total circulating blood volume and only one patient with asymptomatic vasospasm had below-normal red blood cell volumes or total circulating blood volumes. This study not only served to confirm the relationship between hypovolemia and symptomatic vasospasm but also suggested that, in addition to the factors proposed by Maroon and Nelson (28), hyperactivity of the sympathetic nervous system due to hypothalamic dysfunction following subarachnoid hemorrhage was an important factor in inducing hypovolemia.

Hypervolemic Hypertension

More recently, with the ability of the neurosurgical intensivist to assess cardiovascular and cerebrovascular parameters, volume expansion and induced hypertension have become more widely accepted as a modality for the prevention and subsequent treatment of cerebral ischemia resulting from subarachnoid hemorrhage. Brown *et al.* (6) reported favorable results for four patients who, in addition to undergoing volume expansion and pressure support with dopamine, received a continuous infusion of mannitol. Favorable results have also been documented for the treatment of ischemia due to cerebral vasospasm with the use of isoproterenol or Isoprel and aminophylline combination therapy (12–14, 46, 48). Although the assumption was made that the mechanism of reversal of symptomatic vasospasm in these cases was based upon relaxation of spastic arterial smooth muscle cells, in fact, increases in cardiac output secondary to the cardiac-stimulant effect of these agents and the copious intravenous volume administered to maintain steady state levels were more likely the operative factors.

Kassell *et al.* (20) in 1982 reported on one of the largest series of patients with neurological deterioration following cerebral vasospasm secondary to subarachnoid hemorrhage. A protocol of volume expansion, vaso-blockade, and pressor agents resulted in complete reversal of neurological deficits in 43 of 58 patients studied. Success in their study was predicated on prompt treatment before cerebral infarction was manifest and aggressive maintenance of arterial blood pressure for at least a 7-day period, to enhance continued cerebral perfusion above the ischemic threshold. The authors relied on the use of hemodynamic monitoring, including Swan-Ganz catheterization and central venous pressure monitoring, to avoid potential cardiac and pulmonary complications associated with aggressive hypertensive hypervolemic therapy. The observation of Kassell *et al.* (20) that neurological improvement could occur in the early stages of fluid replacement, before mean arterial pressure became elevated, lent further credence to the reports of previous investigators, who felt that rheological phenomena or improved cardiodynamics could contribute to improved CBF (1, 7).

Pritz, *et al.* (40) documented reversal of ischemic neurological deficits in two patients with subarachnoid hemorrhage-induced vasospasm by maximizing cardiac output using the pressure-volume or Starling output curve as a guideline. The important contribution of this study was the use of the pressure-volume curve to maximize cardiac output, with volume expansion based on data obtained using Swan-Ganz catheterization.

Pritz (39) further described in detail the use of Swan-Ganz catheterization in monitoring patients treated for cerebral vasospasm following subarachnoid hemorrhage. Starling pressure-volume curves were generated to determine pulmonary artery wedge pressures resulting in the greatest cardiac outputs. Neurological deficits were reversed in these patients, and no complications associated with hypervolemic therapy or increased intracranial pressure were documented. Simultaneously with the development of clinical protocols for the management of cerebral vasospasm, the physiological impact of subarachnoid hemorrhage and its sequelae was being studied using various indices of CBF. It has been subsequently documented by many investigators that CBF progressively decreases in poor-grade patients or those with vasospasm (3, 17, 23, 32, 33, 37, 38, 45).

Grubb *et al.* (16) showed that reductions in CBF occur in the presence of increased cerebral blood volume. What remained to be determined was the impact of hypertension and hypervolemia on CBF in patients with vasospasm. Rosenstein *et al.* (41) used bedside CBF determinations in the management of patients with subarachnoid hemorrhage. The authors documented reversal of neurological deficits associated with increases in CBF following hypervolemic therapy. The seemingly rational basis for such treatment of vasospasm and the immediate and complete improvement seen in many patients treated in this manner support further studies regarding hypervolemic hypertension as an effective treatment in reversing neurological deficits secondary to subarachnoid hemorrhage-induced vasospasm.

Origitano *et al.* (36) have utilized a treatment of hypertensive hypervolemic hemodilution ("triple H") therapy and have studied its effect on CBF, using the xenon inhalation technique, in the treatment of subarachnoid hemorrhage. They concluded that such therapy is a safe and effective modality for elevating and sustaining CBF after subarachnoid hemorrhage and that it can minimize delayed ischemia and improve outcome (36).

Blood Viscosity

Further analysis of the factors which might increase blood flow led some to evaluate the contribution of blood viscosity to the problem of vasospasm in addition to ischemia (1, 6). Wood *et al.* (57), using an animal stroke model, documented that nondilutional hypervolemia with autologous whole-blood transfusions did not increase perfusion in ischemic regions or reduce the volume of infarcted tissue. A subsequent study by Wood *et al.* (56) reported that hypervolemic hemodilution with expansion of peripheral vascular volume increased cardiac output more than CBF in nonischemic brain. Marked increases in intracranial pressure were noted in their animal model, as well as increases in the cardiac output of up to 71% without attendant changes in mean arterial blood pressure. Muizelaar and Becker (35) in 1986 reported that CBF remained constant despite changes in blood pressure or viscosity, suggesting that autoregulatory adjustments in vascular diameter were present in response to both changes in cardiovascular function and alterations in serum viscosity. More recently, those authors reported that, in patients with impaired autoregulation, CBF seemed to be regulated more by viscosity then by blood pressure (4).

Isovolemic Hemodilution

Most recently, Tu *et al.* (51, 52) proposed that isovolemic hemodilution would potentially be a more appropriate therapeutic regimen in the treatment of focal cerebral ischemia. Given the potential adverse effects associated with volume expansion, *i.e.*, exacerbation of cerebral edema and increases in intracranial pressure, it was proposed that isovolemic as opposed to hypervolemic hemodilution might circumvent these potential problems. In splenectomized dogs that underwent occlusion of the carotid and middle cerebral arteries, isovolemic hemodilution led to a significant reduction in viscosity, which correlated linearly with reductions in hematocrit values and improved neurological outcome.

The foregoing studies lend credence to the concept that alterations in blood rheology may have salutory effects on regional CBF in ischemic states. The relative contributions of cardiodynamic changes *vs.* rheological alterations in the improvement seen in patients treated by volume expansion for cerebral vasospasm remain to be elucidated. However, this body of work led some to investigate the possibility that subarachnoid hemorrhage may result in hemorheological alterations that could contribute to the pathogenesis of cerebral vasospasm. Fisher *et al.* (11) followed serial determinations of hematocrit, whole-blood and plasma viscosity, red cell aggregation, fibrinogen levels, and ζ sedimentation rates in 12 patients with ruptured intracranial aneurysms. Day 4 to day 7 following SAH saw fibrinogen, plasma viscosity, and ζ sedimentation levels reach their maximum levels, which were statistically significantly elevated, compared to controls. Hung *et al.* (18) showed similar findings with 26 patients, also correlating elevated whole-blood viscosities and fibrinogen levels with vasospasm and coma. Thus,

hemorrheological alterations may play a role in ischemic complications from ruptured aneurysms, and secondary improvement in such abnormalities with hemodilutional or volume expansion therapies may be of theoretical benefit.

Relationship of CBF to Cardiac Output

McGillicuddy *et al.* (30), in a primate model of cerebral vasospasm, found a significant increase in CBF with elevations in the animals' central venous pressure in the presence of stable systemic arterial pressures. Of note is the finding that CBF increased only in regions of ischemia and remained unchanged in the nonischemic control hemisphere, where autoregulation was presumably intact. It could not be determined from their data whether increased regional CBF was due to altered cardiovascular dynamics or a dilutional effect on viscosity.

Davis and Sundt (8) maintained stable arterial blood pressures in an animal model while decreasing cardiac output via exsanguination and/or the use of β-blockers. They demonstrated a significant decrease in CBF despite maintenance of stable mean arterial pressures. Thus, there seemed to be a critical link between cardiac function and augmentation in blood flow in ischemic areas of brain. The data of Keller *et al.* (22), using a stroke model, supported this concept, demonstrating that increased cardiac output could improve microcirculatory flow without changes in mean arterial pressure or blood viscosity.

Tranmer *et al.* (50) and others (25, 26), with primate models of ischemia, have documented a profound loss of regulatory control in ischemic brain in response to alterations in cardiac output. They evaluated the effect of volume expansion with colloid and exsanguination to base-line cardiac output on local CBF. They found that local CBF in regions of ischemic brain varied directly with cardiac output, whereas flow in nonischemic brain was not affected by changes in cardiac output ($p < 0.001$). This suggests that variations in blood volume may cause significant changes in the intensity of ischemia. Data from the studies of Matsui and Asano (29), using prolonged albumin administration, support the concept that hyperdynamic hemodilution can have a positive impact on CBF in animal models of vasospasm.

From the above discussion and numerous clinical observations, it is likely that a complex relationship exists between cardiac output and cerebral perfusion, over and above the simple concept of cerebral perfusion pressure. In addition, the pulsatility of blood flow has been reported to contribute significantly to cerebral perfusion in disautoregulated brain (49). The β-agonist dobutamine has also been reported to increase the pulsatility of blood flow, in addition to markedly increasing cardiac output. Benedikter and Mey (2) reported that dobutamine caused significant reductions in the pre-ejection period, in the duration of the electromechanical systole, and in the ratio of the pre-ejection period to the left ventricular ejection time.

Dobutamine

We have been interested recently in devising therapeutic options that could provide for the reversal of clinical vasospasm refractory to hypervolemic treatment. The choice of a β-agonist is based upon the concept that enhancing cardiac output and pulsatility of blood flow can result in increased perfusion of disautoregulated brain. In addition, we decided upon the agent that was associated with the fewest potential cardiac or systemic side effects. A recent study of a series of 47 patients treated with prophylactic hypervolemia reported an unacceptably high complication rate associated with hypervolemia (31). Sixteen patients developed pulmonary edema and one died. The results of this study must be carefully evaluated, given that cardiac performance was not maximized in a large proportion of patients.

The use of pressors, including dopamine and isoproterenol, in the treatment of vasospasm following subarachnoid hemorrhage is well documented in the literature (5, 6, 12, 13, 14, 20, 21, 47, 48, 54, 55). Although the assumption was made that the mechanism of reversal of symptomatic vasospasm in these latter studies was based upon relaxation of spastic arterial smooth muscle cells, in fact, increases in cardiac output secondary to the cardiac-stimulant effect of these agents and the intravenous volume administered to maintain steady state levels were more likely the operative factors.

At our institution, dobutamine is the pressor of choice for the treatment of patients with vasospasm. The use of dobutamine in the postoperative care of patients following cardiothoracic surgery or in the presence of cardiac failure has been widespread for more than a decade (9, 43, 58). Dobutamine is a synthetic sympathomimetic amine that functions as a potent inotrope by stimulating β_1-receptors in the myocardium. Stimulation of peripheral β_2-receptors (which overwhelm its minimal α effects) and reflexive responses to the increases in cardiac output result in vasodilatation and afterload reduction. The net hemodynamic effects of dobutamine are similar to those of combination therapy with dopamine and a vasodilator (Fig. 6A.2). Thus, a reduction in the patients' peripheral vascular resistance following the initiation of dobutamine is expected and the addition of agents such as α-agonists is not indicated. In addition, we have found that dobutamine reduces pulmonary artery wedge pressure, compared to dopamine, which increases pulmonary artery wedge pressure (Fig. 6A.3). We believe that cardiac output and pulsatility are important determinants of flow to disautoregulated brain.

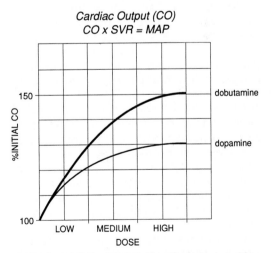

Figure 6A.2. Enhancement of cardiac output resulting from infusions of either dopamine or dobutamine. SVR, systemic vascular resistance; MAP, mean arterial pressure.

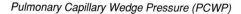

Pulmonary Capillary Wedge Pressure (PCWP)

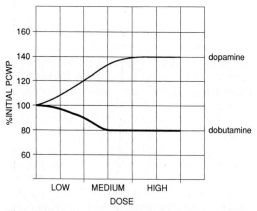

Figure 6A.3. Response of pulmonary capillary wedge pressure to continuous infusions of either dopamine or dobutamine.

In our most recent experience with the protocol described above, dobutamine increased heart rate by only 11% in hyperdynamic therapy in the absence of volume loading and 7% in hyperdynamic therapy in the presence of volume loading. This is due to the increased coronary blood flow that accompanies its positive inotropic effect. Unlike dopamine, the beneficial effects of dobutamine on hemodynamics and the lack of induction of endogenous norepinephrine minimize any negative effects on myocardial oxygen demand. Thus, cardiac function can be maximized while avoiding ischemic cardiac injury in patients with either normal or compromised cardiac function. Finally, the potential arrhythmiogenicity of isoproterenol at high infusion rates is avoided with the use of dobutamine (19). We have reported a 35% increase in CI in hyperdynamic therapy with dobutamine in the presence of volume loading, with only minimal increases (11%) in blood pressure. This leads us to question the efficacy of the use of pure α-agonists, with the intent of markedly increasing blood pressure (at the expense of cardiac output), in the treatment of vasospasm.

We have evaluated only clinical manifestations of cerebral vasospasm and the potential reversal of such in our current study. Future efforts are being directed at evaluating responses in CBF to both ischemic and nonischemic regions following the initiation of therapy, as determined by positron emission tomography scanning. In addition, changes in velocity, as determined by transcranial Doppler scanning, in response to treatment are also being pursued. We recommend that, with careful observation of cardiac parameters in addition to proper fluid management, the complications of fluid overload, congestive heart failure, and cardiac ischemia can be avoided.

Conclusions

We have found that a comprehensive management program for patients with post-subarachnoid hemorrhage cerebral vasospasm requires the therapeutic manipulation and meticulous monitoring of a number of physiological determinants of cardiac function. The factor most significantly influenced by hypervolemic therapy is ventricular pre-load. Pre-load can be rapidly increased by volume infusion, with a subsequent direct effect on cardiac stroke volume and stroke work index, according to the Frank-Starling mechanism. Pre-load of both left and right ventricles is most easily assessed by diastolic pressures, namely the PCWP in the left ventricle and central venous pressure in the right ventricle; however, only pulmonary artery wedge pressures have been found to correlate effectively with cardiac output (43). In the classical description by Sarnoff and Berglund (42), ventricular pre-load is related to the end diastolic fiber length, to which end diastolic volume is related.

Clinically this factor is irrelevant but, since end diastolic volume closely approximates end diastolic pressure, hypervolemia can be managed by critical assessment of PCWP. In normal resting humans, the ventricular function curve is at its peak at a left ventricular end diastolic pressure of approximately 10–14 mm Hg. Below this point there is a strong direct relationship between filling pressure and stroke work, while at higher filling pressures a plateau occurs, according to the Frank-Starling curve. Thus, significant elevation of pulmonary artery wedge pressure above 10–14 mm Hg is not generally associated with further increases in

CI and, in fact, may be associated with decreased cardiac function. Alternatively, catecholamines can be used to maximize cardiac output without the associated risks of hypervolemia. Dobutamine therapy most notably increases stroke output and CI while decreasing systemic vascular resistance, with an attendant increase in heart rate. PCWP can decrease by up to 28%, whereas stroke output may increase above 90% (34).

A basic understanding of cardiac physiology with appropriate monitoring and implementation of methods to increase cardiac performance can measurably improve the outcome of patients with cerebral ischemia from vasospasm. Success is predicated on early recognition of the evolving syndrome, with rapid introduction of measures to improve cerebral perfusion pressure and hemorrheology.

Acknowledgments

The authors wish to thank Karen M. Levy, B.S.R.N., for her assistance in the preparation and statistical analysis required for the completion of this manuscript.

REFERENCES

1. Ackerman, R. H., Burbank, K. M., Buxton, R. B., et al. Relationships between viscosity factors and cerebral blood flow and porous bed viscometry in normal and stroke-prone subjects. In: *Cerebral Ischemia and Hemorheology*, edited by A. Hartmann and W. Kuschinsky, pp. 530–547. Springer-Verlag, Berlin, 1987.
2. Benedikter, L., and Mey, T. Onset and magnitude of cardiovascular response to dobutamine and AR-L 115 BS, a new positive inotropic agent with additional vasodilating activity, in normal subjects. Arzneim.-Forsch. Drug Res. *31*:239–242, 1981.
3. Bergvall, U., Steiner, L., and Forster, D. M. C. Early pattern of cerebral circulatory disturbances following subarachnoid haemorrhage. Neuroradiology *5*:24–32, 1973.
4. Bouma, G. J., and Muizelaar, J. P. The relationship between cardiac output and cerebral blood flow in patients with intact and with impaired autoregulation. J. Neurosurg. *73*:368–374, 1990.
5. Brown, D. D. Treatment of recurrent cardiovascular symptoms and the questions of vasospasm. Med. Clin. North Am. *35*:1457–1474, 1951.
6. Brown, F. D., Hanlon, K., and Mullen, S. Treatment of aneurysmal hemiplegia with dopamine and mannitol. J. Neurosurg. *49*:525–529, 1978.
7. Burke, A. M., Chien, S., McMurtry, J. G., III, et al. Effects of low molecular weight dextran on blood viscosity after craniotomy for intracranial aneurysms. Surg. Gynecol. Obstet. *148*:9–15, 1979.

8. Davis, D. H., and Sundt, T. M., Jr. Relationship of cerebral blood flow to cardiac output, mean arterial pressure, blood volume, and α and β blockade in cats. J. Neurosurg. *52*:745–754, 1980.
9. DiSesa, V., Brown, E., Mudge, G. H., Jr., et al. Hemodynamic comparison of dopamine and dobutamine in the postoperative volume-loaded, pressure-loaded, and normal ventricle. J. Thorac. Cardiovasc. Surg. *83*:256–263, 1982.
10. Farhat, S. M., and Schneider, R. C. Observations on the effect of systemic blood pressure on intracranial circulation in patients with cerebrovascular insufficiency. J. Neurosurg. *27*:441–445, 1967.
11. Fisher, M., Giannotta, S. L., and Meiselman, H. J. Hemorheological alterations in patients with subarachnoid hemorrhage. Clin. Hemorheol. *7*:611–618, 1987.
12. Flamm, E. S., and Ransohoff, J. Treatment of cerebral vasospasm by control of cyclic adenosine monophosphate. Surg. Neurol. *6*:223–226, 1976.
13. Fleischer, A. S., Raggio, J. F., and Tindall, G. T. Aminophylline and isoproterenol in the treatment of cerebral vasospasm. Surg. Neurol. *8*:117–121, 1977.
14. Fleischer, A. S., and Tindall, G. T. Cerebral vasospasm following aneurysm rupture: a protocol for therapy and prophylaxis. J. Neurosurg. *52*:149–152, 1980.
15. Giannotta, S. L., McGillicuddy, J. E., and Kindt, G. W. Diagnosis and treatment of postoperative cerebral vasospasm. Surg. Neurol. *18*:286–290, 1977.
16. Grubb, R. L., Jr., Raichle, M. E., Eichling, J. O., and Mokhtar, H. G. Effects of subarachnoid hemorrhage on cerebral blood volume, blood flow, and oxygen utilization in humans. J. Neurosurg. *46*:446–453, 1977.
17. Heilbrun, M. P., Olesen, J., and Lassen, N. A. Regional cerebral blood flow studies in subarachnoid hemorrhage. J. Neurosurg. *37*:36–44, 1972.
18. Hung, T. L., Konas, H., Butter, O., and Yie, C. L. Rheological abnormalities in patients with subarachnoid hemorrhage. In: *Proceedings of the Annual Meeting of the American Association of Neurological Surgeons.* 1989.
19. Jaffe, A. S. (ed.) *Textbook of Advanced Cardiac Life Support*, Ed. 2, pp. 115–127. American Heart Association, Dallas, 1987.
20. Kassell, N. F., Peerless, S. J., Durward, Q. J., et al. Treatment of ischemic deficits from vasospasm with intravascular volume expansion and induced arterial hypertension. Neurosurgery *11*:337–343, 1982.
21. Kassell, N. F., Sasaki, T., Colohan, A. R. T., et al. Cerebral vasospasm following aneurysmal subarachnoid hemorrhage. Stroke *16*:562–572, 1985.
22. Keller, T. S., McGillicuddy, J. E., LaBond, V. A., et al. Volume expansion in focal cerebral ischemia: the effect of cardiac output on local cerebral blood flow. Clin. Neurosurg. *29*:40–50, 1982.
23. Kindt, G., Youmans, J., and Albrand, O. Factors

influencing the autoregulation of the cerebral blood flow during hypo and hypertension. J. Neurosurg. *36:*299–305, 1967.

24. Kosnik, E. J., and Hunt, W. E. Postoperative hypertension in the management of patients with intracranial arterial aneurysms. J. Neurosurg. *45:*148–154, 1978.

25. Kudo, T., Suzuki, S., and Iwabuchi, T. Importance of monitoring the circulating blood volume in patients with cerebral vasospasm after subarachnoid hemorrhage. Neurosurgery *9:*514–520, 1981.

26. Kuyama, H., Ladds, A., Branston, N. M., *et al.* An experimental study of acute subarachnoid haemorrhage in baboons: changes in cerebral blood volume, blood flow, electrical activity and water content. J. Neurol. Neurosurg. Psychiatry *47:*354–364, 1984.

27. Levy, M. L., and Giannotta, S. L. Cardiac performance and hypervolemic therapy in the treatment of cerebral vasospasm. J. Neurosurg. *75:*27–31, 1991.

28. Maroon, J. C., and Nelson, P. B. Hypovolemia in patients with subarachnoid hemorrhage: therapeutic implications. Neurosurgery *4:*223–226, 1979.

29. Matsui, T., and Asano, T. The hemodynamic effects of prolonged albumin administration in beagle dogs exposed to experimental subarachnoid hemorrhage. Neurosurgery *32:*79–84, 1993.

30. McGillicuddy, J., Kindt, G., Giannotta, S. L., *et al.* Focal cerebral blood flow in cerebral vasospasm: the effect of intravascular volume expansion. Acta Neurol Scand. *60*(suppl. 72)*:*490–491, 1979.

31. Medlock, M. D., Dulebon, S. C., and Elwood, P. W. Prophylactic hypervolemia without calcium channel blockers in early aneurysm surgery. Neurosurgery *30:*12–16, 1992.

32. Meyer, C. H. A., Lowe, D., Meyer, M., *et al.* Progressive change in cerebral blood flow during the first three weeks after subarachnoid hemorrhage. Neurosurgery *12:*58–76, 1983.

33. Mickey, B., Vorstrup, S., Voldby, B., *et al.* Serial measurement of regional cerebral blood flow in patients with SAH using ^{133}Xe inhalation and emission computerized tomography. J. Neurosurg. *60:*916–922, 1984.

34. Mikulic, E., Cohn, J. N., and Frandiosa, J. A. Comparative hemodynamic effects of inotropic and vasodilator drugs in severe heart failure. Circulation *56:*528–533, 1977.

35. Muizelaar, J. P., and Becker, D. P. Induced hypertension for the treatment of cerebral ischemia after subarachnoid hemorrhage: direct effect on cerebral blood flow. Surg. Neurol. *25:*317–325, 1986.

36. Origitano, T. C., Wascher, T. M., Reichman, O. H., and Anderson, D. E. Sustained increased cerebral blood flow with prophylactic hypertensive hypervolemic hemodilution ("Triple H" therapy) after subarachnoid hemorrhage. Neurosurgery *27:*729–740, 1990.

37. Pickard, J. D., Boisvert, D. P. J., Graham, D. I., *et al.* Late effects of subarachnoid haemorrhage on the response of the primate cerebral circulation to drug-induced changes in arterial blood pressure. J. Neurol. Neurosurg. Psychiatry *42:*899–903, 1979.

38. Pitts, L. H., Macpherson, P., Wyper, D. J., *et al.* Cerebral blood flow, angiographic cerebral vasospasm and subarachnoid hemorrhage. Acta Neurol. Scand. *56*(suppl. 64)*:*334–335, 1977.

39. Pritz, M. B. Treatment of cerebral vasospasm: usefulness of Swan-Ganz catheter monitoring of volume expansion. Neurosurgery *3:*364–368, 1984.

40. Pritz, M. B., Giannotta, S. L., Kindt, G. W., *et al.* Treatment of patients with neurological deficits associated with cerebral vasospasm by intravascular volume expansion. Neurosurgery *3:*364–368, 1978.

41. Rosenstein, J., Suzuki, M., Symon, L., *et al.* Clinical use of a portable bedside cerebral blood flow machine in the management of aneurysmal subarachnoid hemorrhage. Neurosurgery *15:*519–525, 1984.

42. Sarnoff, S. J., and Berglund, E. Ventricular function. I. Starling's law of the heart studied by means of simultaneous right and left ventricular function curves in the dog. Circulation *9:*706–718, 1954.

43. Sibbald, W. J., Calvin, J., and Drieoger, H. H. Right and left ventricular pre-load and diastolic ventricular compliance: implications for therapy in critically ill patients. In: *Textbook of Critical Care,* edited by W. C. Shoemaker, W. L. Thompson, and P. R. Holbrook, pp. 367–374. W. B. Saunders, Philadelphia, 1984.

44. Skunhojie, E., Hoeot-Rasmussen, K., Paulsen, D., *et al.* Regional cerebral blood flow and its autoregulation in patients with transient focal cerebral ischemic attacks. Neurology *20:*465–493, 1970.

45. Solomon, R. A., Post, K. D., and McMurtry, J. G., III. Depression of circulating blood volume in patients after subarachnoid hemorrhage: implications for the management of symptomatic vasospasm. Neurosurgery *15:*354–361, 1984.

46. Sundt, T. M., Jr. Management of ischemic complications after subarachnoid hemorrhage. J. Neurosurg. *43:*418–425, 1975.

47. Sundt, T. M., Jr. (ed.) *Surgical Techniques for Saccular and Giant Intracranial Aneurysms.* Williams and Wilkins, Baltimore, 1990.

48. Sundt, T. M., Jr., Szurzewski, J., and Sharbrough, F. W. Physiological considerations important for the management of vasospasm. Surg. Neurol. *7:*259–267, 1977.

49. Tranmer, B. I., Gross, C. E., Kindt, G. W., *et al.* Pulsatile versus nonpulsatile blood flow in the treatment of acute cerebral ischemia. Neurosurgery *19:*724–731, 1986.

50. Tranmer, B. I., Keller, T. S., Kindt, G. W., *et al.* Loss of cerebral regulation during cardiac output variations in focal cerebral ischemia. J. Neurosurg. *77:*253–259, 1992.

51. Tu, Y. K., Heros, R. C., Karacostas, O., *et al.* Isovolemic hemodilution in experimental focal cerebral ischemia. I. Effects on hemodynamics,

hemorheology, and intracranial pressure. J. Neurosurg. *69:*72–81, 1988.

52. Tu, Y. K., Heros, R. C., Karacostas, O., *et al.* Isovolemic hemodilution in experimental focal cerebral ischemia. 2. Effects on regional cerebral blood flow and size of infarction. J. Neurosurg. *69:*82–91, 1988.

53. Waltz, A. Effect of blood pressure on blood flow in ischemic and non-ischemic cerebral cortex: the phenomena of autoregulation and luxury perfusion. Neurology *18:*613–621, 1968.

54. Wilkins, R. H. Attempts at prevention or treatment of intracranial arterial spasm: an update. Neurosurgery *18:*808–825, 1986.

55. Wilkins, R. H. Vasospasm: prevention and treatment. In: *Cerebral Arterial Spasm,* edited by R. H. Wilkins, pp. 691–692. Williams and Wilkins, Baltimore, 1980.

56. Wood, J. H., Simeone, F. A., Kron, R. E., *et al.* Experimental hypervolemic hemodilution: physiological correlations of cortical blood flow, cardiac output, and intracranial pressure with fresh blood viscosity and plasma volume. Neurosurgery *14:*709–723, 1984.

57. Wood, J. H., Snyder, L. L., and Simeone, F. A. Failure of intravascular volume expansion without hemodilution to elevate cortical blood flow in region of experimental focal ischemia. J. Neurosurg. *56:*80–91, 1982.

58. Zimpfer, M., Khosropour, R., and Lackner, F. Effect of dobutamine on cardiac function in man: reciprocal roles of heart rate and ventricular stroke volume. Crit. Care Med. *10:*367–370, 1982.

Management of Vasospasm: Calcium Channel-Blocking Agents

CRAIG M. KEMPER, M.D., GEORGE S. ALLEN, M.D., Ph.D.

INTRODUCTION

Medical therapy for control of vasospasm due to subarachnoid hemorrhage has been proposed since the 1960s. The basis for this therapy was the belief that a vasoactive compound in hemorrhagic cerebrospinal fluid caused arterial vasospasm. The time course of cisternal clot breakdown and release of vasoactive compounds correlates with the time course of clinical vasospasm due to subarachnoid hemorrhage (5, 18, 26). Serotonin was known to be released from platelets in the cisternal blood clot, causing a Ca^{2+}-mediated arterial smooth muscle contraction in experimental models (5, 8). Research initially focused on serotonin inhibition (47) but later shifted to blockade of the final common messenger for contraction, calcium (3, 4). The development of calcium channel-blocking agents for cardiac use eventually produced compounds which were found to have selective effects on the cerebrovascular system. The result was nimodipine, a lipid soluble 1,4-dihydropyridine which inhibited cerebral arteriolar smooth muscle contraction *in vitro* and *in vivo* (14).

These findings were applied clinically, and a reduction in neurological deficits due to vasospasm was demonstrated in patients receiving dihydropyridine calcium channel-blocking agents after subarachnoid hemorrhage. However, the mechanism of this protection was controversial, since the incidence of arteriographic spasm was not universally diminished in treated patients. Basic

research has supported a neuroprotective role for Ca^{2+} channel blockade. These findings have also been applied clinically, producing effective protection in ischemic stroke. The following discussion presents both basic science and clinical research that has formed the basis of current pharmacological therapy for vasospasm due to subarachnoid hemorrhage.

Basic Science

Initial studies supporting the role of serotonin as a vasoactive peptide and a cause of arteriolar vasospasm in subarachnoid hemorrhage were presented by Zervas *et al.* (47). Prophylactically reserpinized dogs showed prevention of experimentally produced vasospasm, implicating serotonin as a principle agent in the production of vasospasm. It was felt that the cisternal blood clot from subarachnoid hemorrhage underwent eventual breakdown and the resultant clot lysis released serotonin and other compounds. Vasoconstriction is a Ca^{2+}-mediated event and has been studied in different models. Peripheral vascular constriction was shown by the lanthanum method to be dependent upon an intracellular source of Ca^{2+} (44). When lanthanum was applied to cerebral vascular structures, no contraction was seen. Thus, the cerebral vascular constriction was dependent upon an extracellular source of Ca^{2+} (8). The method by which serotonin actually caused arterial vasoconstriction was discovered to be Ca^{2+}

dependent (2). Further investigation showed that serotonin caused extracellular Ca^{2+} influx in the canine basilar artery (8). Additional research suggested evidence of vasoactive substances in cerebrospin fluid which could contribute to vasospasm, namely prostaglandin F_2 (7) and thromboxane A_2 (30). These substances cause vasoconstriction by a channel - mediated transmembrane Ca^{2+} flux in the smooth muscle cells of cerebral arteries (2, 6, 8, 30).

Smooth muscle contraction is based on two types of Ca^{2+}. The first type is an intracellular pool that is sequestered in the endoplasmic reticulum of the sarcomere. Its release is messenger dependent, via a cAMP phosphodiesterase system, and this is primarily α-adrenergic. The second type of Ca^{2+} originates from an extracellular source in the interstitial compartment (45). This Ca^{2+} is responsible for transmitter release and Ca^{2+} influx during depolarization in smooth muscle, and is voltage dependent (43). Ca^{2+} availability is controlled by a receptor-sensitive channel for the intracellular source and by a potential-sensitive channel for the extracellular source. The difference between receptor-sensitive channels and potential-sensitive channels has been exploited to achieve selective Ca^{2+} blockade. Extracellular Ca^{2+} flux is thought to be primarily responsible for cerebral vasoconstriction (8) and is caused by activation of the potential-sensitive channel, while the intracellular Ca^{2+} flux is dependent upon the receptor-sensitive channel (43). Ca^{2+} flux into the cell therefore has multiple modes of entry that are controlled by separate agonists. The potential-sensitive channel has been shown to be selectively blocked by dihydropyridine calcium channel-blocking agents (43). Thus, the effectiveness of this novel class of calcium channel-blocking agents is due to blockade of extracellular Ca^{2+} flux through potential-sensitive channels.

Calcium channel-blocking agents are divided into three classes (21, 27). Class I agents are the lipid-soluble 1,4-dihydropyridines nifedipine, nimodipine, nitrendipine, and nicardipine (Fig. 6B.1) Class II agents include verapamil and methoxyverapamil and class III agents include diltiazem. The pharmacokinetics of these calcium channel-

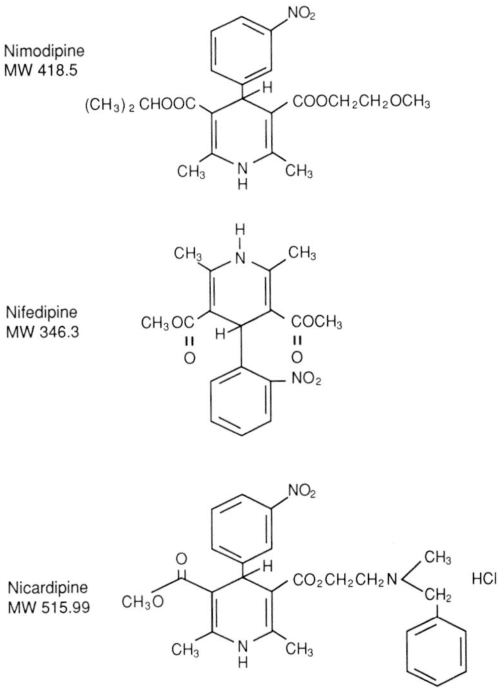

Figure 6B.1. Structures of dihydropyridine class calcium channel-blocking agents.

blocking agents are different (28, 33, 42). Washout studies show a longer time needed for recovery from vasodilation produced by class I calcium channel-blocking agents, compared to either class II or III agents, when used on intracerebral arterioles. (Fig. 6B.2a). Log-dose curves show nifedipine and nimodipine to be effective at 10 and 100 times lower concentrations, respectively, than diltiazem or verapamil (42) (Fig. 6B.2b). This dissimilarity in wash-out recovery and receptor affinity has been attributed to the lipid solubility of class I calcium channel-blocking agents. Additionally, radioligand studies show inhibition of dihydropyridine binding by [^{3}H]nimodipine, while class II agents decrease ^{3}H-labeled calcium channel-blocking agent binding and class II agents increase ^{3}H-labeled calcium channel-blocking agent receptor binding (33).

Class I calcium channel-blocking agents were effective in the treatment of experimentally produced vasospasm in canine basilar artery models. These studies were performed initially with nifedipine (3) and eventually with nimodipine (15). Additional *in vivo*

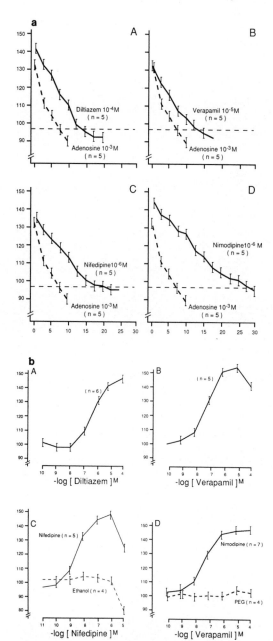

models (27, 42) of experimental vasospasm revealed the potential clinical usefulness of nimodipine. The clinical application of the class I calcium channel-blocking agents then led to the currently available drugs used in the treatment of subarachnoid hemorrhage-induced vasospasm.

Nifedipine was the first calcium channel-blocking agent of the dihydropyridine class that was shown to have effective antivasospastic properties *in vitro* and *in vivo*. Allen and co-workers (3, 4) were able to prevent angiographic vasoconstriction in response to intracisternally injected autologous blood with orally administered nifedipine in dogs. The mechanism of action of nifedipine was thought to be the blockade of extracellular Ca^{2+} flux in cerebral vascular smooth muscle. Results of the *in vivo* studies in dogs encouraged the initiation of clinical studies in humans. Nimodipine, another dihydropyridine, was found to be more effective at an even lower dose than nifedipine *in vitro* and *in vivo* (14) (Table 6B.1).

Nimodipine met the requirements for a compound with potential uses in vasospasm. Because of its lipid solubility it crosses the blood-brain barrier, it has selective cerebrovascular efficacy, it is nontoxic and has minimal side effects, and it is easy to administer. Nimodipine has a half-life of 2 hours and is 95% protein bound, with a high level of first-pass metabolism. The cerebrospinal fluid concentration of nimodipine at clinically effective doses is known to be within the range of its affinity for its receptor in human brain

Figure 6B.2. (*a*) Time courses after washout for recovery from dilation produced by calcium antagonists, compared with adenosine. The minimum dose of each drug sufficient to induce maximum dilation was used. Time for return to resting diameter (100 ± 5%; mean ± standard error) was significantly longer with diltiazem (*A*) ($p < 0.05$), nifedipine (*C*), and nimodipine (*D*) ($p < 0.01$) than with adenosine. Recovery time was also significantly longer with nimodipine than with the calcium antagonists ($p < 0.01$). (From Takayaso, M., Basset, J. E., and Dacey, R. G. Effects of calcium antagonists on intracerebral penetrating arterioles in rats. J. Neurosurg. *69:* 204–209, 1988.) (*b*) Cumulative diameter dose response curves for calcium antagonists. Significant dilation began at concentrations of 10^{-6} mol/liter diltiazem (*A*), 10^{-7} mol/liter verapamil (*B*), 10^{-8} mol/liter nifedipine (*C*), and 10^{-9} mol/liter nimodipine (*D*) ($p < 0.01$). Solvents had essentially no effect on vessel diameter at concentrations corresponding to those used with nifedipine or nimodipine between 10^{-12} and 10^{-6} mol/liter (*C* and *D*). Ethanol significantly constricted vessels only at the highest concentration, corresponding to 10^{-5} nifedipine (analysis of variance, $p < 0.001$). Nifedipine at 10^{-5} mol/liter significantly constricted vessels, when compared to 10^{-6} mol/liter ($p < 0.05$), and this constriction was comparable to that obtained with the solvent alone (*C*), *PBG*, polyethylene glycol 400.

TABLE 6B.1
Changes in Cross-sectional Area (Radius^2/Control Radius^2) of Basilar and Ventral Spinal Arteries of Dogs after the Subarachnoid Injection of Blood and Treatment with Nifedipine or Nimodipine[a]

Animal Group	Drug and Dose	Time of Angiogram	No. of Dogs	Cross-sectional Area (% of control value)	
				Basilar Artery	Ventral Spinal Artery
1	None	Control	3	100	100
		30 min after SAH[b]		73 ± 7	50 ± 10
		80 min after SAH		71 ± 7	48 ± 15
2	Nifedipine (1 mg/kg)	Control	4	100	100
		30 min after SAH		52 ± 9	50 ± 10
		80 min after SAH and 30 min after nifedipine		133 ± 27	122 ± 17
3	Nifedipine (0.28 mg/kg)	Control	4	100	100
		30 min after SAH		50 ± 5	41 ± 3
		80 min after SAH and 30 min after nifedipine		61 ± 10	64 ± 10
4	Nimodipine (0.28 mg/kg)	Control	4	100	100
		30 min after SAH		64 ± 10	69 ± 1
		80 min after SAH and 30 min after nimodipine		97 ± 9	105 ± 21

[a] From Cohen, R. J., and Allen, G. S. Cerebral arterial spasm: the role of calcium in *in vitro* and *in vivo* analysis of treatment with nifedipine and nimodipine. In: *Cerebral Arterial Spasm*, edited by R. H. Wilkins, pp. 527–532. Williams and Wilkins, Baltimore, 1980.
[b] SAH, subarachnoid hemorrhage (subarachnoid injection of 2.5 ml of blood).

tissue (11, 33). An unpublished Bayer study showed, by dose escalation, that nimodipine is most effective at 60 mg orally every 4 hours.

Subsequent clinical studies using nimodipine have demonstrated that clinical outcome of patients is improved in aneurysmal subarachnoid hemorrhage (9, 35, 36, 37). The degree of angiographic vasospasm was reduced, along with the severity of neurological deficits from vasospasm, in patients receiving nimodipine in the initial trial. The incidences of symptomatic vasospasm were not statistically different between treatment and control groups in these studies, however. This led some investigators to propose a neuroprotective role for nimodipine in subarachnoid hemorrhage victims; this has been offered as an alternative explanation for the improved outcome. It is thought that a neuronal level of Ca^{2+} blockade is responsible for the neuroprotective properties of the dihydropyridines (22, 24, 25, 41).

Many physiological changes are induced by subarachnoid hemorrhage. Notable is the decrease in cerebral metabolic rate of O$_2$ and cerebral blood flow, with a rise in cerebral blood volume. These changes correlate directly with the severity of subarachnoid hemorrhage, in terms of patient presentation, and may cause ischemia and infarction (16, 26). Cerebral ischemia and anoxia in humans cause endogenous excitatory amino acid release (39), primarily glutamate and asparate, which produces a cascade of neuronal injuries (15, 40). Choi (13) showed that neurons exposed to glutamate underwent an initial excitotoxic phase of injury due to Na$^+$ and K$^+$ flux. The predominant cell death, however, was delayed and dependent on extracellular Ca^{2+}. Neurons exposed to glutamate in the absence of Ca^{2+} showed a decrease in neuronal loss at 24 hours. When Ca^{2+} was returned to the solution, marked cell dropout occurred. The glutamate-dependent Ca^{2+} reuptake is a critical event in cellular death and injury and is not of an "excitotoxic" nature. The channels through which Ca^{2+} enters could be multiple (13, 32) and may cause neuronal damage through Ca^{2+}-dependent proteases, lipases, and phosphodiesterases (20, 34, 41). BAY K8644 is a dihydropyridine Ca^{2+} channel agonist that produces increases in Ca^{2+} uptake and transmitter release, providing evidence for a dihydropyridine-sensitive channel (32). Dihydropyridine binding sites in human brain have been established previously (33). The possibility, therefore, exists that Ca^{2+}-mediated neurotoxicity might be reduced by pharmacological blockade of such sites. *In vivo* studies have shown that the ischemic deficit caused by occlusion of the rat middle cerebral artery (38, 46), due to Ca^{2+}-mediated neurotoxicity, is prevented by the presence of dihydropyridines. The clinical application of this finding has been studied in stroke (19). Thus, dihydropyridine Ca^{2+} channel blockade has produced both *in vitro* and *in vivo* protection from Ca^{2+}-mediated ischemic neuronal injury. The use of an effective calcium channel-blocking agent provides another weapon in the armamentarium for treatment of cerebral ischemia.

Clinical Studies

The challenge of medically altering the outcome of vasospasm in victims of subarachnoid hemorrhage was first evaluated in 1979 in a United States trial of nimodipine (9). In this multicenter, randomized, double-blinded, placebo-controlled study, 116 patients were studied. Treated patients received a 0.7 mg/kg loading dose and 0.35 mg/kg orally every 4 hours. The study was controlled relative to age/sex, initial presentation, and amount of blood evident on computerized tomography (CT) scans. Only good and moderate grade (Hunt and Hess grade I and II) patients were entered into the study. Results were tabulated in terms of good outcome and poor outcome (severe neurological or death) due to vasospasm. Spasm was found to be directly related to the amount of blood evident on CT scans. Although the frequency of spasm was not different, treated patients had less severe arterial narrowing and improved outcome. No side effects were reported for patients receiving nimodipine. In 1986 Philippon *et al.* (36) showed, in a controlled study, improvement in a series of patients receiving nimodipine (60 mg) orally every 4 hours after subarachnoid hemorrhage. Although the frequency of vasospasm was not different between placebo and treatment groups, the frequency of extensive and diffuse vasospasm was lower in the treated group. No side effects attributable to nimodipine were reported. A subsequent study was done in Canada on poor-grade aneurysm patients; it differed from the study in the United States by inclusion of poor- and severe-grade patients (Hunt and Hess grade III-V) (35). This study used a dose of 90 mg orally every 4 hours and was designed in a fashion similar to that of the study in the United States. The results showed improvement in patients in the poor and vegetative classes, from ischemic deficits due to vasospasm, while mortality rates were not changed. The incidence and severity of angiographically apparent vasospasm were not significantly different between control and treatment groups. Side effects were reported in 25% of the placebo-treated patients and in 21% of those receiving nimodipine. A British study in 1989 included subarachnoid hemorrhage victims of all grades and tested a much larger population (37). Patients were treated with 60 mg of nimodipine orally every 4 hours. Significantly improved outcome was seen in the poor and severe neurological grade groups receiving treatment. The incidence of vasospasm was unchanged between treatment and control groups; however, no attempt was made to quantify the severity of vasospasm. Moreover, the results were not selective for delayed ischemic deficits due to vasospasm alone. Side effects were uncommon and occurred in 5% of nimodipine-treated and 4% of placebo-treated patients. The cumulative results of these trials are presented in Table 6B.2.

Several open trials have demonstrated improved outcomes in patients receiving calcium channel-blocking agent treatment, compared with historical controls (1). Alternative delivery methods for dihydropyridine calcium channel-blocking agents (10) have been explored and include intravenous, intra-arterial, and intracisternal administration. Auer (10) and Ljunggren *et al.* (31) in 1984 reported improved outcomes in patients receiving intracisternal nimodipine followed by intravenous administration. The overall results were similar to those of Allen *et al.* (9) in 1983. Intra-arterially administered nimodipine has produced inconclusive results (12, 23), but these results were obtained from trials using small populations.

TABLE 6B.2
Results of Clinical Trials

Investigators	No. of Patients	Dose	Outcome		
			Death	Poor	Good
Allen et al. (9)[a]	N[b] 56	0.35 mg/kg, every 4	1	0	12
	P 60	hours for 21 days	3	5	8
Philippon et al. (36)[a]	N 31	60 mg, orally, every	2	0	2
	P 39	4 hours for 21 days	4	6	1
Pickard et al. (37)	N 278	60 mg, orally, every	43	12	223
	P 276	4 hours for 21 days	60	31	185
Petruk et al. (35)	N 72	90 mg, orally, every	34	10	28
	P 82	4 hours for 21 days	32	22	28

[a] Results are tabulated in terms of deficits due to vasospasm alone.
[b] N, nimodipine; P, placebo.

A controlled study using nimodipine administered intravenously at 0.15 mg/kg/hour showed a trend toward reduced rates of morbidity and mortality secondary to our vasospasm (29). Adverse reactions in patients receiving nimodipine have been minimal. Liver toxicity and hypotension are the most commonly reported side effects, but the incidence was not significant, compared with controls. In no study was hypersensitivity a problem.

The results of the controlled and open studies are consistent. A significant improvement in outcome due to a decrease in delayed ischemic deficits is seen. In the studies from the United States and Canada, a decrease in deficit due to vasospasm alone was demonstrated. Overall mortality rates do not appear to be affected, but reduction of death due to vasospasm is difficult to show in a statistical manner. Furthermore, the design of these studies would not allow the determination of all the factors which may be affected by calcium channel-blocking agents. Symptomatic vasospasm does appear to be directly related to the amount of blood evident on initial CT scans, and this has been confirmed with subsequent angiography (9, 35). Although the two groups in the American trial had equal numbers of patients developing deficits due to spasm, both the severity and the progression to fixed deficit were diminished in the treatment group. Patients in the Canadian study all initially had a greater degree of blood evident

on CT scans, thus predicting a much higher incidence of vasospasm in these patients. Treated patients, however, had improved outcomes. Philippon et al. (36) showed improved outcome for treated patients and a trend of lessened severity of vasospasm. The British trial treated vasospasm as a factor in delayed ischemia but did not study it in regard to nimodipine. Although the severity of angiographic vasospasm was decreased in some studies, a major criticism of these studies is that the incidence of angiographic vasospasm itself was never shown to be diminished. A likely explanation for this is that the dose-response curve for angiographically evident vasospasm was not shifted far enough by nimodipine. A second explanation may be that the calcium channel-blocking agents act on vessels too small to be seen angiographically (42). The antivasospastic effects of nimodipine on small penetrating arterioles have been shown in animal studies (11, 42) and confirmed in humans (11).

Alternatively, it may be the neuroprotective effects of nimodipine which caused the improved clinical outcome. Clinical evidence supporting the protective effect of calcium channel-blocking agents is seen in studies of stroke. Flamm (17) showed decreases in infarct size when the Ca^{2+} concentration was diminished by intravenous dihydropyridine in the rat ischemia model. The efficacy of calcium channel-blocking agents in humans has been studied by Gelmers et al. (19), who showed that patients receiving

30 mg of nimodipine orally every 4 hours after ischemic stroke had a better outcome than placebo-treated controls.

Nicardipine, another 1,4-dihydropyridine (Fig. 6B.1), has also been studied in the treatment of vasospasm. A dose-escalation study of nicardipine has been completed in the United States, using seven different dosages of intravenous nicardipine from 0.01 to 0.15 mg/kg/hour, giving total doses of 27–375 mg/24 hours (18). The results revealed a higher incidence of improved outcome among those receiving the higher dosages and a lower incidence of angiographically apparent vasospasm among those receiving the highest dose. However, this dose also caused a noticeable decrease in systolic and diastolic blood pressure. Currently, a controlled study using intravenous nicardipine is being completed.

Conclusion

It appears that use of a 1,4-dihydropyridine class I calcium channel-blocking agent improves the outcomes for a population of subarachnoid hemorrhage victims by reducing delayed ischemic deficits due to vasospasm. The results of the clinical studies are consistent. The method by which calcium channel-blocking agents protected against ischemia remains controversial. Laboratory and clinical investigations support roles for vasodilatory effects on small penetrating arterioles as well as a cellular neuroprotective Ca^{2+} channel antagonism. Careful analysis of the clinical studies suggests antivasospastic effects on large vessels, as seen *in vitro*. Routes of administration for these calcium channel-blocking agents have been explored; however, oral therapy seems to be as effective as intravenous. Intra-arterial and intracisternal deliveries have failed to show improved efficacy, but further controlled studies will be required. Nicardipine has been introduced as a possible drug for use in cerebral vasospasm; its clinical trial, currently in progress, will evaluate its potential benefit, compared to standard therapy.

The use of calcium channel-blocking agents in other ischemic conditions has been proposed as well. Outcomes for epilepsy, anoxia, and cardiac and carotid artery surgery could be improved by a pharmacological therapy protective for ischemia. Currently, ischemia has been rigorously studied with nimodipine and the results show benefits for treated patients. The perioperative use of nimodipine in subarachnoid hemorrhage is a standard of care in our institution. It is likely that it will become standard therapy for other conditions involving cerebral ischemia, and further research will provide even more effective compounds for use.

We currently recommend administration of nimodipine (60 mg orally) every 4 hours once aneurysmal subarachnoid hemorrhage is established. Patients unable to cooperate with this regimen are treated sublingually or via nasogastric tubes. Treatment should continue for 21 days.

REFERENCES

1. Adams, H. Calcium antagonists in the management of patients with aneurysmal subarachnoid hemorrhage: a review. Angiology *41:*1010–1016, 1990.
2. Allen, G. S. Cerebral arterial spasm: a discussion of present and future research. Neurosurgery *1:*142–148, 1977.
3. Allen, G. S., and Bahr, A. L. Cerebral arterial spasm. 10. Reversal of acute and chronic spasm in dogs with orally administered nifedipine. Neurosurgery *4:*43–47, 1979.
4. Allen, G. S. and Banghart, S. B. Cerebral arterial spasm: 9. *In vitro* effects of nifedipine on serotonin-, phenylephrine-, and potassium induced contractions of canine basilar arteries. Neurosurgery *4:*37–42, 1979.
5. Allen, G. S., Gold, L. H., Chou, S. N., and French, L. A. Cerebral arterial spasm. 3. *In vivo* intracisternal production of spasm by serotonin and blood and its reversal by phenoxybenzamine. J. Neurosurg. *40:*451–458, 1974.
6. Allen, G. S., and Gross, C. J. Cerebral arterial spasm. 7. *In vitro* effects of α-adrenergic agents on canine arteries from six anatomical sites and six blocking agents on serotonin-induced contractions of the canine basilar artery. Surg. Neurol. *6:*63–70, 1976.
7. Allen, G. S., Gross, C. J., French, L. A., and Chou, S. N. Cerebral arterial spasm. 5. *In vitro* contractile activity of vasoactive agents including human CSF on human basilar and anterior cerebral arteries. J. Neurosurg. *44:*594–600, 1976.
8. Allen, G. S., Gross, C. J., Henderson, L. M., and Chou, S. M. Cerebral arterial spasm. 4. *In vitro* effects of temperature, serotonin analogues, large nonphysiological concentrations of serotonin, and extracellular calcium and magnesium on serotonin induced contractions of the canine basilar artery. J. Neurosurg. *44:*585–593, 1976.
9. Allen, G. S., Ahn, H. S., and Preziosi, T. J., *et al.* Cerebral arterial spasm. A controlled trial of

nimodipine in patients with subarachnoid hemorrhage. N. Engl. J. Med. *308:*619–624, 1983.

10. Auer, L. M. Acute operation and preventive nimodipine improves outcome in patients with ruptured cerebral aneurysms. Neurosurgery *15:*57–66, 1984.

11. Auer, L. M., Oberbauer, R. W., and Schalk, H. V. Human pial vascular reactions to intravenous nimodipine infusion during EC-IC bypass surgery. Stroke *14:*210–212, 1983.

12. Boker, D. K., Solymosi, L., and Wassman, H. Immediate post angiographic intra-arterial treatment of cerebral vasospasm after subarachnoid hemorrhage with nimodipine. Neurochirurgia (Stutts.) *28:*118–120, 1985.

13. Choi, D. W. Glutamate neurotoxicity in cortical cell culture is calcium dependent. Neurosci. Lett. *58:*293–297, 1985.

14. Cohen, R. J., and Allen, G. S. Cerebral arterial spasm: the role of calcium in *in vitro* and *in vivo* analysis of treatment with nifedipine and nimodipine. In: *Cerebral Arterial Spasm*, edited by: R. H. Wilkins, pp. 527–532. Williams and Wilkins, Baltimore, 1980.

15. Erecinska, M., Nelson, D., Wilson, D. F., and Silver, I. A. Regional changes in amino acid levels in rat brain during ischemia and perfusion. Brain Res. *304:*9–22, 1984.

16. Fischer, C. M., Robertson, G. H., and Ojemann, R. G. Cerebral vasospasm with ruptured saccular aneurysm: the clinical manifestations. Neurosurgery *1:*245–248, 1977.

17. Flamm, E. S. The potential use for nicardipine in cerebrovascular diseases. Am. Heart J. *117:*236–241, 1989.

18. Flamm, E. S., Adams, H. P., Beck, D. W., et al. Dose escalation study of intravenous nicardipine in patients with aneurysmal subarachnoid hemorrhage. J. Neurosurg. *68:*393–400, 1988.

19. Gelmers, H. J., Gorter, K., de Weerdt, C. J., and Wiezer, J. J. A. A controlled trial of nimodipine in acute ischemic stroke. N. Engl. J. Med. *318:*203–207, 1988.

20. Gilbert, D. S., Newby, B. J., and Anderson, B. H. Neurofilament disguise, destruction and discipline. Nature *256:*586–589, 1975.

21. Glossmann, H., Ferry, D. R., Lubbecke, F., et al. Identification of voltage operated calcium channels by binding studies: differentiation of subclasses of calcium antagonist drugs with ³H-nimodipine radioligand binding. J. Recept. Res. *3:*177–190, 1983.

22. Greenberg, D. A. Calcium channels and calcium channel antagonists. Ann. Neurol. *21:*317–330, 1987.

23. Grotenhuis, J. A., Bettag, W., Fiebach, B. J. O., et al. Intracarotid slow bolus injection of nimodipine during angiography for treatment of cerebral vasospasm after subarachnoid hemorrhage. J. Neurosurg. *61:*231–240, 1984.

24. Grotta, J., Pettigrew, C., Rosenbaum, D., et al. Efficacy and mechanism of action of calcium channel blockers after global cerebral ischemia in rats. Stroke *19:*447–454, 1988.

25. Grotta, J., Spydell, J., Pettigrew, C., et al. The effect of nicardipine on neuronal function following ischemic stroke. Stroke *17:*213–219, 1986.

26. Grubb, R. L., Raichle, M. E., Eichling, J. O., and Gado, M. H. Effects of subarachnoid hemorrhage on cerebral blood volume, blood flow and oxygen utilization in humans. J. Neurosurg. *46:*446–453, 1977.

27. Haws, C. W., and Heistad, D. D. Effects of nimodipine on cerebral vasoconstrictor responses. Am. J. Physiol. *247:*H170–H176, 1984.

28. Henry, P. D. Comparative pharmacology of calcium antagonists: nifedipine verapamil and diltiazem. Am. J. Cardiol. *46:*1047–1058, 1980.

29. Jan, M., Buccheit, F., and Tremoulet, M. Therapeutic trial of intravenous nimodipine in patients with established cerebro-vasospasm after rupture of intracranial aneurysms. Neurosurgery *23:*154–157, 1988.

30. Juvela, S., Ohman, J., Servo, A., et al. Angiographic vasospasm and release of platelet thromboxane after subarachnoid hemorrhage. Stroke *22:*451–453, 1991.

31. Ljunggren, B., Brandt, L., Saveland, H., et al. Outcome in 60 consecutive patients treated with early aneurysm surgery and intravenous nimodipine. J. Neurosurg. *61:*864–873, 1984.

32. Miller, R. How many types of calcium channels exist in neurons? Trends Neurosci. *8:*45–47, 1985.

33. Peroutka, S. J., and Allen, G. S. Calcium channel antagonist binding sites labelled by ³H-nimodipine in human brain. J. Neurosurg. *59:*933–937, 1983.

34. Peters, T. Calcium in physiological and pathological cell function. Eur. Neurol. *25*(suppl 1):27–44, 1986.

35. Petruk, K. C., West, M., Mohr, G., et al. Nimodipine treatment in poor-grade aneurysm patients: results of a double-blind placebo controlled trial. J. Neurosurg. *68:*505–517, 1988.

36. Philippon, J., Grob, R., Dagreou, F., et al. Prevention of vasospasm in subarachnoid hemorrhage: a controlled study with nimodipine. Acta Neurochir. (Wien) *82:*110–114, 1986.

37. Pickard, J. D., Murray, G. D., Illingworth, R., et al. Effect of oral nimodipine on cerebral infarction and outcome after subarachnoid hemorrhage: British Aneurysm Nimodipine Trial. B. Med. J. *298:*636–642, 1989.

38. Rappaport, Z. H., Young, W., and Flamm, E. S. Regional brain calcium changes in rat middle cerebral artery occlusion model of ischemia. Stroke *18:*760–764, 1987.

39. Rothman, S. M., and Olney, J. W. Glutamate and the pathophysiology of hypoxic-ischemic brain damage. Ann. Neurol. *19:*105–111, 1986.

40. Schanne, F. A. X., Kane, A. B., Young, E. E., and Farber, J. L. Calcium dependence of toxic cell death: a final common pathway. Science *206:*700–702, 1979.

41. Siesjo, B. K. Calcium and ischemic brain damage. Eur. Neurol. *25*(suppl. 1):45–56, 1986.

42. Takayasu, M., Basset, J. E., and Dacey, R. G. Effects of calcium antagonists on intracerebral penetrating arterioles in rats. J. Neurosurg.

69:204–209, 1988.

43. Towart, R. The selective inhibition of serotonin induced contractions of rabbit cerebrovascular smooth muscle by calcium antagonistic dihydropyridines: an investigation of the mechanism of action of nimodipine. Circ. Res. 48:650–657, 1981.

44. Van Breeman, C., Farinas, B. R., Gerba, P., and McNaughton, E. D. Excitation-contraction coupling in rabbit aorta studies by the lanthanum method for measuring cellular calcium flux. Circ. Res. 30:44–54, 1972.

45. Van Breeman, C., Farinas, B. R., Casteels, R., et al. Factors controlling cytoplasmic Ca^{++} concentration. Philos. Trans R. Soc. Lond. [Biol.] 265:57–71, 1973.

46. Young, W., Rappaport, Z. H., Chalif, D. J., and Flamm, E. S. Regional brain Na^+, K^+, and water changes in the rat middle cerebral artery occlusion model of ischemia. Stroke 18:751–759, 1987.

47. Zervas, N. T., Kuwayama, A., Rosoff, C. B., et al. Cerebral arterial spasm: modification by inhibition of platelet function. Arch. Neurol. 28:400–404, 1973.

Management of Vasospasm: Angioplasty

PETER D. LE ROUX, M.D., MARC R. MAYBERG, M.D.

INTRODUCTION

Approximately 30% of patients who survive rupture of a cerebral aneurysm develop symptoms of ischemia secondary to vasospasm (17, 23). Numerous pharmacological agents and therapies have been used in an attempt to prevent or ameliorate the severity of arterial narrowing associated with subarachnoid hemorrhage (SAH). These include early surgery and clot removal, intracisternal thrombolytic agents, antiplatelet agents, steroids and anti-inflammatory agents, adrenergic antagonists, parasympathomimetics, phosphodiesterase or prostaglandin inhibitors, calcium channel or serotonin antagonists, rheological agents, and hypervolemia with enhanced cardiac output (see Ref. 48 for review). Although clinical benefits have been observed with some of these treatments, particularly calcium channel blockers and hypertensive hypervolemic therapy (40, 46), vasospasm continues to be a major cause of mortality and morbidity after SAH. The International Cooperative Study on the Timing of Aneurysm Surgery indicated that 13.5% patients died or were disabled by ischemic stroke related to vasospasm (16, 24).

The inconsistent results of medical therapies for vasospasm are in part related to their lack of efficacy once a neurological deficit occurs. By contrast, recent experience with percutaneous transluminal angioplasty indicates that this technique can benefit a subgroup of patients who demonstrate progressive clinical deterioration despite maximal medical therapy and can reverse a delayed ischemic deficit after it has developed

(11, 18, 20, 31, 38, 39, 47). This chapter reviews the history, mechanism of action, indications, technique, results, and complications of angioplasty in the treatment of intracranial arterial vasospasm after SAH.

Historical Background

Angioplasty refers to the mechanical dilatation of a vessel by an inflatable intravascular balloon navigated under fluoroscopic guidance. Invasive radiology dates back to the introduction of cardiac catherization in the 1920s, but it was not until 1964 that Dotter and Judkins (9) described the use of transluminal dilatation for obstructive, atherosclerotic, peripheral vascular disease. The development of an inflatable balloon catheter by Gruntzig and Hopff in 1974 (14) led to the subsequent description of percutaneous transluminal angioplasty for coronary artery disease (15) and its widespread use in the treatment of atherosclerotic disease. Despite the rapid technical improvements that followed, there has been limited application of angioplasty to cerebrovascular disease, primarily for fibromuscular hyperplasia or atherosclerotic disease of the common carotid or vertebrobasilar arteries.

Endovascular treatment for vasospasm after SAH was introduced in 1984 by Zubkov et al. (52), who used a latex balloon to treat 33 patients with generally favorable results. Over the next several years, Heishima and colleagues developed a silicone elastomer balloon specifically to treat cerebral vasospasm and first reported the use of this technique in the United States in 1989 (1). Two reports of larger series, from Hieshima and colleagues in San Francisco (18) and Eskridge and co-workers in Seattle (39), appeared later the same year and clearly demonstrated that balloon dilatation was effective in both reversing vessel narrowing and improving cerebral blood flow associated with vasospasm. Furthermore, significant clinical improvement was observed in the majority of these patients, indicating that angioplasty could be a viable therapeutic option in patients with symptomatic vasospasm refractory to maximal medical therapy. These encouraging initial results have led to more widespread use of the technique to treat vasospasm after SAH. As more experience has been gained, continued assessment of the results has better defined the indications, limitations, overall effectiveness, and safety of angioplasty.

Mechanism of Action for Angioplasty

Despite numerous clinical and experimental studies, the pathogenesis of vasospasm remains elusive, although it is certain that prolonged contact between cerebral vessels and constituents of red blood cells (in particular, oxyhemoglobin) is a key factor in the development of delayed arterial narrowing (30). Inflammation, imbalance in endothelium-derived vasoactive factors, free radical generation, and activation of second messenger protein kinases may all contribute to initial vasoconstriction and vessel damage (10, 30, 35). However, vasoconstriction is not solely responsible for the persistent effects of vasospasm. There is compelling evidence that an arteriopathy with distinct ultrastructural changes develops coincident with arterial narrowing, possibly as a response to earlier vessel injury (7, 21, 32, 44). Light and electron microscopic examinations of vasospastic human cerebral arteries, obtained either at autopsy or intraoperatively, demonstrate intimal thickening, myonecrosis, and fibrosis of the medial layer with collagen deposition throughout the vessel wall (21, 44). These histological changes parallel the development of clinically significant vasospasm in humans. A similar spectrum of morphological changes has been observed in experimental animal models after continuous exposure of cerebral vessels to blood (7, 32). Other studies indicate that

vessels chronically exposed to periadventitial blood are less compliant. When canine cerebral arteries are exposed to repeated intracisternal hemorrhage, vasospastic vessels exhibit both a decreased response to endothelium-dependent relaxation and increased stiffness of the noncontractile component of the vessel (25, 26). Consistent with these observations are findings by Bevan et al. (2), who noted that primate cerebral vessels in vitro are less distensible and less sensitive to vasoactive agents after exposure to subarachnoid blood.

The structural changes described above may produce a stiff nondistensible vessel. In part, this may account for the inconsistent response of vasospastic arteries to pharmacological or medical therapy aimed at vasodilatation and may form the basis of the action of mechanical balloon dilatation. In addition, the reported effectiveness of angioplasty in relieving arterial narrowing after SAH is consistent with two proposals regarding vasospasm: 1) narrowing of the large basal arteries, rather than the effects of subarachnoid blood on smaller, more distal vessels, is the primary cause of cerebral ischemia and 2) smooth muscle constriction is not solely responsible for the pathophysiological alterations observed in vasospastic vessels. If smooth muscle constriction alone were responsible for vasospasm, mechanically dilated vessels would be expected to reconstrict. By contrast, both short- and long-term follow-up angiographic evaluation of vessels undergoing balloon dilatation demonstrated persistent restoration of vessel patency (11, 20, 37, 38, 52). Furthermore, studies using transcranial Doppler (TCD) scanning showed persistent amelioration of arterial narrowing after angioplasty, whereas spasm persisted in nondilated vessels (37).

It is not entirely clear how angioplasty works. In atherosclerotic disease, the balloon acts to disrupt and fracture the plaque present in both the intima and media (3). The histological correlate of angioplasty for vasospasm, however, is different. First, only minimal balloon pressure (0.5 atm) is required to dilate vasospastic cerebral vessels, whereas relatively large pressures (4–8 atm) are necessary for a satisfactory result in atherosclerotic disease. Second, no angiographic evidence for intimal disruption or dissection has been observed on either immediate or follow-up angiograms of dilated cerebral vessels (11, 20, 38, 39, 47, 52); this observation has been confirmed histologically (27, 41). Konishi *et al.* (27) evaluated human cadaveric cerebral vessels that were dilated either *in vitro* or *in vivo* after implantation into canine carotid arteries. Examination with both light and scanning electron microscopy demonstrated compression of the intima and a stretched internal elastic lamina but no intimal disruption. Newell *et al.* (39) proposed that angioplasty is effective because it disrupts the increased collagenous and fibrous deposition observed in vasospasm. Support for this hypothesis is provided by scanning electron microscopic studies of human middle cerebral arteries obtained at autopsy and mechanically dilated *in vitro* and of cat femoral arteries dilated *in vivo*, which demonstrated disruption and stretching of collagen fibers (45, 50).

A second compelling question is why mechanically dilated cerebral vessels do not subsequently resume a narrowed configuration. Although untreated vessels remain in spasm and can develop further arterial narrowing, restenosis of mechanically dilated vessels has not been reported by either angiographic or TCD evaluation (20, 37, 39, 52). By contrast, nearly 30% of coronary vessels restenose following angioplasty (33). Several possible factors may explain this phenomenon. First, simple disruption of connective tissue may prevent transmission of contractile forces in the vessel wall (50). Second, Chavez *et al.* (6) have postulated that mechanical damage to muscle cells within the media contributes to the persistent effect of angioplasty. This proposal was based on observations in normal canine basilar arteries mechanically dilated to 130% of their original size. Light microscopic examination demonstrated endothelial denudation, stretching of the internal elastic lamina, and distinct morphological alterations of individual muscle cells. However, these morphological changes disappeared within 7 days and so are unlikely to explain the persistent effects of balloon dilatation. Third, even though endothelial denudation is observed in experimental studies, platelet deposition is not found (6). This may be due in part to the use of systemic heparinization during angioplasty. Finally, mechanically dilated vessels may not respond to vasoactive substances. Pile-Spellman *et al.* (41) found that canine basilar artery did not respond to vasoconstrictive pharmacological agents following balloon dilatation.

Balloon and Catheter Technology

The basic principle underlying angioplasty for vasospasm is that the vessel should not be dilated beyond its prestenotic normal diameter. Therefore, the single most important factor determining the safety of angioplasty is the correct choice of the balloon, in particular the balloon size. Latex balloons, as used by Zubkov *et al.* (52) in the original report on angioplasty for vasospasm, are no longer in use. Instead, most practitioners currently employ two types of custom-designed microballoons made of either polyethylene (Target Therapeutics, San Jose, CA) or silicone (Interventional Therapeutics, San Francisco, CA) (11, 19, 20, 38, 39).

Silicone microballoons have several inherent advantages that make them uniquely suited to this technique (19, 34, 49). First, these balloons are soft and exhibit a conformational structure that allows placement in a restricted area without excess lateral stress being exerted. This minimizes the risk of endothelial damage. Second, a low inflation pressure is required to inflate the microballoon; therefore, the likelihood of both endothelial damage and vessel rupture are decreased. Third, silicone balloons expand with gradual enlargement, whereas the pressure build-up in balloons made of other materials results in sudden expansion. Furthermore, the silicone microballoon expands in a proximal-to-distal direction and is designed to elongate if overinflated. In this manner, the balloon can be advanced by sequential inflations without the advantage of flow. These properties also attenuate the risk of vessel rupture. Finally, silicone materials appear to be stable, inert, and biocompatible with vascular structures. It is important that the balloon be sterilized with ethylene oxide gas to avoid damage to the silicone elastomers which results from other means of sterilization.

Silicone microballoons are currently available in two sizes (Fig. 6C.1). The vast majority of basal intracranial arteries (supraclinoid internal carotid, middle cerebral, anterior cerebral, posterior cerebral, and basilar arteries can be dilated with the smaller balloon. This balloon measures 0.85×3.5 mm when uninflated and 3.5×12 mm when fully expanded. The balloon accepts a volume of 0.1 ml and requires an inflation pressure of 0.5 atm. Experimental studies indicate that, in most instances, adequate dilatation of cerebral vessels can be achieved with low inflation pressures. Furthermore, to enhance the effect, a longer inflation time or repeated inflation, rather than greater pressure, provides satisfactory results (6, 27, 50). For example, Konishi *et al.* (27) compared various expansion times and pressures required to mechanically dilate spastic human middle cerebral arteries obtained at autopsy, both *in vivo* (by grafting the vessels into canine carotid arteries) and *in vitro*. Sufficient dilatation, demonstrated angiographically and using histological techniques, was achieved with a pressure of 1 atm for 10 sec. Higher inflation pressures (3 atm) result in greater destruction of collagen (50). This is consistent with clinical observations suggesting that a higher inflation pressure increases the risk of vessel rupture (11).

Despite the low inflation pressure needed

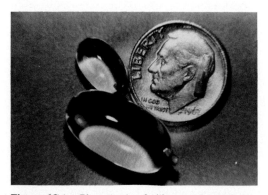

Figure 6C.1. Photograph of silicone microballoons used for angioplasty (Interventional Therapeutics). It is critical that the diameter of the balloon does not exceed the normal luminal diameter of the vessel to be dilated.

for silicone balloons, as described above, microballoons should not be placed beyond the A1 or M2 segments, since the balloon diameter greatly exceeds the normal diameter of these vessels (11). Therefore, angioplasty in distal branches of the cerebral arteries carries an unacceptably high risk of vessel rupture. For larger vessels such as the internal carotid or vertebral arteries, a slightly larger silicone balloon is available. This balloon measures 1.5×4.0 mm when uninflated and expands to 7.5×12.5 mm. Although it requires a volume of only 0.5 ml for inflation, it must be used with caution, even in these larger vessels. Occasionally a stiffer, higher pressure balloon is necessary to dilate more chronic vasospasm where fibrosis is more pronounced (11). A polyethylene balloon (Target Therapeutics) is available for this purpose. A slightly higher pressure (5 atm) is necessary to inflate this balloon; therefore, it must be used with extreme care. For optimal results, a selection of balloons should be available before angioplasty is attempted.

A second important factor in the safety of angioplasty is navigation. In general, it is difficult to negotiate sharp angles (*e.g.*, the origin of A1 from the internal carotid). Similarly, it is difficult to selectively enter narrowed vessels at a bifurcation or trifurcation after one of the branches has been dilated. The ability to precisely steer the balloon depends on both the delivery catheter and the balloon. For example, polyethylene balloons more readily accept guidewires. Two types of coaxial microcatheter guidance systems are currently in use. Both are 150 cm in length and can be inserted from a transfemoral approach that allows rapid access to all major intracranial vessels. First, silicone microballoons can be chemically bonded to a 2.0-French polyethylene catheter (Interventional Therapeutics). Although polyethylene can be steam-shaped into a variety of curves, it lacks the advantage of a steerable guidewire. By contrast, the 2.2-French coaxial tracker catheter (Target Therapeutics) has a softer distal segment that can be used with a steerable guidewire (11, 20, 31, 47). Therefore, the balloon can be guided into less accessible vessels, such as from the supraclinoid carotid into the A1 segment. When the guidewire is advanced beyond the tip of the inflated balloon, the balloon is deformed into a curve. Rotation of the wire then allows the balloon to be steered (5, 11, 47). In some instances, the presence of a guidewire can limit access to very narrow vessels. To overcome this potential drawback and also to improve steering, the guidewire can be advanced through the tip of the balloon. Two distinct disadvantages, however, limit the application of this technique. First, the hole in the balloon enlarges with time and therefore extra balloons are necessary. Second, to expand the balloon, larger volumes of contrast are required, which may have a deleterious effect on ischemic brain areas.

Although a variable-stiffness microcatheter and guidewire may improve access to vasospastic vessels, it must be emphasized that the limiting factor to more distal catheterization is balloon size, not the microcatheter. Beyond the proximal segments of the intracranial vessels (*i.e.*, the A1 or proximal M2 segments), the balloon diameter exceeds the vessel diameter and the balloon should never be inflated. When smaller balloons become available, distal angioplasty may become feasible.

Indications for Angioplasty

Angioplasty is not intended to be used in isolation; rather, it should complement and be used in conjunction with other medical and surgical modalities to optimally treat vasospasm in patients with ruptured cerebral aneurysms. The following protocol has been developed for application of angioplasty for patients with vasospasm at the University of Washington (Fig. 6C.2). Immediately upon admission, patients undergo full radiological evaluation, including computed tomography (CT) scan and four-vessel angiography. Surgery and obliteration of the aneurysm responsible for the SAH are performed as soon after rupture as possible (preferably within 72 hours). In the immediate postoperative period the following studies provide a useful base-line for further care: 1) TCD, 2) cranial CT, 3) single-photon emission computed tomography (SPECT), and 4) repeat angiography. During angiography it is particularly important to examine clip placement, confirm aneurysm obliteration,

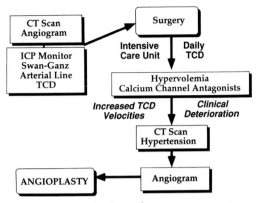

Figure 6C.2. Protocol for management of patients with SAH (see text). Angioplasty is utilized only after maximal medical therapy for vasospasm has been unsuccessful in reversing the neurological deficit.

and determine the caliber of intracranial vessels. All these studies should be available for direct comparison if angioplasty becomes indicated later. For the first 7–10 days after SAH, patients are managed in an intensive care unit with continuous monitoring of hemodynamic parameters (arterial and Swan-Ganz catheters) and intracranial pressure, daily TCD scanning, and frequent neurological evaluation. Hypervolemic therapy is initiated prophylactically using colloid, crystalloid intravenous fluid and if necessary blood products to maintain left ventricular end diastolic pressure in the range of 10–15 mm Hg. Calcium channel antagonists are routinely administered.

Mechanical dilatation of vasospastic vessels can produce dramatic clinical improvement in carefully selected patients, but it is an invasive and potentially hazardous procedure. Therefore, comprehensive management of SAH, such as that described above, should provide a basis from which patients requiring angioplasty are selected. When a new neurological deficit, such as a decrease in the level of consciousness or focal motor weakness, develops, the patient is first given a fluid bolus to further augment cardiac output (left ventricular end diastolic pressure = 16–18 mm Hg) and systolic blood pressure is increased with ionotropic agents. Angioplasty is indicated if the deficit persists despite maximal medical and pharmacological therapy. Three additional criteria should be met prior to angioplasty. First, other causes of clinical deterioration, such as hypoxia, sepsis, an intracranial hemorrhage, or hydrocephalus, must be excluded. Second, there should be no evidence of infarction or recent hemorrhage on head CT or magnetic resonance imaging scans. Third, severe vascular spasm, compatible with the neurological deficit, should be confirmed by angiography. Finally, it is preferable that the aneurysm causing the SAH be adequately obliterated.

One of the most important factors in the success of the procedure is early intervention (11, 20, 38, 47). Therefore, a critical issue is the early and accurate diagnosis of vasospasm. Although angiography is the standard method used to evaluate vasospasm, it is invasive and cannot be repeated each time a neurological deficit develops. By contrast, sequential TCD represents an ideal noninvasive means to diagnose and follow the development of spasm and to predict the likelihood of symptomatic ischemia. Therefore, in our protocol patients undergo a baseline TCD study at admission and daily evaluations thereafter. Changes in blood flow velocity demonstrated by TCD correlate well with the severity of vasospasm (8, 13, 37, 43). For example, middle cerebral artery velocity in excess of 120 cm/sec indicates spasm, whereas velocity greater than 200 cm/sec is invariably associated with symptomatic ischemia (43). Similarly, a rapid increase in velocity (>50 cm/sec increase in 1 day) indicates a patient at high risk for ischemic stroke (13). It is important to assess relative flow velocity of cerebral arteries, because hyperdynamic therapy may contribute to generalized increased flows. Therefore, the ratio of middle cerebral artery to extracranial internal carotid artery velocity is calculated; ratios greater than 8 are associated with existing or imminent symptomatic ischemia due to vasospasm (38).

Additional techniques which supplement and complement TCD in the evaluation of vasospasm are various noninvasive assessments of regional cerebral blood flow (rCBF) (12, 28, 38, 42, 51). These measurements can indicate relative restriction of blood flow and the degree of compensation in the microcirculation associated with vasospasm. SPECT is a widely available means to determine qualitative changes in rCBF. Lewis et al. (28) evaluated patients with severe spasm diagnosed by TCD and those undergoing angioplasty for symptomatic spasm. When severe symptomatic spasm was present, the SPECT study was abnormal in 70% of patients. By contrast, all patients who had a normal neurological exam, despite severe vasospasm by TCD, had normal SPECT scans. Similarly, xenon enhanced CT (Xe/CT) (12, 41, 51) is useful for identifying patients at risk for infarction and provides quantitative assessment of rCBF. In patients with vasospasm, neurological deficit was associated with rCBF of <15 ml/100 g/min; rCBF of <12 ml/100 g/min was indicative of infarction. By contrast, patients with neurological deficits and rCBF of >18 ml/100 g/min usually recovered (12, 51). In contrast to TCD, SPECT and Xe/CT are less easy to repeat and may not be as useful for providing early warning of an impending deficit. However, when these studies are used in conjunction with TCD, frequent neurological evaluation, and regular CT scans; patients at particular risk for symptomatic spasm can be reliably predicted and diagnosed, often before the critical ischemic time threshold is exceeded. Ultimately, it may be possible to identify patients who will benefit from angioplasty prior to the development of symptoms. Although prophylactic angioplasty has been attempted in some institutions, it has yet to be widely applied and should not be considered a standard treatment for vasospasm. Perhaps the most useful role for noninvasive studies, in particular TCD, is to monitor vessels not in spasm at the time of angioplasty which may later develop critical spasm. Newell et al. (37) performed daily TCD evaluations on patients undergoing angioplasty; although there was a dramatic and sustained decrease in the velocity of the vessel undergoing balloon dilatation, nondilated vessels often demonstrated a subsequent increase in velocity, indicative of worsening spasm.

Angioplasty Technique

The procedure is best performed in a dedicated, interventional, neurovascular suite that is equipped for high-resolution subtraction angiography and road mapping. In addition, provision should be made for ventilatory support and continuous invasive monitoring. Many patients with vasospasm are comatose or critically ill, due to either vasospasm or direct effects of the SAH, and require intensive care. Also, it is essential to have a still and cooperative patient to safely perform angioplasty. If this is not possible, general anesthesia or muscular paralysis and sedation are necessary, even though this precludes neurological assessment. In patients who are fully cooperative, neuroleptic analgesia can be given.

A transfemoral percutaneous approach is used. First, a complete four-vessel angiogram should be obtained and compared to the pre- and postoperative studies. This is essential for several reasons: 1) the diagnosis of vasospasm can be confirmed and its location and severity correlated with the clinical findings, 2) the correct balloon size can be chosen, 3) the length and luminal diameter of the vasospastic segment requiring angioplasty can be measured to guide subsequent balloon dilatation, and 4) the status of the aneurysm and the clips occluding it can be examined. It is preferable that the aneurysm be completely obliterated before proceeding to angioplasty (11, 29, 38, 39, 47). In general, only symptomatic vessels should undergo mechanical dilatation. The most symptomatic vessel is treated first. However, we and others (47) have recently performed angioplasty in vessels that are not contributing to symptoms but are associated with a perfusion defect on SPECT scan and demonstrate severe spasm by TCD and angiogram. Whether this approach will decrease the incidence of delayed ischemic neurological deficit has yet to be determined; we do not advise the routine use of prophylactic angioplasty.

The femoral artery is punctured with an 18-gauge needle using the Seldinger technique, and a 7.5-French sheath is inserted. Prior to insertion of the guiding catheter, the patient undergoes systemic anticoagulation with intravenous heparin to prevent thrombus formation. At the conclusion of the procedure, reversal can be achieved with protamine. The guiding catheter (*e.g.*, a non-

tapered 7.3-French polyethylene catheter) is then positioned in the internal carotid or vertebral artery using a 5-French inner catheter and guide wire (0.035 inch) if necessary. A correctly sized microballoon, affixed to an appropriate coaxial delivery system (2.0- or 2.2-French catheter), is then introduced through the 7.3-French sheath. Heparinized saline should be perfused into the dead space between the two catheters. When the balloon is observed beyond the guiding catheter, it can be inflated and then positioned by advancing the coaxial catheter or by using flow direction; progress can be monitored radiologically by digital subtraction road mapping after injection of contrast through the 7.3-French catheter.

Once the balloon is correctly positioned at the site of vasospasm, mechanical dilatation is performed by gentle inflation and deflation of the balloon under continuous fluoroscopic control. To visualize the balloon and control the injection volume, the balloon is best inflated with Metrizamide (200 mg/ml). A small volume (0.05–0.5 ml) is usually all that is required. Furthermore, short inflation times (5–10 sec) and relatively low pressures (0.5 atm) are sufficient to dilate the vessel. Several inflations of short duration may be necessary for an effect and are preferable to prolonged inflation, which may aggravate cerebral ischemia. Following restoration of the vasospastic segment to normal diameter (compared to the preoperative angiogram), or when severe narrowing is effaced, the balloon is further advanced under fluoroscopic control and dilatation is performed in a stepwise fashion from the proximal to the distal end of the narrowed vessel.

Technical difficulties can be encountered under the following circumstances. First, very severe narrowing may prevent balloon entry. This can occasionally be overcome by advancing the guidewire preceding the balloon. Second, access to vessels forming sharp corners, *e.g.*, the A1 takeoff, is often limited. Again, a guidewire or curved balloon may improve the chances of entering these vessels. Third, after one vessel of a bifurcation or trifurcation is dilated it can be difficult to enter the other branches, because preferential flow and vessel shape direct the balloon into the first branch. Finally, it can often be difficult to determine whether spasm observed more distally is a primary event or secondary to decreased flow through more proximal and not necessarily severe vascular spasm. In general, after the proximal segment is dilated, distal narrowing may resolve (5, 52). Distal dilatation beyond the A1 and proximal M2 segments should not be attempted with materials currently available.

Following angioplasty, an angiogram is again obtained to evaluate vessel caliber and determine whether structural damage has occurred to the vessels. In addition, this provides a base-line for subsequent care. The procedure usually takes 2–6 hours to perform, depending on the number and severity of vessels in spasm that require dilatation. At the completion of the procedure, the patient is returned to the intensive care unit. Hypervolemic therapy, calcium channel blockers, and intensive monitoring should be continued and repeat TCD and SPECT studies obtained. A follow-up angiogram is obtained 1 week later.

Results

Angioplasty for the treatment of symptomatic vasospasm is still in its infancy; despite this, generally favorable outcomes have been reported. The results of several large series are summarized in Table 6C.1. These data illustrate that angiographic resolution of vasospasm can be achieved in virtually all

vessels in which balloon dilatation is attempted. By contrast, untreated vessels remain in spasm for the usual course of 5–20 days. Follow-up angiograms, obtained immediately after the procedure and up to 18 months later, indicate that vessel injuries, including endothelial damage, intimal disruption, thrombosis, and dissection, are rarely encountered (11, 18, 20, 38, 39, 47). Furthermore, repeat angiographic evaluation demonstrates that the vessel caliber obtained by mechanical dilatation persists in both short- and long-term follow-up (Figs. 6C.3 and 6C.4) (11, 18, 20, 38, 39, 47).

In addition to the restoration of normal vessel caliber, improved angiographic perfusion is often observed following angioplasty. Both TCD (Fig. 6C.5) and SPECT (Fig. 6C.6) studies correlate with improved cerebral perfusion. Newell et al. (37) evaluated 31 patients undergoing angioplasty, using TCD assessment. Twenty-three patients demonstrated distinct clinical improvement. In all but one of the patients showing clinical improvement, TCD blood flow velocities decreased and remained below preangioplasty levels. By contrast, velocities continued to increase in untreated vessels, some of which became symptomatic at later times. Improvement in cerebral perfusion (as demonstrated by SPECT or xenon-133 evaluation), which correlates with clinical improvement, has been noted in the majority of patients undergoing angioplasty (27, 28, 31, 38).

TABLE 6C.1
Results of Angioplasty for Cerebral Vasospasm

Series	No. of Patients	No. of Vessels	Angiographic Improvement (%)	Clinical Improvement	Complications
Zubkov et al. (52)	33	105	99	Unknown	None from procedure, 21 deaths
Newell et al. (39)	10	33	100	8/10	1 branch occlusion, 2 rebleeds (unclipped aneurysms)
Brothers and Holgate (5)	4	27	100	4/4	
Nemoto et al. (36)	10	18	83	4/10	
Takahashi et al. (47)	22	48	100	14/20[a]	1 rebleed (unclipped aneurysm)
Konishi et al. (27)	8	19	100	5/8	1 rebleed (unclipped aneurysm)
Higashida et al. (20)[b]	28	99	100	17/28	Hemorrhagic infarct, 2 vessel ruptures (latex balloon)
Eskridge, 1992[c]	45	135	98	31/45	1 branch occlusion, 2 rebleeds, 1 vessel rupture

[a] Series included two asymptomatic patients.
[b] Includes 13 patients reported by Higashida et al. (18).
[c] Current series at the University of Washington (Seattle, WA); inlcudes 10 patients reported by Newell et al. (39).

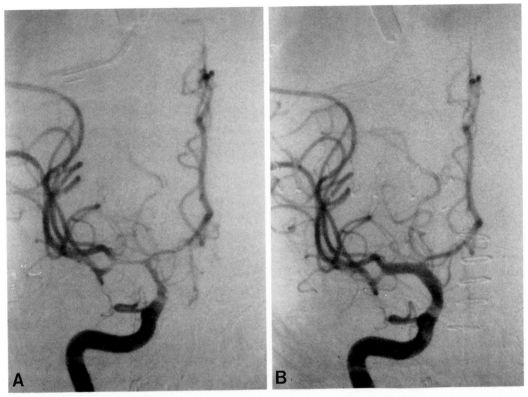

Figure 6C.3. (*A*) Right internal carotid angiogram obtained shortly after the patient developed a left hemiparesis, demonstrating severe vasospasm in the supraclinoid internal carotid, middle cerebral (M1), and anterior cerebral arteries. (*B*) Angiogram obtained following angioplasty. The normal diameters of the internal carotid and middle cerebral arteries have been restored. The patient's hemiparesis resolved over 30 min following angioplasty.

Approximately 60–70% of patients undergoing balloon dilatation for vasospasm demonstrate clinical improvement. The symptomatic improvement in this group of patients is particularly significant since nearly all had vasospasm that was refractory to other treatments. Furthermore, most patients in these series have sustained their improvements and continued to do well (11, 18, 20, 38, 39, 47). Amelioration of the neurological deficit has been generally observed within minutes to hours after the procedure, although it can be seen up to 48 hours later. Most studies suggest that the likelihood of reversing an ischemic deficit is greater with earlier treatment. Takahashi *et al.* (47) performed angioplasty in 22 patients; among 14 patients treated within 6 hours of the onset of symptoms, 11 made an excellent recovery and there were no reported deaths.

By contrast, of eight patients who underwent the procedure after >6 hours of ischemia, only two made an excellent recovery and three died. In most other series, 12–18 hours appeared to be the critical period that determined success (11, 20, 31, 38, 39). There is a suggestion that it is generally easier to dilate the vessel early in the course of vasospasm, thereby reducing the risk of vessel rupture. These results emphasize the need for early diagnosis of vasospasm.

Despite angiographic resolution of spasm, 30–40% of patients do not demonstrate clinical improvement, perhaps due to the presence of a completed infarct or intracranial hypertension (36). As discussed above, angioplasty after a delay of 48 hours from the onset of symptoms is usually associated with a poor clinical result (11, 20, 31). In addition, most of the patients who have failed

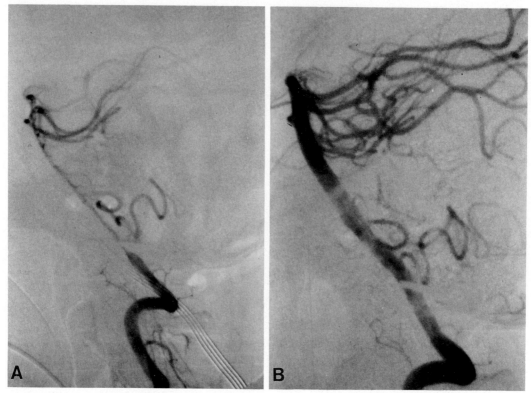

Figure 6C.4. (*A*) Lateral vertebrobasilar angiogram illustrating severe vasospasm in the basilar artery. (*B*) Angiogram following successful balloon dilatation, demonstrating a widely patent basilar artery; note the augmented flow throughout the basilar circulation.

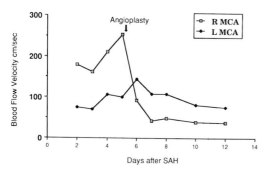

Figure 6C.5. Graph illustrating serial blood flow velocities measured by TCD. The patient developed a left hemiparesis and underwent angioplasty of the right internal carotid and middle cerebral arteries, with subsequent resolution of the neurological deficit. Following balloon dilitation (*arrow*) there was a dramatic and persistent decrease in velocities in the treated right middle cerebral artery (*R MCA*). By contrast, TCD velocities remained elevated in the untreated left middle cerebral artery (*L MCA*).

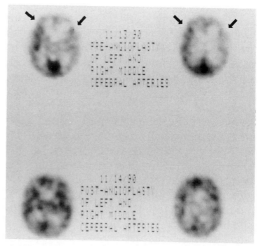

Figure 6C.6. SPECT scan before (*top*) and after (*bottom*) bilateral middle cerebral artery angioplasty, demonstrating resolution of bilateral perfusion defects (*arrows*).

angioplasty have been in poor-grade groups (Hunt and Hess grades IV and V). Therefore, the lack of clinical response may reflect the severity of the initial hemorrhage or may be due in part to the difficulty of diagnosing a new ischemic deficit in this subgroup of patients. Poor-grade patients are at very high risk for vasospasm; it is possible that these patients may benefit most from prophylactic vessel dilatation when noninvasive evidence of severe spasm is identified.

Complications

Complications resulting directly from transluminal angioplasty are uncommon. In general, complications result from three technical problems: 1) overdistention of the balloon, 2) distal balloon dilatation, or 3) angioplasty in the presence of an unclipped or inadequately clipped aneurysm. In most centers, these events have occurred early in the acquisition of experience with the procedure (11, 20, 37, 38). Initial promising reports describing angioplasty have generated widespread use of balloon dilatation for vasospasm, accompanied by anecdotal reports of fatalities ascribed to the technique. However, when the procedure is performed by properly trained and experienced individuals, it is a safe and effective therapeutic modality. As more individuals gain experience in the use of angioplasty, complication rates will likely decrease. The results compiled from several large series describing balloon dilatation for vasospasm after SAH indicate that complications are encountered in <5% of procedures (Table 6C.1). These complications include hemorrhage into an infarct (18, 20), vessel rupture (18, 20, 29), rebleeding from unclipped aneurysms (11, 38, 39, 47), and vessel occlusion (11, 38, 39).

The complications noted above have further defined specific indications for angioplasty. Higashida *et al.* (18) described one patient who developed a hemorrhage into a region of basal ganglion infarction 24 hours after vessel dilatation. Therefore, it is recommended that angioplasty should not be attempted if a cerebral infarct is identified on CT or magnetic resonance imaging scans, particularly if it is in the distribution of the vessel due to be dilated. By contrast, it may be safe to perform angioplasty if a small infarct in another vascular distribution is identified (5). Second, the presence of an unsecured ruptured aneurysm is cause for concern with angioplasty (11, 38, 39, 47). Rebleeding can occur both at the time of angioplasty and following the procedure. Hemorrhage in this setting may result indirectly from increased flow, rather than direct mechanical disruption of the aneurysm. Eskridge *et al.* (11) described fatal rupture of a posterior cerebral artery mycotic aneurysm 72 hours after dilatation of both internal carotid arteries. Therefore, it is critical to occlude the aneurysm responsible for the SAH before angioplasty is attempted. In addition, aneurysm occlusion must be confirmed by careful inspection of the postoperative angiogram. Linskey *et al.* (29) described fatal rupture of the intracranial internal carotid artery at the neck of an aneurysm, possibly related to an unclipped segment of the aneurysm. In this case, both fluoroscopic and histopathological examinations demonstrated that balloon dilatation did not displace the aneurysm clip blades. Experience with angioplasty in the presence of unsecured unruptured aneurysms is limited, but no hemorrhages have thus far been reported in this setting. Vessel rupture (recognized by a change in balloon configuration or dye extravasation) usually results from attempted distal dilatation or use of an inappropriate balloon. Higashida *et al.* (18, 20) described rupture of the internal carotid and posterior cerebral arteries during balloon dilatation with a latex balloon. When distal dilatation is attempted, the elongating effect of the balloon does not seem to provide protection against rupture (4). A single instance of delayed M2 branch occlusion 6 weeks following dilatation with a high-pressure balloon has been reported (11); damage to the endothelium may have predisposed the vessel to thrombosis in this case.

Conclusions

The overall results of angioplasty indicate that, in selected cases, balloon dilatation of arteries with delayed narrowing after SAH can offer marked improvement for patients with an ischemic deficit that is refractory to conventional modalities of therapy. Despite the success of this new technique, many issues remain unresolved. Little is known regarding the mechanism by which angioplasty affects cerebral arteries in spasm or the optimal time to offer treatment. The role for prophylactic angioplasty in patients with significant asymptomatic spasm remains uncertain. The patient with severe symptomatic spasm and an unclipped ruptured aneurysm presents a challenging clinical dilemma. Whether angioplasty affects only large-capacitance arteries at the circle of Willis or indirectly augments flow through smaller perforating arteries has not been determined. Similarly, it is not clear whether successful restoration of proximal flow by angioplasty always results in improved distal perfusion. Finally, new adjuncts to the endovascular treatment of vasospasm, such as local intra-arterial papaverine infusion (22), may provide additional means to treat these patients.

As further experience is accumulated, the role of angioplasty in vasospasm will be further defined and better understood. Current experience indicates that angioplasty is a viable therapeutic tool in the comprehensive management of SAH and can lead to dramatic neurological improvement in selected patients who otherwise would progress to a severe and disabling stroke or death.

REFERENCES

1. Barnwell, S. I., Higashida, R. T., Halbach, V. V., et al. Transluminal angioplasty of intracerebral vessels for cerebral arterial spasm: reversal of neurological deficits after delayed treatment. Neurosurgery 25:424–249, 1989.
2. Bevan, J. A., Bevan, R. D., and Frazee, J. G. Functional arterial changes in chronic cerebrovasospasm in monkeys: an in vitro assessment of the contribution of arterial narrowing. Stroke 18:472–481, 1987.
3. Block, P. C., Baughman, K. L., Pasternak, R. C., and Fallon, J. T. Transluminal angioplasty: correlation of morphologic and angiographic findings in an experimental model. Circulation 61:778–785, 1980.
4. Brothers, M. F., Hedlund, L. W., and Friedman, A. H. Arterial rupture during "distal" vasospasm angioplasty. Neuroradiology 33:S155, 1991.
5. Brothers, M. F., and Holgate, R. C. Intracranial angioplasty for treatment of vasospasm after subarachnoid hemorrhage: technique and modifications to improve branch access. AJNR 11:239–247, 1990.
6. Chavez, L., Takahashi, A., Yoshimoto, T., et al. Morphological changes in normal canine basilar arteries after transluminal angioplasty. Neurol. Res. 12:12–16, 1990.
7. Clower, B. R., Smith, R. R., Haining, J. L., et al. Constrictive endarteropathy following experimental subarachnoid hemorrhage. Stroke 12:501–508, 1981.
8. Davis, S. M., Andrews, J. T., Lichtenstein, M., et al. Correlations between cerebral arterial velocities, blood flow, and delayed ischemia after subarachnoid hemorrhage. Stroke 23:492–497, 1992.
9. Dotter, C. T., and Judkins, M. P. Transluminal treatment of arteriosclerotic obstruction: description of a new technique and a preliminary report of its application. Circulation 30:654–670, 1964.
10. Edwards, D. H., Byrne, J. V., and Griffith, T. M. The effect of chronic subarachnoid hemorrhage on basal endothelium-derived relaxing factor activity in intrathecal cerebral arteries. J. Neurosurg. 76:830–837, 1992.
11. Eskridge, J. M., Newell, D. W., Mayberg, M. R., and Winn, H. R. Update on transluminal angioplasty of vasospasm. Perspect. Neurol. Surg. 1:120–126, 1990.
12. Fukui, M. B., Johnson, D. W., Yonas, H., et al. Cerebral blood flow evaluation of delayed symptomatic cerebral ischemia after subarachnoid hemorrhage. AJNR 13:265–270, 1992.
13. Grosset, D. G., Straiton, J., du Trevou, M., and Bullock, R. Prediction of symptomatic vasospasm after subarachnoid hemorrhage by rapidly increasing transcranial Doppler velocity and cerebral blood flow changes. Stroke 23:674–679, 1992.
14. Gruntzig, A., and Hopff, H. Perkutane Rekanalisation chronischer arterieller Verschlusse mit einem neuen Dilatationskatheter Modifikation der Dotter-technik. Dtsch. Med. Wochenschr. 99:2502–2510, 1974.
15. Gruntzig, A. R., Senning, A., and Seigenthaler, W. E. Non-operative dilation of coronary artery stenosis: percutaneous transluminal coronary angioplasty. N. Engl. J. Med. 301:61–68, 1979.
16. Haley, E. C., Jr., Kassell, N. F., and Torner, J. C. The International Cooperative Study on the timing of aneurysm surgery: the North American experience. Stroke 23:205–214, 1992.
17. Heros, R. C., Zervas, N. T., and Varsos, V. G. Cerebral vasospasm after subarachnoid hemorrhage: an update. Ann. Neurol. 14:599–608, 1983.
18. Higashida, R. T., Halbach, V. V., Cahan, L. D., et al. Transluminal angioplasty for treatment of intracranial arterial vasospasm. J. Neurosurg. 71:648–653, 1989.
19. Higashida, R. T., Halbach, V. V., Dormandy, B., et al. New microballoon device for transluminal angioplasty of intracranial arterial vasospasm. AJNR 11:233–238, 1990.
20. Higashida, R. T., Halbach, V. V., Dowd, C. F., et al. Intravascular balloon dilatation therapy for intracranial arterial vasospasm: patient selection, technique, and clinical results. Neurosurg. Rev. 15:89–95, 1992.
21. Hughes, J. T., and Schianchi, P. M. Cerebral artery spasm: a histological study at necropsy of the

blood vessels in cases of subarachnoid hemorrhage. J. Neurosurg. 48:515–525, 1978.

22. Kassell, N. F., Helm, G., Simmons, N., et al. Treatment of cerebral vasospasm with intra-arterial papaverine. J. Neurosurg. 77:848–852, 1992.

23. Kassell, N. F., Sasaki, T., Colohan, A. R. T., et al. Cerebral vasospasm following aneurysmal subarachnoid hemorrhage. Stroke 16:562–572, 1985.

24. Kassell, N. F., Torner, J. C., Haley, E. C., et al. The International Cooperative Study on the Timing of Aneurysm Surgery. J. Neurosurg. 73:18–46, 1990.

25. Kim, P., Sundt, T. M., Jr., and Vanhoutte, P. M. Alterations in endothelium-dependent responsiveness of the canine basilar artery after subarachnoid hemorrhage. J. Neurosurg. 69:239–246, 1988.

26. Kim, P., Sundt, T. M., Jr., and Vanhoutte, P. M. Alterations of mechanical properties in canine basilar arteries after subarachnoid hemorrhage. J. Neurosurg. 71:430–436, 1989.

27. Konishi, Y., Maemura, E., Shiota, M., et al. Treatment of vasospasm by balloon angioplasty: experimental studies and clinical experiences. Neurol. Res. 14:273–281, 1992.

28. Lewis, D. H., Hsu, S., Eskridge, J., et al. Brain SPECT and transcranial Doppler ultrasound in vasospasm-induced delayed cerebral ischemia after subarachnoid hemorrhage. J. Stroke Cerebrovasc. Dis. 2:12–21, 1992.

29. Linskey, M. E., Horton, J. A., Rao, G. R., and Yonas, H. Fatal rupture of the intracranial carotid artery during transluminal angioplasty for vasospasm induced by subarachnoid hemorrhage. J. Neurosurg. 74:985–990, 1991.

30. Macdonald, R. L., Weir, B. K. A., Runzer, T. D., et al. Etiology of cerebral vasospasm in primates. J. Neurosurg. 75:415–424, 1991.

31. Mayberg, M., Eskridge, J., Newell, D., and Winn, H. R. Angioplasty for symptomatic vasospasm. In: Cerebral Vasospasm, edited by K. Sano, K. Takakura, N. F. Kassell, and T. Sasaki, pp. 433–436. University of Tokyo Press, Tokyo, 1990.

32. Mayberg, M. R., Okada, T., and Bark, D. H. The significance of morphological changes in cerebral arteries after subarachnoid hemorrhage. J. Neurosurg. 72:626–633, 1990.

33. McBride, W., Lange, R. A., and Hillis, L. D. Restenosis after successful coronary angioplasty: pathophysiology and prevention. N. Engl. J. Med. 318:1734–1737, 1988.

34. Miller, F. Elastomers in medicine: selecting the right elastomer for the right application. Elastomerics 117:15–20, 1985.

35. Minami, N., Tani, E., Maeda, Y., et al. Effects of inhibitors of protein kinase C and calpain in experimental delayed cerebral vasospasm. J. Neurosurg. 76:111–118, 1992.

36. Nemoto, S., Abe, T., Tanaka, H., et al. Percutaneous transluminal angioplasty for cerebral vasospasm following subarachnoid hemorrhage. In: Cerebral Vasospasm, edited by K. Sano, K. Takakura, N. F. Kassell, and T. Sasaki, pp. 437–439. University of Tokyo Press, Tokyo, 1990.

37. Newell, D. W., Eskridge, J., Lewis, D., and May-berg, M. Transcranial Doppler usefulness in balloon angioplasty. In: Advances in Neurosurgery, edited by M. Oka et al., pp. 101–103. Elsevier Science Publishers, New York, 1992.

38. Newell, D. W., Eskridge, J., Mayberg, M., et al. Endovascular treatment of intracranial aneurysms and cerebral vasospasm. Clin. Neurosurg. 39:348–360, 1992.

39. Newell, D. W., Eskridge, J. M., Mayberg, M. R., et al. Angioplasty for the treatment of symptomatic vasospasm following subarachnoid hemorrhage. J. Neurosurg. 71:654–660, 1989.

40. Pickard, J. D., Murray, G. D., Illingworth, R., et al. Effect of oral nimodipine on cerebral infarction and outcome after subarachnoid haemorrhage: British Aneurysm Nimodipine Trial. Br. Med. J. 298:636–642, 1989.

41. Pile-Spellman, J., Berenstein, A., Bun, T., et al. Angioplasty of canine cerebral vessels. AJNR 8:938, 1987.

42. Pistoia, F., Horton, J. A., Sekhar, L., and Horowitz, M. Imaging of blood flow changes following angioplasty for treatment of vasospasm. AJNR 12:446–448, 1991.

43. Seiler, R. W., and Newell, D. W. Subarachnoid hemorrhage and vasospasm. In: Transcranial Doppler, edited by D. W. Newell, and R. Aaslid, pp. 101–107. Raven Press, New York, 1992.

44. Smith, R. R., Clower, B. R., Grotendorst, G. M., et al. Arterial wall changes in early human vasospasm. Neurosurgery 16:171–176, 1985.

45. Smith, R. R., Connors, J. J., III, Yamamoto, Y., and Bernanke, D. H. Balloon angioplasty for vasospasm: theoretical and practical considerations. In: Cerebral Vasospasm, edited by K. Sano, K. Takakura, N. F. Kassell, and T. Sasaki, pp. 415–420. University of Tokyo Press, Tokyo, 1990.

46. Solomon, R. A., Fink, M. E., and Lennihan, L. Early aneurysm surgery and prophylactic hypervolemic hypertensive therapy for the treatment of aneurysmal subarachnoid hemorrhage. Neurosurgery 23:699–704, 1988.

47. Takahashi, A., Yoshoto, T., Mizoi, K., et al. Transluminal balloon angioplasty for vasospasm after subarachnoid hemorrhage. In: Cerebral Vasospasm, edited by K. Sano, K. Takakura, N. F. Kassell, and T. Sasaki, pp. 429–432. University of Tokyo Press, Tokyo, 1990.

48. Wilkins, R. H. Attempts at prevention of treatment of intracranial arterial spasm: an update. Neurosurgery 18:808–825, 1986.

49. Wright, J. Rubber in medicine: the past, present, the future. Elastomerics 114:28–32, 1982.

50. Yamamoto, Y., Smith, R. R., and Bernanke, D. H. Mechanisms of action of balloon angioplasty in cerebral vasospasm. Neurosurgery 30:1–6, 1992.

51. Yonas, H., Sekhar, L., Johnson, D. W., et al. Determination of irreversible ischemia by xenon-enhanced computed tomographic monitoring of cerebral blood flow in patients with symptomatic vasospasm. Neurosurgery 24:368–372, 1992.

52. Zubkov, Y. N., Nikiforov, B. M., and Shustin, V. A. Balloon catheter technique for dilatation of constricted cerebral arteries after aneurysmal SAH. Acta Neurochir. (Wien) 70:65–79, 1984.

Management of Vasospasm: Tissue Plasminogen Activator

R. LOCH MACDONALD, M.D., BRYCE K. WEIR, M.D.

INTRODUCTION

Cerebral vasospasm can be detected on 30–70% of cerebral angiograms obtained from patients who have suffered aneurysmal subarachnoid hemorrhage (SAH) within the prior 4–14 days (32). Previous work indicated that neurological deficit resulting in morbidity and mortality develops in 20–30% of patients with angiographic vasospasm (32). In the most recent Cooperative Study on the Timing of Aneurysm Surgery, however, vasospasm caused only 13.5% of death and disability following aneurysmal SAH (37). There are no data to suggest that the incidence of angiographic vasospasm has changed, and the decrease in complications due to vasospasm is usually attributed to advances in treatment, including nimodipine and hypervolemic/hemodilution/hypertensive therapy.

Another promising therapy for vasospasm is subarachnoid clot lysis with tissue plasminogen activator (t-PA) after early surgical clipping of the ruptured aneurysm(s) (18). This represents a major departure from previous management of aneurysmal SAH, when antifibrinolytic drugs were given to retard clot lysis and keep the hole in the ruptured aneurysm sealed until surgery could be performed 1 or 2 weeks later (28, 33, 72, 73). Prevention of vasospasm in experimental animals by rapid lysis and clearance of SAH by t-PA has been reported (18, 21) and has profound implications for the etiology and pathogenesis, in addition to the treatment, of vasospasm. These findings may be generalizable to humans.

Etiology and Pathogenesis of Vasospasm

The most common cause of cerebral vasospasm is SAH from an intracranial aneurysm (75). SAH from other causes may also be associated with vasospasm (78). Cerebral angiography and transcranial Doppler measurements in head trauma patients, who commonly have SAH, suggest that vasospasm develops in 5–34% of severe head injuries and has a time course similar to that of spasm after aneurysmal SAH (74, 75, 78). Cases of vasospasm following surgery in the basal cisterns for unruptured aneurysms or pituitary adenomas are most likely due to unrecognized bleeding into the subarachnoid space. Many of these cases were reported prior to the computed tomography (CT) era, and postoperative bleeding into the basal cisterns cannot be ruled out (78). Inflammatory processes in the subarachnoid space may be associated with "vasospasm." Arterial narrowing in purulent or tuberculous meningitis is due to inflammatory cell infiltration and damage to subarachnoid arteries and probably differs in mechanism from vasospasm after aneurysmal SAH (75).

Further evidence for a role of subarachnoid blood clot in generating vasospasm may be derived from CT studies of aneurysmal SAH. Following SAH, the best predictors of the location and severity of vasospasm are the location and quantity of subarachnoid blood as seen on CT scan within 5 days of hemorrhage (26, 41). Arteries coursing through thick blood clots are most prone to narrow several days after SAH. In other conditions associated with SAH, such as head injury, thick basal cistern blood clots rarely develop and, hence, severe symptomatic vasospasm is less common. This fact, in addition to the observation that patients rarely develop vasospasm if their aneurysm ruptures primarily into the cerebral parenchyma or ventricular system (26), supports the theory that spasmogenic compounds are released from subarachnoid blood clot and are responsible for maintaining arterial narrowing. The actual rupture of the aneurysm or accompanying acute increase in intracranial pressure seems less likely to be important in vasospasm, because these events accompany other processes not associated with vasospasm, such as arterial dissection and intraparenchymal aneurysm rupture.

The mechanism by which subarachnoid blood causes vasospasm remains a matter of conjecture, although there is a large body of literature implicating spasmogens released by red blood cell breakdown (19, 44, 75). Studies in experimental animals show that vasospasm does not develop if blood devoid of erythrocytes is placed in the subarachnoid space (15, 45). Intact erythrocytes are not particularly vasoactive but, upon lysis, red cells release a spasmogenic chemical which, when analyzed, appears to be oxyhemoglobin or a related peptide (44, 62). Oxyhemoglobin appears in cerebrospinal fluid (CSF) of humans during the time vasospasm develops (7, 44, 70). Oxyhemoglobin causes many of the changes which have been documented to occur in vasospastic arteries, such as vasoconstriction, generation of endothelin, free radical production and lipid peroxidation, release of eicosanoids, inhibition of endothelium-dependent relaxation, and damage to smooth muscle cells and perivascular nerves (18, 44). Oxyhemoglobin is metabolized by cells in the subarachnoid space to bilirubin, another potentially spasmogenic substance (14, 55). When SAH is created in monkeys by placing blood clot in the subarachnoid space, vasospasm does not develop if the clot is removed before red cell lysis occurs to any substantial degree (about 48 hours) (31, 48). Antifibrinolytic drugs increase the risk of ischemic complications after aneurysmal SAH, presumably because more subarachnoid erythrocytes remain in the subarachnoid space to hemolyze and release oxyhemoglobin (28, 72, 76).

Treatment of Vasospasm

From the above discussion, it is evident that vasospasm depends to a substantial degree on the presence of subarachnoid blood. Vasospasm could theoretically be prevented by removing subarachnoid blood clot before the onset of vasospasm. Experiments in monkeys and rats support this hypothesis (6, 31, 48). With humans, Suzuki *et al.* (66) operated within the first days after aneurysm rupture to try to lessen the risk of rebleeding. They also recognized that removal of subarachnoid blood clots within 48 hours of SAH might prevent vasospasm. Analysis of their cases showed that early aneurysm surgery with aggressive removal of clots decreased the percentage of patients developing vasospasm to about 35% if clot removal was performed within 48 hours. If clot removal was performed >2 days after SAH, about 62% of patients developed vasospasm. Other surgeons substantiated these results, although opinion about the efficacy of early clot removal is not unanimous (35, 47, 50, 69, 77). Ohta *et al.* (50) reported that extensive clot evacuation within 48 hours of SAH reduced the severity of vasospasm but did not prevent it. In their hands, thorough cisternal dissection and clot removal sometimes aggravated brain swelling and actually induced more bleeding. A better method of riding the subarachnoid space of blood was required, and the use of genetic engineering to produce pure human recombinant t-PA may have answered that need.

Once established, narrowed vasospastic arteries are usually considered to be temporarily fixed in diameter and unresponsive to infusion of vasodilator drugs (75). There is, however, evidence that at least part of the narrowing is pharmacologically reversible with, for example, nicardipine (27). Intra-arterial infusions of papaverine also have been effective in some cases (36). The arteries may also be mechanically dilated by balloon angioplasty (19). Cerebral blood flow can also be augmented by a combination of increasing blood pressure, decreasing blood viscosity, and increasing circulating blood volume (19). Finally, nimodipine could exert its beneficial effects in SAH by protecting neurons from ischemia or by dilating the microcirculation, although it does not seem to affect the lumen size of the major basal arteries of the circle of Willis (52).

Fibrinolysis, Coagulation, and Subarachnoid Clot Clearance

Blood coagulation prevents bleeding by producing a fibrin plug which forms a matrix and enmeshes red blood cells, platelets, and white blood cells. The body also possesses a fibrinolytic system capable of breaking down blood clots (11). Plasmin or fibrinolysin, the major fibrinolytic enzyme, breaks fibrin down into several fibrin degradation products (11). Plasmin circulates in blood as an inactive proenzyme, plasminogen, which is activated by plasminogen activators. Plasmin has a high affinity for fibrin and is incorporated into the fibrin blood clot as it forms. Plasminogen activators are of two types, tissue-type (t-PA) and urokinase-type (urokinase) plasminogen activators. Like plasmin, t-PA has specific affinity for fibrin and is partly sequestered in clotting blood. t-PA is relatively inefficient at activating free plasminogen unless the t-PA binds to fibrin, where it rapidly forms plasmin from plasminogen already incorporated into the clot. Some types of urokinase have lower affinity for fibrin and may theoretically activate circulating as well as fibrin-bound plasminogen. Under normal circumstances, however, fibrinolysis is effectively localized to the area of blood clotting by the enhanced activity of t-PA when it is bound to fibrin and by circulating plasmin inactivators such as α_2-antiplasmin which inactivate any plasmin which diffuses away from the clot. Plasmin inactivators are not attracted to fibrin and tend to remain in circulating blood.

Endothelial cells, which are thought to be the main source of t-PA, release t-PA in response to many stimuli, including injury, ischemia, and occlusion (11, 21, 33). Very little free t-PA circulates in blood, because it is rapidly bound to a circulating inhibitor protein and cleared by the liver. Urokinase-type plasminogen activators have a variety of sources, including fibroblasts, pneumocytes, and epithelial cells. Leukocytes and platelets may also be sources of plasminogen activators (21, 33).

The blood-brain barrier normally excludes higher molecular weight serum proteins from CSF, resulting in levels of coagulation proteins in normal CSF about 1–5% as high as those in blood (18, 54). With breakdown of the blood-brain barrier, serum proteins including coagulation cascade components leak into the CSF. Normal CSF is generally believed to be devoid of plasminogen activators and fibrinolytic activity (53, 54, 67). At least one investigator, however, has reported that normal CSF contains a complete plasminogen activator (13). The leptomeninges contain more fibrinolytic activity than does CSF or brain tissue and, with the hemogenic meningitis accompanying SAH, they may act as a source of plasminogen activators (54). Furthermore, the breakdown of the blood-brain barrier, with leaching of protein into CSF, after SAH allows some t-PA into CSF, although t-PA is present in only very low levels in blood (11, 18, 54).

Aneurysmal SAH introduces variable amounts of blood into the subarachnoid space and produces some degree of leakiness of the blood-brain barrier (57). If bleeding is minimal, the clotting proteins in whole blood are diluted out by CSF and clotting does not occur. With large volumes of SAH, coagulation is activated by collagen fibers in the arachnoid trabeculae and by release of thromboplastins from brain tissue and the meninges (18, 38). Plasminogen which flowed into the subarachnoid space with the arterial blood is incorporated into the fibrin clot. A small amount of t-PA accompanies the SAH and more may be released from inflamed meningeal vessels, breakdown of the blood-brain barrier, platelets deposited with the SAH, and leukocytes associated with the inflammatory response (18, 53, 67, 71). Despite the multiple potential sources of t-PA, fibrinolysis in the subarachnoid space after SAH is limited (33). The appearance of fibrin degradation products in CSF after SAH suggests that minimal subarachnoid clot fibrinolysis occurs (29, 33, 64, 73). This has been studied largely in relation to the use of antifibrinolytic drugs to prevent lysis of clot sealing the rent in the aneurysm. Vermuelen *et al.* (73) studied patients treated with antifibrinolytic drugs after SAH and found that, despite a reduction in aneurysm rebleeding with antifibrinolytic agents, CSF fibrin degradation products were not decreased. They believed that, in the second week after SAH, fibrin degradation products represented damage to the blood-CSF barrier rather than subarachnoid fibrinolysis. In support of this, fibrin degradation products increase in CSF in other inflammatory conditions of the subarachnoid space, such as bacterial and viral meningitis (10). It is not surprising that CSF fibrin degradation product levels correlate with the development of vasospasm after SAH, because vasospasm, the volume of subarachnoid clot, and meningeal inflammation are all correlated (29). They probably do not play a direct role in generating vasospasm, particularly in view of literature reviewed below suggesting that vasospasm can be prevented by augmenting subarachnoid fibrinolysis, a process which should elevate CSF fibrin degradation products (29).

Because of the relative inefficiency of fibrinolysis in the subarachnoid space, other mechanisms are probably more important in the removal of subarachnoid blood. Studies of the subarachnoid space after experimental SAH show that about 75% of erythrocytes injected into the cisterna magna of dogs become trapped in the arachnoid cisterns (1). The remaining red cells, floating free in CSF, are cleared through the arachnoid villi and possibly along cranial nerve arachnoid sheaths and into cervical lymphatics. The relative contributions of these mechanisms have not been established in animals and appear to be species dependent (4, 16, 60, 61). Even less is known in humans. The majority of the red cells, imprisoned in the complex arachnoid cisterns, hemolyze slowly in the hypotonic CSF, spilling their spasmogenic contents next to the major subarachnoid cerebral arteries. Spectrophotometric examinations of CSF after SAH show that oxyhemoglobin, a major protein within erythrocytes, appears within hours, peaks 3–4 days after SAH, and disappears by about the 10th day after SAH (7, 70). Higher and more prolonged oxyhemo-

globin levels occur with larger SAH and, therefore, with vasospasm. The emergence of methemoglobin, the oxidation product of oxyhemoglobin, lags several days behind. Bilirubin appears at 3–4 days and disappears by 3 weeks (7).

Another mechanism by which clotted blood is removed after SAH is phagocytosis by macrophages which probably traverse the inflammed leptomeningeal vessels and infiltrate the clot (5, 18, 21, 30). Phagocytosis of erythrocytes by macrophages and arachnoid cells may also take place in the arachnoid villi (4). Again, little is known about the roles of these processes in humans.

If t-PA or urokinase were instilled into the subarachnoid space shortly after SAH, plasminogen in the clot would be activated. Fibrinolysis would free erythrocytes and release them into CSF. Experimental data reviewed in the next section indicate that clots are rapidly lysed with intrathecal t-PA, although the sites and mechanisms of removal of these cells from CSF, presumably involving arachnoid villi and cranial nerve sheaths, remain undefined. The dependence of vasospasm on subarachnoid clot suggests, however, that if, red blood cells disappear from the subarachnoid space before they are lysed vasospasm may be prevented.

Experimental Studies

Several investigators have experimented with the use of thrombolysis to prevent vasospasm. Findlay and colleagues, however, provided the major impetus for the use of fibrinolytic therapy, based on experiments conducted in the monkey model of SAH and vasospasm developed at the University of Alberta. In 1988, they conducted a blinded, randomized, placebo-controlled trial of intrathecal t-PA in this model (24). Twenty-four monkeys underwent placement of 5 ml of blood clot against the middle cerebral artery. Twelve received placebo and 12 received three t-PA injections of 0.5 mg each, via an Ommaya reservoir and subarachnoid catheter. All placebo-treated animals had subarachnoid clot present 7 days later, and all developed moderate to severe vasospasm (>30% reduction in vessel caliber). Eleven animals treated with t-PA had complete clot clearance by day 7 after SAH and vasospasm did not develop to a significant degree, except in the anterior cerebral artery, where it was mild (14% vessel caliber reduction). Systemic fibrinolysis did not develop, there were no intracranial bleeding complications, and intrathecal t-PA did not cause meningoencephalitis. The dose of t-PA was estimated from studies *in vitro* which found that 1 mg of t-PA completely lyzed 5 ml of whole clotted monkey blood. A higher dose of t-PA was administered *in vivo* to account for dilution by CSF after intrathecal injection. Subsequently, the safety of intrathecal thrombolytic therapy was tested in the same model by administering a much larger intrathecal dose (10 mg of t-PA) after craniectomy, arachnoid dissection, and subarachnoid clot placement (20). Seven days later, clot clearance was complete and vasospasm was prevented, without producing alterations in systemic coagulation parameters or inflammation in the subarachnoid space. Two monkeys developed minor wound hemorrhages, however, which persisted for 24 hours. The effect of time of administration of t-PA after SAH in the monkey model was then assessed (22). Thirty monkeys were randomly allocated into five equal groups to receive 0.75 mg of intrathecal t-PA at 0, 24, 48, or 72 hours after subarachnoid clot placement; the fifth group underwent subarachnoid clot placement only. If t-PA was given between 0 and 48 hours after clot placement, vasospasm was prevented, whereas at 72 hours significant arterial narrowing was noted, although to a milder degree than seen in controls. The safety and efficacy of t-PA demonstrated in these studies in the monkey model led these investigators to use t-PA in humans.

Other investigators have experimented with thrombolysis after SAH. Kennady (40) is recognized as the first to instill a fibrinolytic agent into the subarachnoid space. He labeled erythrocytes with a radioactive tracer and injected them into the cisterna magna of dogs. Clearance of blood from CSF could be augmented by adding fibrinolysin (t-PA) to the irrigating solution. Angiography was not done. Peterson *et al.* (51), working on the premise that degeneration of clotted subarachnoid blood somehow caused vasospasm, administered a mixture of streptokinase and streptodornase to cats who had undergone injection of blood into the cisterna magna 1 hour earlier. When animals were allowed to survive for 4 hours, complete clot lysis was observed in the absence of subarachnoid inflammation. If the animals were observed for 24 or more hours, severe malaise, opisthotonic posturing, and shallow rapid breathing developed and pathological examination of the brains showed diffuse meningoencephalitis. Angiography was not done. Espinosa *et al.* (17), believing that the inflammation might be due to streptodornase, conducted a trial of intracisternal streptokinase to lyse subarachnoid blood clot and prevent vasospasm in a dog model of SAH. This regimen was not effective, because significant vasospasm developed in both streptokinase- and saline-treated animals.

Alksne *et al.* (2) studied the effect of intrathecal plasmin on proliferative vascular changes in subarachnoid arteries of pigs subjected to SAH. At the time of killing, 10 days after intrathecal injection of plasmin or saline, all animals demonstrated complete subarachnoid clot clearance. Plasmin-treated animals, however, had less severe intimal proliferation and fewer necrotic smooth muscle cells in the basilar arteries than did animals given intrathecal saline. Angiography was not done and, since none of the animals had clot remaining at 10 days, the effect of plasmin on clot lysis could not be assessed. The authors subsequently reported on the time course of the effect of intracisternal plasmin in the pig model (3). A correlation was present between increasing time from SAH to plasmin injection and worsening intimal proliferation.

Further evidence of the efficacy of t-PA against experimental vasospasm was obtained by Seifert *et al.* (58) in a study using the double-hemorrhage dog model of SAH. Intracisternal t-PA (25 μg) prevented angiographic vasospasm, cleared subarachnoid clot, and diminished electron microscopic evidence of vascular damage. These authors suggested that t-PA be incorporated into the clinical armamentarium against vasospasm. Yamakawa *et al.* (80), using the same model, found that 25 μg of t-PA partially prevented vasospasm and that doses as high as 250 μg were necessary to reliably lyse clot and prevent spasm.

Clinical Studies of t-PA

Published case series of patients with aneurysmal SAH treated with t-PA are summarized in Table 6D.1 Lamond and Alksne (43) administered 25–50 mg of t-PA to eight poor-grade patients operated upon early after aneurysmal SAH. Clot clearance was observed at 24 and 48 hours in two cases each. Three patients developed vasospasm, and this was symptomatic in one. Three patients had good outcomes, two were left in poor condition, one patient died, and the fate of the other two cases was not stated. Tanabe *et al.* (68) treated 12 patients with varying doses of intracisternal t-PA, amikacin, and "CBPC." All patients had Fisher grade 3 SAH on CT scan (26) and were clinically of grade 2 or 3, according to the scale of Hunt and Kosnik (34). From 10 to 75 mg of t-PA were injected into the basal cisterns over several days, as guided by the color of CSF drainage from a cisternal catheter. There was one case of symptomatic vasospasm. The authors stated that simultaneous administration of intravenous tranexamic acid prevented subgaleal hematoma formation in their last two cases. Seven patients eventually required permanent CSF diversion, and overall outcome was described as excellent in 11 cases and fair in one.

Mizoi *et al.* (46) studied 10 patients with SAH graded as 3 by the Fisher scale on CT scan (26). From the published CT scans, some patients appeared to have associated intracerebral hemorrhages. Bilateral craniotomy was performed and multiple subarachnoid catheters were placed for subsequent daily infusions of t-PA, in total doses between 4 and 26 mg over up to 9 days. Based on detailed angiographic, CT, and clinical follow-up, no patient developed vasospasm or delayed ischemic neurological deficit and there were no hemorrhagic complications attributed to t-PA. There were four good and six excellent outcomes. Fifteen patients were operated upon within 48 hours of SAH by Findlay *et al.* (23). Most were of grades 3–5 (12), and 13 patients had diffuse or localized thick subarachnoid hematomata (Fisher grade 3). Tissue plasminogen activator was given as a single intraoperative intracisternal bolus injection of 7.5–15 mg. Only one patient did not have complete clot clearance on CT scan 24 hours later. This patient, who went on to die, developed the only case of symptomatic vasospasm in the series. The remaining patients had good recoveries (12 cases) or were moderately (one case) or severely (one case) disabled. Complications included one larger extradural hematoma requiring surgery and resulting in permanent morbidity. There was no evidence of systemic fibrinolysis. The method of t-PA administration which was settled upon involved giving 10 mg of t-PA in the basal cisterns after clipping of the aneurysm. The t-PA was allowed to diffuse through the subarachnoid space and bind to the fibrin clot for 15 min, after which the subarachnoid cisterns were irrigated with 1–2 liters of saline to wash away the unbound t-PA. It was hoped that this method would prevent free t-PA from leaking out through the dura closure and causing bleeding. With this system, which is much simpler than several other published procedures, clot clearance, for which excellent documentation was provided, was rapid and the results were comparable to those in other series.

Ten patients with thick subarachnoid clots after aneurysmal SAH were treated with between 1.5 and 5 mg of intracisternal t-PA (82). In five cases, a subarachnoid catheter was left in place for repeated administration of small doses (0.5 mg) of t-PA. A smaller dose was used after patients treated with 5 mg developed local bleeding complications. Mild to moderate vasospasm developed in nine patients. Overall outcome was classified as good in six cases, moderately disabled in two cases, and dead in two cases. Cisternal and ventricular CSF t-PA levels were measured, and cisternal levels were found to be much higher. Support for use of small doses of t-PA was suggested by observations that cisternal levels of t-PA 6 hours after administration of 5 mg t-PA were about 7–70 times higher than necessary for systemic fibrinolysis.

Ohman *et al.* (49) treated 30 patients consecutively with t-PA. Ten patients each received direct intracisternal applications of 3,

TABLE 6D.1
Summary of Reports of Patients Treated with t-PA for Prevention of Vasospasm after SAH

Authors	No. of Cases	Admission Grade	CT Grade	SAH to Surgery	t-PA Dose	Clot Clearance	Patients developing Vasospasm		Complications	Outcome and Comments
							Angiographic	Clinical		
Lamond and Alksne (43)	8	Botterell (8) 3 and 4	a	a	25–50 mg intraoperatively	≤24 hours (n = 2), ≤48 hours (n = 2)	3	1	None requiring surgery	3 good, 2 poor, 1 death
Tanabe et al. (68)	12	Hunt and Kosnik (34) 2 (n = 8), 3 (n = 4)	Fisher grade 3 (26)	≤48 hours	10–70 mg over 1–4 days	a	4	1	3 subgaleal hematomas, ? hemorrhagic infarct	11 excellent, 1 good, 7 shunted
Findlay et al. (23)	15	WFNS[b] (12) 2 (n = 1), 3 (n = 5), 4 (n = 8), 5 (n = 1)	Diffuse thick, 11; diffuse thin, 2; localized thick, 2	≤48 hours	7.5–15 mg intraoperatively	≤24 hours (n = 14)	9	1	1 extradural hematoma	12 good, 1 moderate disability, 1 severe disability, 1 death
Mizoi et al. (46)	10	Hunt and Kosnik 2 (n = 5), 3 (n = 4), 4 (n = 1)	Fisher grade 3	≤48 hours	4–26 mg over 2–9 days	a	1	0	None	6 excellent, 4 good, bilateral craniotomy, multiple catheters
Zabramski et al. (82)	10	Hunt and Kosnik 3 (n = 7), 4 (n = 3)	Fisher grade 3	≤72 hours	1.5–5 mg over ≤48 hours postoperatively	a	10	a	Incisional bleeding in 4 patients, 1 extra-axial hematoma	6 good, 2 moderate disability, 2 deaths; CSF t-PA levels
Ohman et al. (49)	30	Hunt and Kosnik 1 (n = 11), 2 (n = 14), 3 (n = 3), 4 (n = 2)	Diffuse severe, 10; thick, 10; thin, 10.	≤72 hours	3–13 mg intraoperatively	≤24 hours (n = 12)	16	1	Subgaleal hematoma, facial bruising in 21 cases, extradural hematoma, ? increase in 1 intracerebral hemorrhage	21 good, 7 moderate disability, 1 severe disability, 1 death; dosage study
Stolke and Seifert (65)	20	a	Fisher grade 3	≤72 hours	10 mg intraoperatively	Usually within 3 days	a	1	None	16 good recovery, 2 moderate disability, 2 deaths

a Information not provided.
b WFNS, World Federation of Neurological Surgeons SAH scale (12).

10, or 13 mg of t-PA after early surgery for clipping of their aneurysms. Severe vasospasm did not occur, and there was a decline in the severity of vasospasm with increasing t-PA dose. Only one of 30 patients developed delayed cerebral ischemia. Wound swelling and hematoma were common and sometimes extensive, although they always resolved without sequelae. Outcomes at 3 months were similar between groups.

A series of 20 patients was reported by Stolke and Seifert (65). All patients had thick subarachnoid clots, surgery within 72 hours of ictus, and 10 mg of t-PA instilled into the cisterns after aneurysm clipping. Unlike other series, angiography was not mandatory during the time of vasospasm. Instead, transcranial Doppler ultrasound results were presented. One patient died of delayed deterioration attributed to vasospasm. There were no complications due to t-PA, and these authors noted that increased Doppler velocities frequently developed, suggesting that some degree of vasospasm was present. They recommended that more rapid and complete blood removal, which presumably would entirely prevent vasospasm, might require higher drug doses or multiple postoperative cisternal t-PA injections.

In summary, at least 105 patients have been treated with t-PA after SAH (Table 6D.1). The majority had diffuse or localized thick subarachnoid hematomata and, hence, were in higher clinical grades. A variety of doses and administration regimens were reported. Overall, however, the incidence of severe and symptomatic vasospasm was about 5%. Mild or moderate arterial narrowing was more frequent, occurring in about 50% of cases. Although concurrent control patients were not reported, these results are remarkably better than those, for example, for the patients with thick SAH included in a study of Nimodipine (52). Ninety-four percent of those patients developed vasospasm and in 61% it was severe and diffuse. Furthermore, the overall outcome for patients treated with t-PA was better than that for this "historical control" group. Mortality due to t-PA did not occur, and morbid complications developed in about 3%. With these favorable safety and efficacy studies, a prospective, double-blind,

placebo-controlled trial of t-PA for prevention of vasospasm has been started.

Figures 6D.1 and 6D.2 compare the CT scans and angiograms of two patients, one of whom received t-PA and who did not develop significant vasospasm.

Clinical Studies of Urokinase

As discussed above, there are two classes of enzymes which activate plasminogen, tissue-type and urokinase-type plasminogen activators. Prior to the availability of genetically engineered, human, recombinant, tissue-type plasminogen activator, investigators in Japan administered urokinase intracisternally to patients with aneurysmal SAH. There should be no theoretical differences between the thrombolytic activities of t-PA and urokinase. One advantage of t-PA, however, may be the differing affinities of t-PA and some of the urokinase plasminogen activators for fibrin (11, 81). Some urokinases may indiscriminately activate circulating plasminogen in the absence of fibrin. Activation of plasminogen by t-PA, however, is much more efficient in the presence of fibrin, so that systemic or diffuse fibrinolysis may be a lesser problem with t-PA than with urokinase. This may or may not be important, because circulating blood contains plasmin inhibitors, which are also found in low levels in CSF and which may rapidly inactivate free plasmin in CSF (11). In treatment of myocardial ischemia due to coronary atherothrombosis, t-PA and another fibrinolytic agent, streptokinase, are equally efficacious (59).

Kodama et al. (42) reported results of cisternal irrigation therapy with urokinase and ascorbic acid in 106 patients with aneurysmal SAH. Ascorbic acid was added to the irrigating solution to oxidize ferrous iron in oxyhemoglobin to harmless ferric iron (methemoglobin). All patients had thick subarachnoid clots, most were of clinical Hunt and Kosnik grades 2 and 3, and the mean interval from SAH to surgery was 20 hours. A solution of urokinase and ascorbic acid was infused through two subarachnoid catheters for a mean of 10 days. Symptomatic vasospasm was remarkably rare (2.8% of patients), and most patients had excellent or good outcomes. The authors commented

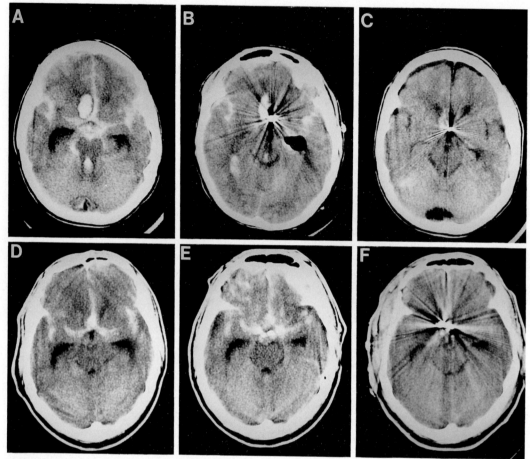

Figure 6D.1. Photographs of CT scans of two patients with diffuse thick SAH. Similar amounts of SAH were present within 24 hours of ictus (*A*, patient 1, *D*, patient 2). Patient 1 received 10 mg of intracisternal t-PA after aneurysm clipping and demonstrated extensive clot clearance, particularly in the midline basal cisterns, on CT scan 24 hours later (*B*). In the second patient, who did not receive t-PA, more clot remained 24 hours later (*E*). By 4 days after SAH, subarachnoid blood was cleared completely in patient 1 (*C*), whereas the basal cisterns still contained resolving blood (*F*) in patient 2.

that the disadvantage of this therapy was the long duration and great energy and care necessary to operate the irrigation system. Kawamura and Ikeda (39) reported on the use of a similar postoperative cisternal irrigation system containing urokinase and sodium nitrite, with favorable results. Although these studies were not prospective, blinded, or controlled, the incidence of symptomatic vasospasm was greatly reduced, compared with historical controls, suggesting that a therapeutic effect is present with urokinase.

A randomized, double-blind comparison of urokinase and t-PA was conducted using

the monkey model of SAH. Urokinase (200,000 units) and t-PA (2 mg) were equally effective at clearing subarachnoid clot, although neither dose significantly ameliorated vasospasm. Urokinase did not inflame the subarachnoid space or leptomeninges. The minimal effect on vasospasm was thought to be due to multiple factors, including small numbers of animals in each group and low dosages of urokinase and t-PA employed. Further work is required before conclusions can be drawn about the relative merits of t-PA *vs.* urokinase.

Cisternal irrigation or drainage without urokinase may also wash away enough spas-

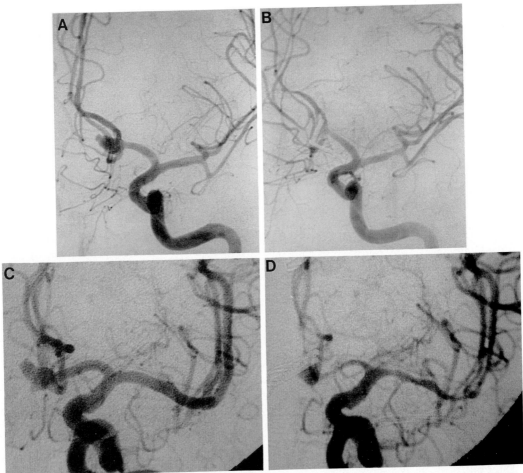

Figure 6D.2. Photographs of angiograms of two patients with diffuse thick SAH (same patients as Fig. 6D.1). The admission left internal carotid angiograms, obtained within 24 hours of SAH, showed that both patients had anterior communicating artery aneurysms (*A*, patient 1; *C*, patient 2). There was no vasospasm. Four days later, left internal carotid angiogram of patient 1 (*B*), who received t-PA, showed only mild vasospasm of proximal middle and anterior cerebral arteries. There was more marked narrowing, however, of the pericallosal arteries. In contrast, left internal carotid angiogram of patient 2 (*D*), who did not receive t-PA, showed severe vasospasm (>50% reduction in lumen diameter) of proximal middle and anterior cerebral arteries as well as narrowing of more peripheral branches. Transluminal angioplasty was performed to prevent cerebral infarction.

mogenic clot from the basal cisterns to diminish vasospasm. Yagishita *et al.* (79) randomly used cisternal drainage in 47 of 205 aneurysmal SAH patients. Although the groups were not comparable in risk factors important for vasospasm, when stratification was made for amount of SAH on CT scan cisternal drainage significantly decreased the incidence of symptomatic vasospasm. In a nonrandomized, nonblinded comparison of cisternal irrigation with and without urokinase, there was no significant

difference between groups in the incidence of delayed ischemic neurological deficits or in outcome (56). These results are consistent with several laboratory investigations showing that irrigating the subarachnoid space may remove enough blood to diminish the incidence and severity of vasospasm (6, 77). A blinded, placebo-controlled trial of t-PA will establish whether cisternal irrigation which is done after intrathecal fibrinolytic therapy accounts for the effect of t-PA on vasospasm.

Fibrinolytic Therapy and Hydrocephalus

In one series of patients admitted with ruptured aneurysms, 29% had acute ventricular enlargement and 20% eventually required some type of shunting procedure (63). The incidence of late hydrocephalus after aneurysmal SAH is increased further by the use of antifibrinolytic agents (28). Presumably, the fibrotic reaction to subarachnoid clot in the subarachnoid space and arachnoid villi is worsened by preventing the already poor ability of CSF to activate fibrinolysis and remove the irritating fibrin-bound erythrocytes. Follow-up on humans with aneurysmal SAH treated with the fibrinolytic agent t-PA is too short and incomplete to indicate whether a reduction in posthemorrhage hydrocephalus will occur. In one series, seven of 12 t-PA-treated patients required CSF shunting (68).

The effect of intracisternal t-PA on acute hydrocephalus was studied after SAH in 11 cats (9). CSF outflow resistance was markedly elevated immediately after SAH, and this increase could be reversed by intracisternal injection of t-PA. Development of late hydrocephalus was not assessed in this acute-phase experiment. Intraventricular injection of t-PA into a patient with intraventricular hemorrhage has been reported (23, 25). Findlay et al. (25) clipped an anterior cerebral artery aneurysm in a patient with SAH and intraventricular hemorrhage. Intracranial pressure rose following surgery and became difficult to control. Intraventricular hematoma was lyzed with 8 mg of intraventricular t-PA, resulting in normalization of the intracranial pressure.

Current Role of Fibrinolytic Therapy

The use of t-PA for prevention of vasospasm following aneurysmal SAH remains experimental. A multicenter randomized study has been started in which patients will be randomized to receive t-PA or placebo at the time of aneurysm clipping, which must be within 72 hours of SAH. All aneurysms must be obliterated, and there are a variety of exclusion criteria. Patients with small intraparenchymal hematomas have received t-PA without precipitating intracranial hemorrhage. Since treatment advances have lowered the incidence of symptomatic vasospasm to about 13%, a properly conducted clinical trial is necessary to ensure that the potential benefits of subarachnoid clot lysis outweigh any risks associated with t-PA. It may be, for example, that nimodipine, hypervolemic/hemodilution/hypertensive therapy, and timely transluminal angioplasty will be as effective as clot lysis for patients at low risk for vasospasm and t-PA will be indicated only in more severe cases of SAH.

Many other questions remain about the use of t-PA for aneurysmal SAH. Little is known about the fate of the erythrocytes released after clot lysis. The effect of t-PA on hydrocephalus and its efficacy in comparison to other thrombolytic agents have not been thoroughly investigated. Plasminogen activators have other biological effects, on, for example, tissue development, cell migration, and remodelling. A major source of t-PA is endothelium, a tissue which is being recognized as important in vasospasm, suggesting that t-PA may affect vasospasm in ways other than by clot lysis (81).

REFERENCES

1. Adams, J. E., and Prawirohardjo, S. Fate of red blood cells injected into cerebrospinal fluid pathways. Neurology 9:561–564, 1959.
2. Alksne, J. F., Branson, P. J., and Bailey, N. Modification of experimental post-subarachnoid hemorrhage vasculopathy with intracisternal plasmin. Neurosurgery 19:20–25, 1986.
3. Alksne, J. F., Branson, P. J., and Bailey, N. Modification of experimental post-subarachnoid hemorrhage vasculopathy with intracisternal plasmin. Neurosurgery 23:335–337, 1988.
4. Alksne, J. F., and Lovings, E. T. The role of the arachnoid villus in the removal of red blood cells from the subarachnoid space: an electron microscopic study in the dog. J. Neurosurg. 36:192–200, 1972.
5. Alpers, B. J., and Forster, F. M. The reparative processes in subarachnoid hemorrhage. J. Neuropathol. Exp. Neurol. 4:262–268, 1945.
6. Aydin, I. H., and Onder, A. The effect of very early cisternal irrigation on basilar artery spasm after SAH in the rat model. Acta Neurochir. (Wien) 113:69–73, 1991.
7. Barrows, L. J., Hunter, F. T., and Banker, B. Q. The nature and clinical significance of pigments in the cerebrospinal fluid. Brain 78:59–80, 1955.
8. Botterell, E. H., Lougheed, W. M., Scott, J. W., and Vandewater, S. L. Hypothermia and interrup-

tion of carotid, or carotid and vertebral circulation, in the surgical management of intracranial aneurysms. J. Neurosurg. *13:*1–42, 1956.

9. Brinker, T., Seifert, V., and Stolke, D. Effect of intrathecal fibrinolysis on cerebrospinal fluid absorption after experimental subarachnoid hemorrhage. J. Neurosurg. *74:*789–793, 1991.

10. Brueton, M. J., Breeze, G. R., and Stuart, J. Fibrin-fibrinogen degradation products in cerebrospinal fluid. J. Clin. Pathol. *29:*341–344, 1976.

11. Collen, D., and Lijnen, H. R. The fibrinolytic enzyme system. In: *Fibrinolysis and the Central Nervous System,* edited by R. Sawaya, pp. 14–25. Hanley and Belfus, Philadelphia, 1990.

12. Drake, C. G. Report of World Federation of Neurological Surgeons Committee on a universal subarachnoid hemorrhage grading scale. J. Neurosurg. *68:*985–986, 1988.

13. Dube, R. K., Dube, B., Ahmad, N., *et al.* Presence of complete plasminogen activator in the cerebrospinal fluid. Indian J. Med. Res. *69:*474–475, 1979.

14. Duff, T. A., Feilbach, J. A., Yusuf, Q., and Scott, G. Bilirubin and the induction of intracranial arterial spasm. J. Neurosurg. *69:*593–598, 1988.

15. Duff, T. A., Louie, J., Feilbach, J. A., and Scott, G. Erythrocytes are essential for development of cerebral vasculopathy resulting from subarachnoid hemorrhage in cats. Stroke *19:*68–72, 1988.

16. Dupont, J. R., Van Wart, C. A., and Kraintz, L. The clearance of major components of whole blood from cerebrospinal fluid following simulated subarachnoid hemorrhage. J. Neuropathol. Exp. Neurol. *20:*450–455, 1961.

17. Espinosa, F. J., Gross, P. M., Tao, J. H., *et al.* Streptokinase in the treatment of cerebral vasospasm after subarachnoid hemorrhage in dogs (Abstract). Can. J. Neurol. Sci. *19:*272, 1992.

18. Findlay, J. M. Intrathecal thrombolytic therapy in the prevention of vasospasm following subarachnoid hemorrhage. In: *Fibrinolysis and the Central Nervous System,* edited by R. Sawaya, pp. 203–212. Hanley and Belfus, Philadelphia, 1990.

19. Findlay, J. M., Macdonald, R. L., and Weir, B. K. A. Current concepts of pathophysiology and management of cerebral vasospasm following aneurysmal subarachnoid hemorrhage. Cerebrovasc. Brain Metab. Rev. *3:*336–361, 1991.

20. Findlay, J. M., Weir, B. K. A., Gordon, P., *et al.* Safety and efficacy of intrathecal thrombolytic therapy in a primate model of cerebral vasospasm. Neurosurgery *24:*491–498, 1989.

21. Findlay, J. M., Weir, B. K. A., Kanamaru, K., *et al.* Intrathecal fibrinolytic therapy after subarachnoid hemorrhage: dosage study in a primate model and review of the literature. Can. J. Neurol. Sci. *16:*28–40, 1989.

22. Findlay, J. M., Weir, B. K. A., Kanamaru, K., *et al.* The effect of timing of intrathecal fibrinolytic therapy on cerebral vasospasm in a primate model of subarachnoid hemorrhage. Neurosurgery *26:*201–206, 1990.

23. Findlay, J. M., Weir, B. K. A., Kassell, N. F., *et al.* Intracisternal recombinant tissue plasminogen activator after aneurysmal subarachnoid hem-

orrhage. J. Neurosurg. *75:*181–188, 1991.

24. Findlay, J. M., Weir, B. K. A., Steinke, D., *et al.* Effect of intrathecal thrombolytic therapy on subarachnoid clot and chronic vasospasm in a primate model of SAH. J. Neurosurg. *69:*723–735, 1988.

25. Findlay, J. M., Weir, B. K. A., and Stollery, D. E. Lysis of intraventricular hematoma with tissue plasminogen activator: case report. J. Neurosurg. *74:*803–807, 1991.

26. Fisher, C. M., Kistler, J. P., and Davis, J. M. Relation of cerebral vasospasm to subarachnoid hemorrhage visualized by computed tomographic scanning. Neurosurgery *6:*1–9, 1980.

27. Flamm, E. S., Adams, H. P., Jr., Beck, D. W., *et al.* Dose-escalation study of intravenous nicardipine in patients with aneurysmal subarachnoid hemorrhage. J. Neurosurg. *68:*393–400, 1988.

28. Fodstad, H., and Ljunggren, B. Antifibrinolytic drugs in subarachnoid hemorrhage. In: *Fibrinolysis and the Central Nervous System,* edited by R. Sawaya, pp. 257–273. Hanley and Belfus, Philadelphia, 1990.

29. Guggiari, M., Dagreou, F., Rivierez, M., *et al.* Prediction of cerebral vasospasm: value of fibrinogen degradation products (FDP) in the cerebrospinal fluid (CSF) for prediction of vasospasm following subarachnoid haemorrhage due to a ruptured aneurysm. Acta Neurochir. (Wien) *73:*25–33, 1984.

30. Hammes, E. M., Jr. Reaction of the meninges to blood. Arch. Neurol. Psychiatry *52:*505–514, 1944.

31. Handa, Y., Weir, B. K. A., Nosko, M., *et al.* The effect of timing of clot removal on chronic vasospasm in a primate model. J. Neurosurg. *67:*558–564, 1987.

32. Heros, R. C., Zervas, N. T., and Varsos, V. Cerebral vasospasm after subarachnoid hemorrhage: an update. Ann. Neurol. *14:*599–608, 1983.

33. Hindersin, P., Heidrich, R., and Endler, S. Hemostasis in cerebrospinal fluid: basic concept of antifibrinolytic therapy of subarachnoid haemorrhage. Acta Neurochir. (Wien) *34*(suppl.)*:*1–77, 1984.

34. Hunt, W. E., and Kosnik, E. J. Timing and perioperative care in intracranial aneurysm surgery. Clin. Neurosurg. *21:*79–84, 1974.

35. Inagawa, T., Yamamoto, M., and Kamiya, K. Effect of clot removal on vasospasm. J. Neurosurg. *72:*224–230, 1990.

36. Kaku, Y., Yonekawa, Y., Tsukahara, T., and Kazekawa, K. Percutaneous transluminal angioplasty for vasospasm: superselective intra-arterial infusion of papaverine (Abstract). Neuroradiology *33*(suppl.)*:*S155, 1991.

37. Kassell, N. F., Torner, J. C., Haley, E. C., Jr., *et al.* The International Cooperative Study on the Timing of Aneurysm Surgery. 1. Overall management results. J. Neurosurg. *73:*18–36, 1990.

38. Kasuya, H., Shimizu, T., Okada, T., *et al.* Activation of the coagulation system in the subarachnoid space after subarachnoid haemorrhage: serial measurement of fibrinopeptide A and bradykinin of cerebrospinal fluid and plasma in

patients with subarachnoid haemorrhage. Acta Neurochir. (Wien) 91:120–125, 1988.

39. Kawamura, T., and Ikeda, S. Prevention of vasospasm by cisternal and ventricular administrations of urokinase and sodium nitrite. In: *Cerebral Vasospasm*, edited by K. Sano, K. Takakura, N. F. Kassell, and T. Sasaki, pp. 326–327. University of Tokyo Press, Tokyo, 1990.

40. Kennady, J. C. Investigations of the early fate and removal of subarachnoid blood. Pacif. Med. Surg. 75:163–168, 1967.

41. Kistler, J. P., Crowell, R. M., Davis, K. R., *et al.* The relation of cerebral vasospasm to the extent and location of subarachnoid blood visualized by CT scan: a prospective study. Neurology 33:424–436, 1983.

42. Kodama, N., Sasaki, T., Kawakami, M., *et al.* Prevention of vasospasm: cisternal irrigation therapy with urokinase and ascorbic acid. In: *Cerebral Vasospasm*, edited by K. Sano, K. Takakura, N. F. Kassell, and T. Sasaki, pp. 292–296. University of Tokyo Press, Tokyo, 1990.

43. Lamond, R. G., and Alksne, J. F. Cisternal rt-PA administration in aneurysmal subarachnoid hemorrhage. In: *Cerebral Vasospasm*, edited by K. Sano, K. Takakura, N. F. Kassell, and T. Sasaki, pp. 302–303. University of Tokyo Press, Tokyo, 1990.

44. Macdonald, R. L., and Weir, B. K. A. A review of hemoglobin and the pathogenesis of cerebral vasospasm. Stroke 22:971–982, 1991.

45. Mayberg, M. R., Okada, T., and Bark, D. H. The role of hemoglobin in arterial narrowing after subarachnoid hemorrhage. J. Neurosurg. 72:634–640, 1990.

46. Mizoi, K., Yoshimoto, T., Fujiwara, S., *et al.* Prevention of vasospasm by clot removal and intrathecal bolus injection of tissue-type plasminogen activator: preliminary report. Neurosurgery 28:807–813, 1991.

47. Mizukami, M., Kawase, T., Usami, T., and Tazawa, T. Prevention of vasospasm by early operation with removal of subarachnoid blood. Neurosurgery 10:301–307, 1982.

48. Nosko, M., Weir, B. K. A., Lunt, A., *et al.* Effect of clot removal at 24 hours on chronic vasospasm after SAH in the primate model. J. Neurosurg. 66:416–422, 1987.

49. Ohman, J., Servo, A., and Heiskanen, O. Effect of intrathecal fibrinolytic therapy on clot lysis and vasospasm in patients with aneurysmal subarachnoid hemorrhage. J. Neurosurg. 75:197–201, 1991.

50. Ohta, H., Ito, Z., Yasui, N., and Suzuki, A. Extensive evacuation of subarachnoid clot for prevention of vasospasm: effective or not? Acta Neurochir. (Wien) 63:111–116, 1982.

51. Peterson, E. W., Choo, S. H., Lewis, A. J., *et al.* Lysis of blood clot and experimental treatment of subarachnoid hemorrhage. In: *Cerebral Arterial Spasm*, edited by R. H. Wilkins, pp. 625–627. Williams and Wilkins, Baltimore, 1980.

52. Petruk, K. C., West, M., Mohr, G., *et al.* Nimodipine treatment in poor grade aneurysm patients: results of a multicenter, double-blind, placebo-

controlled trial. J. Neurosurg. 68:505–517, 1988.

53. Porter, J. M., Acinapura, A. J., Kapp, J. P., and Silver, D. Fibrinolysis in the central nervous system. Neurology 19:47–52, 1969.

54. Ramo, O. J., Sawaya, R., and Zuccarello, M. Fibrinolytic enzymes in the central nervous system. In: *Fibrinolysis and the Central Nervous System*, edited by R. Sawaya, pp. 26–32. Hanley and Belfus, Philadelphia, 1990.

55. Roost, K., Pimstone, N. R., Diamond, I., and Schmid, R. The formation of cerebrospinal fluid xanthochromia after subarachnoid hemorrhage: enzymatic conversion of hemoglobin to bilirubin by the arachnoid and choroid plexus. Neurology 22:973–977, 1972.

56. Saito, I., Segawa, H., Mishima, K., and Sano, K. Prevention of postoperative vasospasm by cisternal irrigation with and without urokinase. In: *Cerebral Vasospasm*, edited by K. Sano, K. Takakura, N. F. Kassell, and T. Sasaki, pp. 297–301. University of Tokyo Press, Tokyo, 1990.

57. Sasaki, T., Kassell, N. F., Yamashita, M., *et al.* Barrier disruption in the major cerebral arteries following experimental subarachnoid hemorrhage. J. Neurosurg. 63:433–440, 1985.

58. Seifert, V., Eisert, W., Stolke, D., and Goetz, C. Efficacy of single intracisternal bolus injection of recombinant tissue plasminogen activator to prevent delayed cerebral vasospasm after experimental subarachnoid hemorrhage. Neurosurgery 25:590–598, 1989.

59. Sherry, S., and Marder, V. J. Streptokinase and recombinant tissue plasminogen activator (rt-PA) are equally effective in treating acute myocardial infarction. Ann. Int. Med. 114:417–423, 1991.

60. Simmonds, W. J. The absorption of blood from the cerebrospinal fluid in animals. Aust. J. Exp. Biol. Med. Sci. 30:261–270, 1952.

61. Simmonds, W. J. The absorption of labelled erythrocytes from the subarachnoid space in rabbits. Aust. J. Exp. Biol. Med. Sci. 31:77–84, 1953.

62. Sonobe, M., and Suzuki, J. Vasospasmogenic substance produced following subarachnoid hemorrhage, and its fate. Acta Neurochir. (Wien) 44:97–106, 1978.

63. Steinke, D., Weir, B., and Disney, L. Hydrocephalus following aneurysmal subarachnoid haemorrhage. Neurol. Res. 9:3–9, 1987.

64. Steinmetz, H., and Grote, E. The fibrinolytic activity of cerebrospinal fluid after subarachnoid hemorrhage. Neurol. Res. 5:59–65, 1983.

65. Stolke, D., and Seifert, V. Single intracisternal bolus of recombinant tissue plasminogen activator in patients with aneurysmal subarachnoid hemorrhage: preliminary assessment of efficacy and safety in an open clinical study. Neurosurgery 30:877–881, 1992.

66. Suzuki, J., Onuma, T., and Yoshimoto, T. Results of early operations on cerebral aneurysms. Surg. Neurol. 11:407–412, 1979.

67. Takashima, S., Koga, M., and Tanaka, K. Fibrinolytic activity of human brain and cerebrospinal fluid. Br. J. Exp. Pathol. 50:533–539, 1969.

68. Tanabe, T., Arimitsu, M., Morimoto, M., *et al.*

The effect of intracranial thrombolytic therapy with tissue-type plasminogen activator on subarachnoid clot and chronic cerebral vasospasm. In: *Cerebral Vasospasm*, edited by K. Sano, K. Takakura, N. F. Kassell, and T. Sasaki, pp. 321–323. University of Tokyo Press, Tokyo, 1990.

69. Taneda, M. Effect of early operation for ruptured aneurysms on prevention of delayed ischemic symptoms. J. Neurosurg. *57:*622–628, 1982.

70. Tourtellotte, W. W., Metz, L. N., Bryan, E. R., and DeJong, R. N. Spontaneous subarachnoid hemorrhage: factors affecting the rate of clearing of the cerebrospinal fluid. Neurology *14:*301–306, 1964.

71. Tovi, D., Nilsson, I. M., and Thulin, C. A. Fibrinolytic activity of the cerebrospinal fluid after subarachnoid haemorrhage. Acta Neurol. Scand. *49:*1–9, 1973.

72. Vermeulen, M., Lindsay, K. W., Murray, G. D., et al. Antifibrinolytic treatment in subarachnoid hemorrhage. N. Engl. J. Med. *311:*432–437, 1984.

73. Vermeulen, M., van Vliet, H. H. D. M., Lindsay, K. W., et al. Source of fibrin/fibrinogen degradation products in the CSF after subarachnoid hemorrhage. J. Neurosurg. *63:*573–577, 1985.

74. Weber, M., Grolimund, P., and Seiler, R. Evaluation of posttraumatic cerebral blood flow velocities by transcranial Doppler ultrasonography. Neurosurgery *27:*106–112, 1990.

75. Weir, B. *Aneurysms Affecting the Nervous System.* Williams and Wilkins, Baltimore, 1987.

76. Weir, B. Antifibrinolytics in subarachnoid hemorrhage. Do they have a role? No. Arch. Neurol. *44:*116–118, 1987.

77. Weir, B. The effect of clot removal on cerebral vasospasm. In: *Cerebral Vasospasm. Neurosurgery Clinics of North America*, edited by M. Mayberg, pp. 377–385. Saunders, Philadelphia, 1990.

78. Wilkins, R. H. Cerebral vasospasm in conditions other than subarachnoid hemorrhage. In: *Cerebral Vasospasm. Neurosurgery Clinics of North America*, edited by M. Mayberg, pp. 329–334. Saunders, Philadelphia, 1990.

79. Yagishita, T., Nukui, H., Kaneko, M., et al. Effect of continuous cisternal drainage for symptomatic vasospasm. In: *Cerebral Vasospasm*, edited by K. Sano, K. Takakura, N. F. Kassell, and T. Sasaki, pp. 311–313. University of Tokyo Press, Tokyo, 1990.

80. Yamakawa, K., Nakagomi, T., Sasaki, T., et al. Effect of single intracisternal bolus injection of tissue plasminogen activator on cerebral vasospasm after subarachnoid hemorrhage. In: *Cerebral Vasospasm*, edited by K. Sano, K. Takakura, N. F. Kassell, and T. Sasaki, pp. 328–329. University of Tokyo Press, Tokyo, 1990.

81. Yamamoto, Y., Clower, B., Haining, J. L., and Smith, R. R. Effect of tissue plasminogen activator on intimal platelet accumulation in cerebral arteries after subarachnoid hemorrhage in cats. Stroke *22:*780–784, 1991.

82. Zabramski, J. M., Spetzler, R. F., Lee, K. S., et al. Phase I trial of tissue plasminogen activator for the prevention of vasospasm in patients with aneurysmal subarachnoid hemorrhage. J. Neurosurg. *75:*189–196, 1991.

CHAPTER 7

Neuroradiological Aspects of Aneurysms

ROBERT W. TARR, M.D., JOHN PERL II, M.D., THOMAS J. MASARYK, M.D.

INTRODUCTION

Aneurysm rupture is the most common cause of nontraumatic subarachnoid hemorrhage (SAH), accounting for approximately 70–80% of cases (88). The incidence of aneurysm rupture in North America is approximately 28,000/year, and the rate of mortality within the first 30 days following rupture is approximately 50% (10). Estimates of the prevalence of unruptured aneurysms in the general population, based on autopsy series, vary between 0.2% and 9% (3, 34, 39, 49). The yearly bleed rate for unruptured aneurysms is approximately 3% (38). The rebleed rate for untreated ruptured aneurysms is approximately 20% within the first 2 weeks (40).

Intracranial aneurysms are most commonly intradural but may arise in extradural locations. Intradural aneurysms most commonly arise at proximal arterial branch points in the vicinity of the circle of Willis. The most common aneurysm locations are the junction of the anterior cerebral artery and arterior communicating artery (30%), the junction of the internal carotid artery and the posterior communicating artery (25%), the middle cerebral artery bi/trifurcation (15%), and the internal carotid artery terminus or carotid-opthalmic artery junction (15%). Approximately 15% of aneurysms arise within the vertebro-basilar system, most commonly at the terminus of the basilar artery or the origin of the posterior inferior cerebellar artery (50). Extradural aneurysms most commonly arise within the cavernous sinus and usually present clinically with cranial nerve palsies or carotid cavernous fistulae rather than SAH.

Aneurysms may be classified morphologically into two general categories: 1) saccular, *i.e.*, an exophytic aneurysm arising from a parent artery, and 2) fusiform, *i.e.*, an aneurysmal dilation of the parent artery. Intracranial aneurysms are most commonly saccular and are felt to have a combined congenital and developmental etiology arising from a combination of intrinsic arterial wall weakness and hemodynamic stress (13, 80). Fusiform aneurysms tend to be secondary to atherosclerosis or arterial dissection. Aneurysms in peripheral or unusual locations may be caused by vasculitis, neoplasm, sepsis, or trauma. In addition, aneurysms may be associated with systemic conditions such as polycystic kidney disease, fibromuscular dysplasia, Marfan's syndrome, or cerebral arteriovenous malformation (6, 31, 53, 57).

Neuroimaging in aneurysm assessment is an important and growing area of radiology. Applications include high-risk or suspected population screening, diagnosis of SAH following rupture, preoperative aneurysm definition, intraoperative assessment, and the detection of complications of aneurysm rupture. In addition, neurointerventional endovascular techniques such as balloon test occlusion, intraoperative aneurysm decompression, parent artery occlusion, endovascular aneurysm occlusion, and angioplasty of vasospasm may be used in appropriate circumstances.

Aneurysm Screening

The role of neuroimaging in screening for aneurysms is evolving at the current time. Certainly, conventional angiography remains the gold standard for aneurysm detection and definition. Noninvasive screening techniques are, however, available for appropriate indications. Patients who have systemic disorders which predispose them to aneurysm formation (6, 31, 53, 57), those with a strong family history of intracranial aneurysms (6, 7, 43, 63, 72), and patients with atypical migraines, changes in patterns of chronic headache, or subacute presentation of sudden onset of headache without documentation of SAH may be candidates for noninvasive aneurysm screening techniques. At this time, however, reliance on noninvasive techniques to screen for intracranial aneurysms must be tempered by the level of clinical suspicion. Noninvasive imaging modalities which can be used to screen for aneurysms include computed tomography (CT), magnetic resonance (MR) imaging (MRI), and MR angiography (MRA).

CT

CT can routinely detect aneurysms larger than 0.7 mm to 1 cm in size; however, the sensitivity and specificity of CT for detecting small aneurysms vary widely in the literature and are undefined at the current time (1, 92). Several techniques can be used to optimize the ability of CT to detect an aneurysm: 1) bolus contrast injection, 2) dynamic scan sequence, and 3) use of thin slices (1.5–2.0 mm) and minimal interslice gap (1.5–2.0 mm) through the circle of Willis (73). Limitations of CT for aneurysm detection include variable resolution on different scanners and single-plane acquisition. The typical CT appearance of an aneurysm is a rounded area of hyperdensity in close proximity to the circle of Willis on the uncontrasted scan which demonstrates contrast enhancement (Fig. 7.1). The entire aneurysm lumen or only a portion of it may be enhanced. The enhancement may be central due to enhancement of a patent central lumen with peripheral thrombus, peripheral due to enhancement of organizing thrombus via the peripheral vasa vasorum, or a combination of both. Calcification may be seen on the uncontrasted CT. The calcification is typically curvilinear and peripheral (73) (Fig. 7.2).

MRI

Conventional spin-echo MRI has several advantages, compared to CT, for aneurysm detection. These include excellent contrast between different tissues and multiplanar acquisition capabilities. Fast-flowing blood is typically seen as a area of absent signal (signal void) on routine spin-echo sequences. This is due to the fact that blood product protons which are excited by the initial 90-degree radiofrequency pulse move out of the imaging plane by the time the readout portion of the MRI sequence is being performed. In addition, fast flow creates random motion of protons, which results in loss of proton phase coherence and causes loss of signal intensity (9).

The typical MRI appearance of an aneurysm is a rounded area of signal void in close proximity to the circle of Willis (Fig. 7.3). The size of a nonthrombosed aneurysm as demonstrated by MRI correlates well with the angiographic size (84). MRI has the advantages of demonstrating portions of the aneurysm which are thrombosed and not visualized at angiography. These thrombosed regions have intermediate or high signal intensity and are typically peripheral in location (Fig. 7.4). Thus, MRI is often more accurate than angiography for determining the true size of the aneurysm. Intermediate or high signal intensity within the aneurysm may be caused by factors other than thrombosis, such as slow inflow/outflow or flow turbulence.

Compared to CT, MRI provides a much better delineation of the location of an aneurysm as well as its relationship to adjacent neural structures (2, 8, 61, 81). Often the artery from which the aneurysm arises is identified on MRI, although the neck of the aneurysm may not be (68).

There are several factors which may result in the false-positive interpretation of an aneurysm on MRI. Transmitted vascular pulsations may result in adjacent areas of cerebrospinal fluid (CSF) hypointensity due to signal mismapping from phase shift (12). Also, pneumatized anterior clinoid processes demonstrate signal void and may mimic a paraclinoid aneurysm (22). In addition, as with CT, aneurysms of <7–10 mm may not be detected on MRI due to the

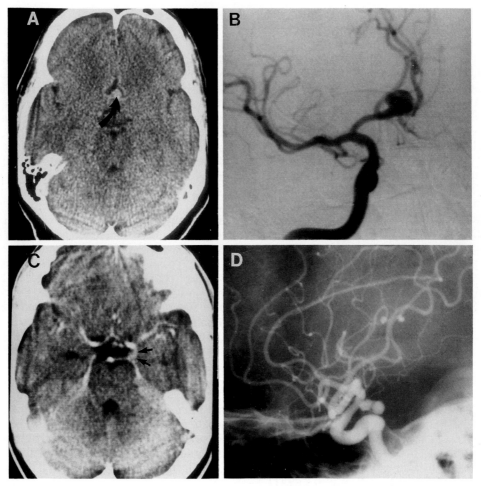

Figure 7.1. (*A*) Uncontrasted CT scan demonstrates a round hyperdense lesion (*curved arrow*), consistent with an anterior communicating aneurysm. (*B*) Anterior oblique right internal carotid artery angiogram demonstrates the anterior communicating aneurysm. (*C*) Contrast-enhanced CT scan through the circle of Willis of a different patient demonstrates an oblong enhanced lesion (*arrows*), consistent with a posterior communicating aneurysm. (*D*) Lateral left internal carotid artery angiogram demonstrates the posterior communicating aneurysm.

interslice gap on most conventional spin-echo images.

MRA

Three-dimensional (3D) time-of-flight (TOF) MRA is a rapidly evolving technique which is currently at the stage of clinical evolution. In general, 3D TOF MRA utilizes the inflow of fully magnetized protons into an imaging volume generated by gradient-echo techniques. The fully magnetized protons in flowing blood thus have much higher signal intensity, compared to partially mag-

netized stationary protons within the imaging volume. A computerized reconstruction algorithm such as maximum intensity projection can be used to subtract background stationary tissue, allowing visualization of vascular structures alone. The vascular distributions can then be displayed in a 3D format with continuous rotating capabilities. Thus, an optimal projection can be chosen which demonstrates the anatomy of the origin of the aneurysm. This information can be used alone or to plan projections for conventional angiography. Saturation pulses over selected vascular distributions may be

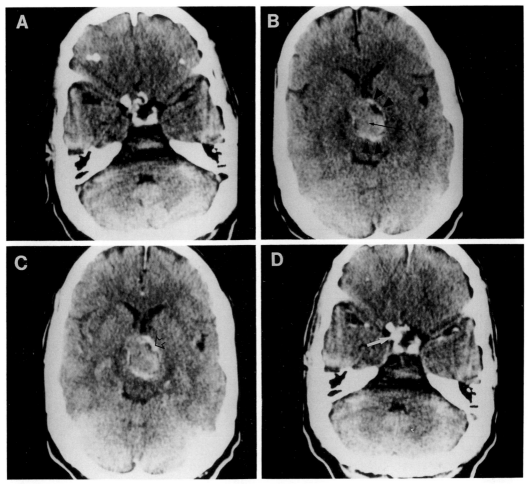

Figure 7.2. (*A* and *B*) Unenhanced CT scan (A and B) through a right internal carotid artery terminus aneurysm. Note hyperdense clot within the center of the aneurysm (*arrow*), as well as peripheral aneurysm wall calcification (*arrowheads*). (*C* and *D*) Contrast-enhanced CT scan (C and D) of the same patient. Note central enhancement of the patent aneurysm lumen (*white arrow*), as well as peripheral enhancement of developing thrombus (*open arrow*).

used when acquiring images, to minimize vessel overlap (Fig. 7.5).

A retrospective study examining the accuracy of the 3D TOF MRA method for the detection of aneurysms demonstrated a sensitivity of 95% and a specificity of 100% (68). Aneurysms as small as 3–4 mm were detected in this study. The sensitivity for aneurysm detection was greatest when the maximum intensity projection MRA data were reviewed in concert with the individual axial slices of the 3D gradient-echo data set, as well as with the multiplanar images from a conventional spin-echo study. These data suggest that the combination of MRI and

MRA may provide a useful screening examination in high-risk populations without documented SAH.

There are, however, several limitations to the 3D TOF MRA method. Flow or turbulent flow in an aneurysm or in vessels from which the aneurysm arises can result in signal dropout and false-negative examination. Signal dropout is a particular problem in the cavernous and supraclinoid segments of the internal carotid artery. The high signal intensity from methemoglobin within an intraparenchymal hemorrhage is displayed on the MRA examination. This may obscure the presence of an adjacent aneurysm or,

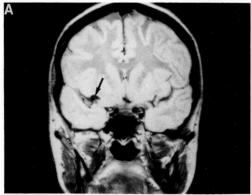

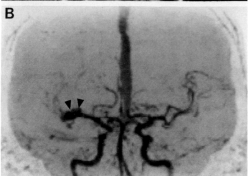

Figure 7.3. (*A*) Coronal spin-echo MRI (T_R = 2500 msec, T_E = 25 msec) demonstrates round signal void in the region of the right middle cerebral artery trifurcation (*arrow*), consistent with an aneurysm. (*B*) Three-dimensional TOF MRA examination (T_R = 40 msec, T_E = 8 msec, flip angle = 15 degrees) demonstrates right middle cerebral artery trifurcation aneurysm (*arrowheads*).

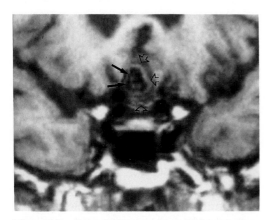

Figure 7.4. Coronal MR scan (T_R = 500 msec, T_E = 2 msec) demonstrates right ophthalmic artery aneurysm. Note signal void within the patent central lumen (*closed arrows*) and laminated heterogeneous signal within peripheral thrombus (*open arrows*).

potentially, mimic an aneurysm (94). Depending on the stage, thrombus within the aneurysm may cause an underestimation of the true aneurysm size in MRA. This may be compensated for if conventional spin-echo MRI is reviewed with the MRA. Lastly, patient motion may cause severe misregistration artifacts which cannot be compensated for on the MRA examination.

Imaging of Aneurysm Rupture

SAH from aneurysm rupture is most commonly an acute event accompanied by severe headache and often followed by loss of consciousness. Uncontrasted CT scanning is the imaging modality of choice to confirm acute SAH. Initially blood is visualized as increased density within the sulci, cisterns, and fissures of the brain. Examination of CT scans at wider window settings and level settings intermediate between those for brain and bone can enable detection of subtle SAH at brain-bone interfaces. Unenhanced CT is approximately 90% sensitive in detecting SAH within the first 24 hours following the initial event and approximately 50% sensitive if examination is performed within 1 week following the initial event (23, 36, 44, 45). More than 1 week following the initial event CT scanning becomes much less sensitive in detecting SAH, due to the fact that, as the hemoglobin is progressively broken down, the blood becomes progressively more isointense to CSF. If increased density is visualized in the subarachnoid space >1 week following the initial event, an episode of rebleeding should be considered. Even in the acute stage, a negative uncontrasted CT scan does not exclude a small amount of SAH from an intracranial source or SAH from a spinal source. Therefore, if there is no contraindication, a lumbar puncture should be performed for patients suspected of having SAH if the uncontrasted CT scan is negative.

MRI is notoriously insensitive for detecting acute SAH (4, 29, 56). The specificity of MRI for detecting extravasated blood products is dependent upon the progressive breakdown of hemoglobin (25, 96, 97). The lack of sensitivity of MRI in the acute stages of SAH relates to the higher partial pressure of oxygen within the CSF, compared to

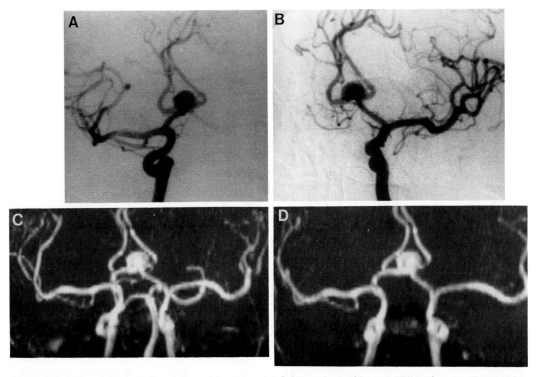

Figure 7.5. (*A* and *B*) Anterior oblique right (A) and left internal carotid artery (B) angiograms demonstrate anterior communicating artery aneurysm. (*C*) Three-dimensional TOF MRA examination (T_R = 40 msec, T_E = 8 msec, flip angle = 15 degrees) demonstrates the aneurysm, comparable to the angiographic views. (*D*) Three-dimensional TOF MRA with saturation pulse applied over the vertebral arteries excludes overlapping vessels from the vertebro-basilar system.

brain parenchyma (29). This higher oxygen partial pressure delays conversion of oxyhemoglobin to deoxyhemoglobin and methemoglobin. This conversion is essential for altering the relaxation rates of neighboring protons, which allows detection of hemorrhage on MRI. Although MRI is not as sensitive as uncontrasted CT in detecting acute SAH, MRI is exquisitively sensitive to the effects of chronic SAH (24, 26). This is due to the subpial deposition of hemosiderin in the chronic stage, which results in superficial hemosiderosis. Chronic subpial deposition of hemosiderin is visualized as marked hypointensity lining the parenchymal surface and is best visualized on long-repitition time (TR), long-echo time (TE) spin-echo or gradient-echo sequences (Fig. 7.6).

Although SAH is the most common imaging finding of acute aneurysm rupture, intraparenchymal hemorrhage (IPH) and intraventricular hemorrhage (IVH) may accompany aneurysm rupture as well. Isolated IVH may be seen with anterior choroidal artery, posterior inferior cerebellar artery, anterior communicating artery, or basilar tip artery rupture. Isolated IPH or IVH without evidence of SAH, however, is uncommon with berry aneurysm rupture, and under these circumstances other causes of intracranial hemorrhage should be considered.

The location of blood on an uncontrasted CT scan may at times be utilized as a general guide to aneurysm location (78). In this regard, the location of SAH is least sensitive in determining the site of origin of an aneurysm, since layering of SAH may be produced by changes in head position following the initial ictus. IPH in association with aneurysm rupture is the most sensitive guide

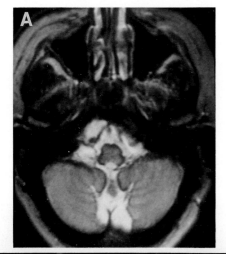

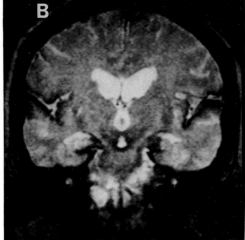

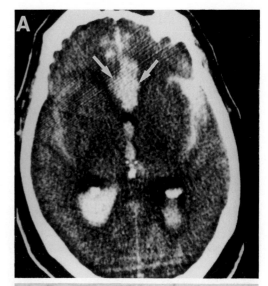

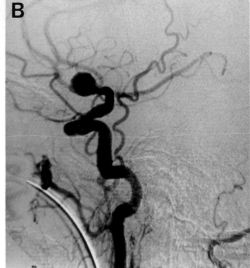

Figure 7.6. (*A* and *B*) Axial (A) and coronal (B) MR scans (T_R = 2500 msec, T_E = 80 msec) demonstrate superficial siderosis, which is evidence of chronic SAH. Subpial deposition of hemosiderin is visualized as hypointensity lining the pial surfaces of the sylvian fissures, the brainstem, and the cerebellum.

to aneurysm location. Hemorrhage dissecting into the septum pellucidum is usually associated with anterior communicating artery aneurysm rupture but may be seen with distal internal carotid artery aneurysm rupture as well (72) (Figs. 7.7 and 7.8). Similarly, inferomedial frontal hematomas are also usually associated with anterior communicating artery aneurysms, although they may be visualized with internal carotid ar-

Figure 7.7. (*A*) Uncontrasted CT demonstrates SAH and IVH as well as hemorrhage in the septum pellucidum (*arrows*). (*B* and *C*) Posterior-anterior (B) and lateral left internal carotid artery (C) angiogram demonstrates anterior communicating artery aneurysm.

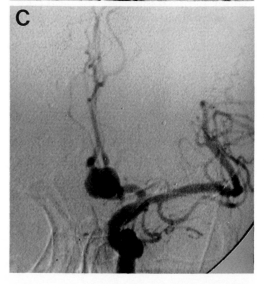

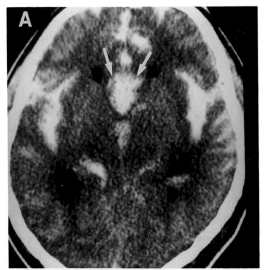

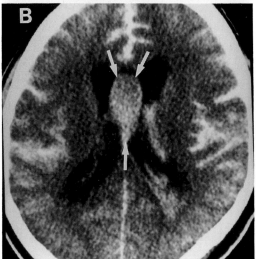

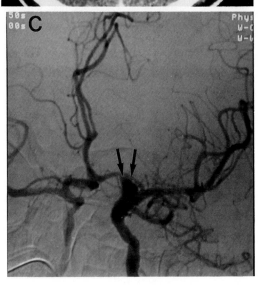

tery rupture as well. Temporal lobe hematomas are usually associated with middle cerebral artery bi/trifurcation aneurysms. However, medial temporal lobe hematomas may be seen with posterior communicating artery or internal carotid artery rupture as well. Corpus callosal hematomas usually indicate pericallosal artery aneurysm rupture. IVH located predominantly within the fourth ventricle, particularly associated with cerebellar IPH, is usually indicative of a posterior inferior cerebellar artery aneurysm. Again, the cisternal location of SAH is a less specific indicator of aneurysm location. However, predominance of perimesencephalic and intrapeducular cistern hemorrhage with slight extension into the sylvian fissures is suggestive of a basilar tip or posterior communicating artery aneurysm rupture. Similarly, isolated or predominant hemorrhage in the sylvian fissure is suggestive of a middle cerebral artery bi/trifurcation aneurysm.

Angiography in Acute Aneurysm Rupture

Conventional film screen and intra-arterial digital subtraction angiography (IADSA) remain the gold standards for the evaluation of intracranial aneurysms. The goals of angiography in the evaluation of aneurysms include determination of location, size, orientation, morphology, and relationship to adjacent vascular structures. In addition, angiography should evaluate for associated vasospasm and multiple aneurysms. Detection of an aneurysm by angiography in the presence of acute rupture is approximately 95% (47).

Although film screen angiography has traditionally been felt to provide superior spatial resolution, compared to IADSA, newer IADSA units with smaller focal spot size and 1024 × 1024 digital matrix provide resolution comparable to that of conventional film screen angiography. IADSA provides several advantages for aneurysm analysis, compared

Figure 7.8. (*A* and *B*) Uncontrasted CT scan (A and B) demonstrates SAH and IVH as well as hemorrhage into the septum pellucidum (*white arrows*). (*C*) Anterior-oblique left internal carotid artery angiogram with cross-compression demonstrates a left ophthalmic artery origin aneurysm. The dome of the aneurysm is oriented medially and superiorly (*black arrows*).

to film screen angiography. Fast frame rate allows assessment of flow dynamics within the aneurysm. By using fast frame rates (4–6 frames/sec), a jet of contrast entering the aneurysm can usually be seen. Visualization of this jet is often useful in determining the morphology of the neck of an aneurysm. Rapid image acquisition allows multiple projections to be obtained in a short time, allowing accurate determination of the aneurysm orientation. Improved contrast resolution often enables less contrast to be used per vessel injection with IADSA. In addition, post-processing capabilities of IADSA, such as use of a delayed-mask technique, can give more specific information regarding the location and direction of an aneurysm neck, as well as the size of the neck relative to the aneurysm (42) (Fig. 7.9). In individual patients, multiple aneurysms occur with a frequency of 15–22% (52). Therefore, when performing angiography in the presence of acute SAH it is imperative to examine all intracranial vessels. If multiple aneurysms are detected by angiography, several factors can be used to determine the aneurysm which ruptured. These include the largest size, irregular shape, lobulation, aneurysm nipple, adjacent mass effect, and focal vasospasm (15, 55, 70, 91). These angiographic signs, in combination with CT scan findings such as location of intraparenchymal hematoma and clinical signs such as third nerve palsy, hemiparesis, or dysphasia, can be used as general guides to the specific site of rupture in cases of multiple aneurysms.

In the event of a negative angiographic examination for aneurysm in the setting of acute SAH, other causes of bleeding into the subarachnoid space should be considered. These include nonvisualized cerebral or spinal vascular malformation, rupture of a small superficial cortical vessel, cerebral or spinal venous thrombosis, neoplastic hemorrhage, blood dyscrasia or anticoagulant therapy, unknown trauma, and traumatic lumbar puncture. The inability of angiography to detect an aneurysm in the presence of SAH due to aneurysm rupture is uncommon. The frequency of detecting an aneurysm on repeat angiography in the event of a negative initial angiogram is approxi-

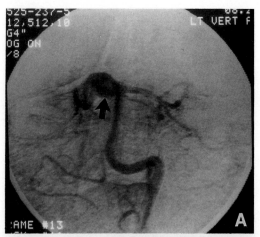

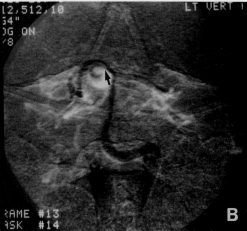

Figure 7.9. (*A*) Transfacial left vertebral artery angiogram demonstrates an aneurysm in the region of the basilar tip (*large arrow*). (*B*) Delayed-mask technique allows improved visualization of the origin of the aneurysm from the inferior surface of the right posterior cerebral artery (*small arrow*).

mately 2% (19, 37). Factors which may lead to false-negative angiographic examinations include severe vasospasm, small aneurysm size (<3 mm), spontaneous aneurysm thrombosis, inadequate angiographic projections, or poor-quality films (37).

Intraoperative Angiography

In the past, postoperative angiograms were frequently obtained to confirm the placement of aneurysm clips. Recently, the availability of mobile IADSA units has allowed accurate intraoperative angiography to be performed. Intraoperative examination enables the adequacy of aneurysm occlusion as well as the patency of parent and adjacent arteries to be determined before closure of the craniotomy (Fig. 7.10). In the event of suboptimal clip position, repositioning can, therefore, be efficiently performed. In a study by Barrow *et al.* (5) which examined intraoperative angiography for neurovascular procedures, approximately

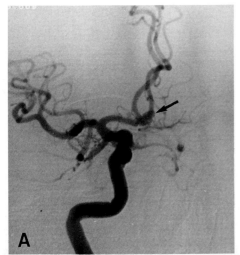

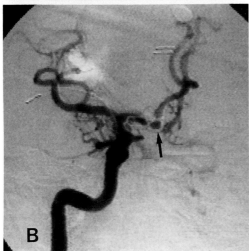

Figure 7.10. (*A*) Preoperative anterior-oblique right internal carotid artery angiogram demonstrates an anterior communicating artery aneurysm (*arrow*). (*B*) Intraoperative right common carotid artery angiogram obtained during open craniotomy demonstrates an aneurysm clip occluding the aneurysm (*arrow*), as well as bilateral patent A2 segments.

10% of aneurysm operations were altered based upon findings on the intraoperative angiogram. The combination of intraoperative angiography and microvascular Doppler analysis of the aneurysm dome increases the confidence regarding adequate clip position prior to craniotomy closure. While residual necks or outpouchings at the site of clips were thought in the past to be inconsequential, recent series have documented that recurrent aneurysms from these sites are not uncommon (14, 46).

Several technical factors should be considered to allow optimal efficiency of intraoperative angiographic procedures. Placement of a femoral artery sheath during anesthesia induction allows rapid arterial access at the time of angiography. A radiolucent head-holder is necessary to provide an unobstructed view of intracranial vascular structures. The table connection arm of the head-holder must be extended to allow positioning of the angiographic C-arm. Also, a radiolucent operating room table or a radiolucent table extender is necessary to enable adequate visualization of the aortic arch during catheterization.

There are several limitations of intraoperative angiography. The number of angiographic projections may be limited due to restricted C-arm rotation. Subtraction artifacts from overlying metal appliances such as retractors may exclude visualization of underlying vascular structures. In addition, patient positioning (such as seated for certain posterior fossa aneurysms) may preclude transfemoral catheterization (5).

Imaging of the Sequela of Sah

Hydrocephalus

The development of hydrocephalus following aneurysm rupture is not an uncommon occurrence. Blood in the subarachnoid space increases CSF protein levels. The excess protein within the CSF obstructs microscopic absorption sites in the pacchionian granulations at the brain surface, resulting in communicating hydrocephalus (86). In addition, hydrocephalus may occur on an obstructive basis if IVH is present. Obstructive hydrocephalus is particularly common if blood is present in the third or fourth ventricles (28).

Obstructive hydrocephalus may result in noncytotoxic nonvasogenic cerebral edema. Distension of the ventricles may damage the ventricle-brain barrier, thereby allowing CSF to spread through the extracellular space within the periventricular white matter (77).

Unenhanced CT scanning is an accurate modality for detecting the presence and degree of hydrocephalus. Also, hydrocephalus-related cerebral edema is visualized as periventricular lucency. If hydrocephalus causes a sufficient rise in intracranial pressure, venous drainage of the hemispheres may be impaired. As the result of impaired venous drainage, venous infarcts may ensue. These are typically visualized on CT scans as focal areas of cortical hemorrhage. Following ventricular shunt placement, CT scanning is useful to document shunt tube position and function.

Rebleeding

For untreated aneurysms one cause of clinical deterioration following SAH is aneurysm rebleeding. The rates of rebleeding following aneurysm rupture vary among different series (38, 40, 48, 51, 58, 62, 69, 85, 93). However, it is agreed that the risk is greatest within the first 2 weeks following the initial rupture. Rebleeding in the first few days may be difficult to determine on CT scans, because hyperdense blood in the subarachnoid space from the initial SAH may mask additional bleeding into the subarachnoid space. Increased volume of SAH or IVH in addition to new or expanding IPH are CT signs which indicate early rebleeding. More than 1 week following the initial SAH, blood in the subarachnoid space should be isointense or almost isointense to parenchymal gray matter. If repeat CT scanning at this time demonstrates hyperintense SAH, rebleeding has probably occurred.

Vasospasm

Vasospasm is one of the main causes of morbidity and mortality following acute aneurysm rupture (89, 90). The arterial spasm may be local or diffuse; mild, moderate, or severe; and symptomatic or asymptomatic. Approximately 40% of patients develop vasospasm following aneurysmal

SAH. Fifty percent of patients with angiographic evidence of vasospasm develop delayed ischemic deficits, and the mortality rate for patients who develop delayed ischemic deficits is approximately 50% (89). Delayed ischemic deficits secondary to vasospasm typically develop between day 3 and day 13 following SAH (17, 90).

In general, the development of clinically significant vasospasm is related to the amount of SAH detected on CT within 4 days of the initial ictus. Patients with large clots within their sylvian fissures or basal cisterns commonly develop delayed ischemic deficits secondary to vasospasm. It is very unusual for patients with only CSF and no CT evidence of SAH to develop symptomatic vasospasm following aneurysm rupture (18, 41, 54, 82).

Uncontrasted CT scanning is essential in patients who develop delayed ischemic deficits following aneurysm rupture. CT scanning in this setting excludes entities other than vasospasm, such as hydrocephalus or rebleed, which may result in delayed ischemic deficits. In addition, CT scanning may detect a vascular distribution of infarction or hemorrhage into a vascular territory of infarction. There are, however, several limitations of CT in the setting of delayed ischemic deficits. Infarcted tissue may not be evident on CT for 24–48 hours following the initial damage. Also, in the postoperative setting it may be difficult to differentiate postoperative edema from infarction. This distinction is made somewhat easier by the fact that postoperative edema tends to conform to the surgical approach and, for most aneurysms, is located at the base of the brain. Infarction secondary to vasospasm occurs mainly in the peripheral cortex and adjacent white matter (60) (Fig. 7.11).

For patients who can tolerate the examination, MRI may be useful in the early detection of infarction secondary to vasospasm. The sensitivity of MRI in detecting infarcts in the first 24 hours is approximately 80%, compared to a sensitivity of approximately 50% for CT (95). The earliest changes of infarction visualized on MRI are enlargement and distortion of cortical gyri due to tissue swelling. These morphological changes are best visualized on short-TE,

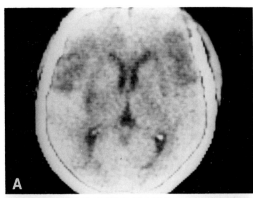

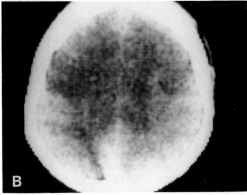

Figure 7.11. (*A* and *B*) Uncontrasted CT scan (A and B) demonstrates bihemispheric infarcts secondary to vasospasm.

short-TR sequences and can be seen within 2–6 hours following infarction (11). Slightly later, increased T_2 signal intensity is visualized in the involved tissue as the result of developing cytotoxic edema.

Although not universally available, noninvasive cerebral blood flow (CBF) analysis using ^{15}o-labeled water and positron emission tomography (PET) scanning, Xe/CT scanning, or technetium exametazime single photon emission computed tomography scanning may provide valuable CBF information in patients with suspected vasospasm (21, 67) PET and Xe/CT CBF methods have the advantages of providing quantitative blood flow measurements. In addition, PET and Xe/CT studies can be repeated in short time intervals, which allows pharmacological or ventilator manipulations between examinations. CBF methods demonstrate areas of brain parenchyma which may be ischemic but not grossly infarcted. These

areas are certainly at risk for developing infarctions but may be undetected on CT or MR examinations. In addition, the ability to manipulate factors between CBF studies is useful. Hypertensive drug dosages and respiratory settings can then be titrated to maximize CBF in the setting of cerebral vasospasm.

Angiography in patients with suspected vasospasm provides morphological information regarding the degree and distribution of vessel narrowing. Angiographically there is typically smooth narrowing of the lumen caliper in vessels involved with vasospasm. The spasm can be focal or diffuse. At times the spasm is segmental, with skip areas of normal-caliber vessel. Diffuse vasospasm indicates an unfavorable prognosis. Sano and Saito (71) documented a fatal outcome in 10 of 22 patients with diffuse vasospasm but in only five of 24 with segmental and two of 20 with focal spasm.

Giant Aneurysms

Giant aneurysms have been defined as aneurysms whose greatest diameter exceeds 2.5 cm (69). These aneurysms constitute approximately 5% of all aneurysms (64). The locations of these aneurysms differ somewhat from those of smaller saccular aneurysms. In general, the most frequent locations of giant aneurysms are the intradural and cavernous segments of the internal carotid artery, followed by the vertebral-basilar artery system, the middle cerebral artery, and the anterior communicating/anterior cerebral artery junction. A review of the literature by Nukui *et al.* (59) documented a distribution of giant aneurysms as follows: intradural internal carotid artery/ophthalmic artery, 21%; middle cerebral artery, 16%; anterior communicating artery/anterior cerebral artery 12%; intradural internal carotid artery bifurcation, 9%; basilar artery/superior cerebellar artery, 8%; basilar artery bifurcation, 7%; cavernous internal carotid artery, 6%; vertebral artery, 4%; vertebral-basilar artery junction, 3%; posterior cerebral artery, 3%; intradural internal carotid artery/posterior communicating artery, 3%; posterior communicating artery, 1%; posterior inferior cerebellar artery, 1%.

Although giant aneurysms are more likely than smaller sacular aneurysms to present with symptoms secondary to mass effect, rupture with resultant intracranial hemorrhage is a not uncommon mode of presentation. Approximately 13–76% (average 35%) of giant aneurysms present with SAH (64).

Partial thrombosis of the lumen of giant aneurysms is not uncommon, because the volume of the aneurysm sac is often large in relation to the size of the orifice to the parent artery. This results in slowed and turbulent flow within the aneurysm, which increases platelet adherence to the wall (64). Thrombus within a giant aneurysm usually begins peripherally and progresses centrifugally in a laminated manner. Often the majority of thrombus accumulates on the wall opposite the orifice to the parent artery. This is most likely due to the jet effect of blood entering the aneurysm and resultant turbulent flow at this location.

The appearance of giant aneurysms on imaging studies is dependent on the degree of thrombosis as well as the blood flow characteristics within the aneurysm (Fig. 7.12). Three CT patterns have been described for giant aneurysms (66). Nonthrombotic giant aneurysms are slightly hyperdense to gray matter on uncontrasted CT scans, and the lumen of the aneurysm is markedly enhanced with contrast. The aneurysm typically has a round configuration and is located in close proximity to the parent artery of origin. At times, especially if the aneurysm is lobulated, it may be difficult to differentiate the aneurysm from other sellar and parasellar masses such as meningiomas, craniopharyngiomas, or pituitary adenomas. Dynamic contrast CT scanning may aid in this differential diagnosis; there is usually more rapid transit of contrast through an aneurysm than through other parasellar masses (65). If aneurysm remains a diagnostic consideration after CT or MR examination, angiography should be performed for definitive diagnosis.

Partially thrombosed giant aneurysms demonstrate a rim of peripheral hyperdensity on uncontrasted CT scans. Often, peripheral curvilinear calcification is present. If calcification is present it is important to

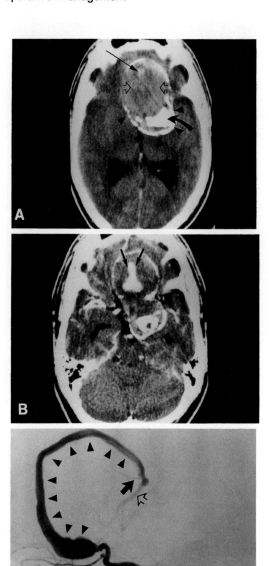

Figure 7.12. (*A*) Uncontrasted CT scan demonstrates giant aneurysm. Note central hyperdense patent lumen (*arrow*), peripheral thrombus (*open arrows*), and rim calcification (*arrowheads*), as well as large calcifications within thrombus (*curved arrow*). (*B*) Contrast-enhanced CT scan. Note enhancement of central lumen (*arrows*). (*C*) Lateral left internal carotid artery angiogram demonstrates fusiform distal internal carotid artery aneurysm (*arrowheads*, distal left internal carotid artery; *closed arrow*, left A1 segment; *open arrow*, left M1 segment).

define the relationship of the calcification to the surgical neck. Calcification of the surgical neck may be a contraindication to neurosurgical clipping (23) (Fig. 7.13). Following contrast administration, partially thrombosed aneurysms may be enhanced centrally, peripherally, or both. Central enhancement is due to contrast accumulating in the residual patent lumen of the aneurysm. Peripheral enhancement is due to enhancement of developing thrombus via the vasa vasorum.

Completely thrombosed giant aneurysms are hyperdense to gray matter on uncontrasted CT. Calcification may be present and can be either peripheral, central, or both. The thrombus may be enhanced mildly following contrast administration, but no in-

tense enhancement of a central lumen is visualized.

MRI is complementary to CT in the examination of giant aneurysms. The majority of giant aneurysms are not completely thrombosed at the time of examination. Flow void within the residual lumen, which is usually visualized on MRI, increases diagnostic certainty of a giant aneurysm. The superior tissue contrast and multiplanar capabilities of MRI allow the distinction between extradural and intradural location to be made more easily (61). In addition, MRI is often superior to CT in defining the mass effect of the aneurysm on adjacent structures. Calcification within the wall of the aneurysm is more readily detected by CT.

On MRI nonthrombosed giant aneurysms usually demonstrate flow void within the patent lumen. Even with nonthrombosed aneurysms, however, some signal heterogeneity within the aneurysm may be seen because of slow flow within the aneurysm. Therefore, signal heterogeneity within the aneurysm does not necessarily imply thrombosis. If the luminal flow void is not well visualized on spin-echo sequences due to slow flow, gradient-echo techniques may be useful to document flow and differentiate flow from thrombus (86). Often bands of pulsation artifact are visualized on both sides of the aneurysm. Visualization of this artifact aids in the differential diagnosis of giant aneurysms.

Partially thrombosed giant aneurysms have been reported to have a characteristic appearance on MRI (2). Signal void can be seen in the patent residual aneurysm lumen. At the periphery of the aneurysm the thrombus has a laminated appearance, with intervening layers of hemosiderin and methemaglobin (Fig. 7.14). The hemosiderin appears dark on both long-T_R and short-T_R spin-echo pulse sequences, whereas the methemaglobin appears bright on both sequences.

As with smaller berry aneurysms, MRA provides adjunctive information regarding giant aneurysm morphology and the relationship of the aneurysm to the parent artery. MRA technique selection for giant aneurysms is crucial. Techniques which are not sensitive to slowly flowing blood may suggest complete aneurysm thrombosis for

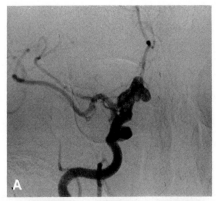

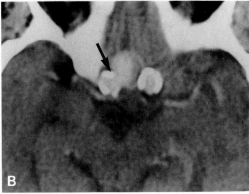

Figure 7.13. (*A*) Anterior-oblique right internal carotid artery angiogram demonstrates a giant right ophthalmic artery origin aneurysm with an irregular patent lumen. (*B*) Enhanced CT scan through the origin of the aneurysm. Note calcification extending to the neck of the aneurysm (*arrow*).

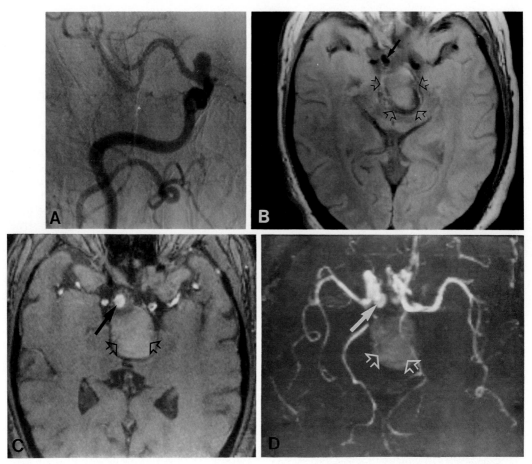

Figure 7.14. (*A*) Anterior-oblique right common carotid artery angiogram demonstrates patent lumen of a giant right carotid terminus aneurysm. (*B*) MRI (T_R = 2500 msec, T_E = 15 msec). Note signal void in patent aneurysm lumen (*closed arrow*) and peripheral laminated thrombus (*open arrows*). (*C* and *D*) Three-dimensional TOF MRA (T_R = 35 msec; T_E = 8 msec, flip angle = 15 degrees) before (*C*) and after (*D*) post-processing. Note flow within patent aneurysm lumen (*closed arrow*). The peripheral thrombus is visualized as hyperintense signal due to extracellular methemaglobin (*open arrows*). This hyperintense signal may mimic flowing blood.

giant aneurysms with slow outflow. In addition, high signal intensity from methemaglobin within aneurysm thrombus can be mistaken for flow within the aneurysm with certain MRA techniques. Also, motion artifact from aneurysm pulsations can degrade the post-processed MRA images.

In general, TOF MRA techniques provide the best vessel resolution. Two-dimensional TOF MRA techniques have the advantage over 3D TOF techniques of being more sensitive to slowly flowing blood. However, with both TOF techniques signal from methemaglobin within thrombus appears bright and can mimic flowing blood (68) (Fig. 7.15). As

with two-dimensional TOF techniques, phase-contrast MRA techniques are sensitive to slow flow. In addition, strong signal from methemaglobin is subtracted from the data set during phase-contrast image post-processing. However, phase-contrast techniques are hampered by low signal-to-noise ratio and poor vessel resolution, compared to TOF techniques.

Angiography remains the gold standard for assessment of the morphology of giant aneurysms as well as the relationship of the aneurysm to the parent artery. Because of aneurysm size it may be difficult to accurately define the neck of the aneurysm at

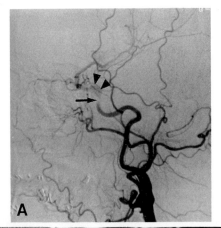

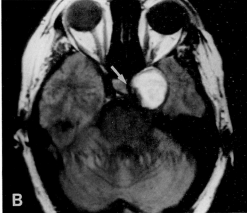

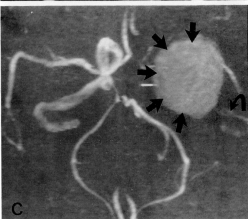

angiography. Again, rapid film rates as well as delayed-mask post-processing techniques can aid in defining the anatomy of the aneurysm neck (42). Also, especially with internal carotid artery giant aneurysms, injection of the opposite carotid artery or a vertebral artery while the ipsilateral carotid artery is compressed may allow a jet of contrast to enter the aneurysm via the circle of Willis and aid in defining the orifice of the aneurysm. If these techniques fail to identify the anatomy of the aneurysm neck, a aneurysmogram can be performed. This involves gently positioning a steam-curved microcatheter into the aneurysm lumen and injecting contrast. If aneurysm catheterization is performed, care must be taken not to puncture the wall of the aneurysm with catheter or guidewire. Also, care must be taken not to dislodge any mural thrombus. The injection of contrast should be rather slow and gentle, so as not to injure the aneurysm wall.

Aspects of Endovascular Therapy for Aneurysms

In the early 1970s Serbinenko (75, 76) first described the use of latex balloons in the treatment of complex neurovascular disorders such as arteriovenous malformations, carotid cavernous fistulas, and aneurysms. Initial treatment of aneurysms involved proximal occlusion of the aneurysm and parent vessel using detachable latex balloons introduced via direct puncture of the cervical internal carotid artery. Research in the past two decades has yielded major advances in microcatheter, microballoon, and detachable coil technology. These advances have made it presently feasible to treat appropriate aneurysms using endovascular methods via a transfemoral approach. Endovascular therapy is an alternative to conventional neurosurgery for aneurysms which, because of size, location, neck anatomy, or medical

Figure 7.15. (*A*) Oblique left common carotid artery angiogram demonstrates small residual patent lumen of a giant left cavernous carotid artery aneurysm (*arrowheads*). Note proximal left internal carotid artery stenosis due to mass effect from the aneurysm (*arrow*). (*B*) MR (T_R = 2500 msec, T_E = 15 msec) demonstrates strong signal within thrombosed portion of giant left cavernous carotid aneurysm. Note small size of left cavernous carotid artery (*arrow*). (*C*) Three-dimensional TOF MRA (T_R = 35 msec, T_E = 8 msec, flip angle = 13 degrees). The thrombosed aneurysm is visualized with strong signal intensity due to extracellular methemaglobin (*arrows*). Note minimal flow detected in petrous segment of left internal carotid artery (*curved arrow*).

condition of the patient, are difficult or unsafe to treat by craniotomy (32). Endovascular embolization of aneurysms may be broadly divided into two categories: 1) occlusion of the aneurysm and parent artery and 2) occlusion of the aneurysm with parent artery preservation.

Parent Artery Occlusion

Aneurysms which are fusiform or giant and do not have a well defined neck may necessitate parent artery occlusion for treatment. Prior to permanent parent artery occlusion a test occlusion of the involved artery must be performed. The most accurate method to test the adequacy of the circle of Willis during arterial occlusion is to perform a balloon test occlusion (16). The balloon test occlusion procedure involves catheterizing the involved artery with a nondetachable balloon catheter system. Immediately prior to test occlusion the patient undergoes systemic anticoagulation. The balloon is inflated with contrast medium to an occlusive position. Serial neurological examinations are performed during the 30 min of test occlusion. If the patient develops a deficit during test occlusion the balloon is immediately deflated. To further test cerebrovascular reserve during arterial occlusion, the balloon test occlusion should be combined with either a CBF study or a hypotensive challenge (16). Patients who cannot tolerate the test occlusion or demonstrate marginal vascular reserve require an external carotid artery to middle cerebral artery bypass or vein graft reconstruction to improve cerebral perfusion prior to parent vessel occlusion (74, 79).

Once tolerance to arterial occlusion is established, parent artery occlusion can be performed using detachable balloons. Ideally the balloons should be positioned so that the aneurysm is trapped, thereby preventing aneurysm filling via collateral routes. However, if the neck of the aneurysm is wide compared to the diameter of the parent artery it may not be possible to position the distal balloon beyond the aneurysm. In this instance the parent artery can be sacrificed immediately proximal to the aneurysm (Fig. 7.16). As opposed to open surgical parent artery occlusion, patients may undergo anticoagulation following endovascular parent artery occlusion, to prevent thrombotic or embolic complications resulting from rapid thrombus progression. In two recent series examining a total of 136 aneurysms treated successfully by endovascular parent artery occlusion, the total morbidity rate was approximately 15%, the permanent morbidity rate averaged approximately 3%, and there were no deaths (20, 33).

Direct Aneurysm Occlusion

In patients who demonstrate a well defined aneurysm neck, it is possible to directly occlude the aneurysm with detachable balloons or coils and preserve the parent artery (Fig. 7.17). Correlation with CT and MRI is essential to evaluate for the presence of intraluminal thrombus. In non-acutely ill patients direct endovascular occlusion should be delayed in the presence of fresh thrombus within the aneurysm, to reduce the risk of embolic complications. If detachable balloons are used care must be taken not to overexpand the aneurysm during balloon inflation, due to risk of aneurysm rupture. Whereas during parent artery occlusion the detachable balloons may be filled with isotonic contrast medium, a permanent solidifying agent such as hydroxyethylmethacrylate must be used to fill the detachable balloons during direct aneurysm occlusion (27, 35, 83). This is to prevent balloon deflation should the valve fail or the outer balloon shell deteriorate over time and allow recanalization. A recent series reported experience with direct aneurysm balloon occlusion of 84 patients in whom aneurysm occlusion could not be obtained by conventional neurosurgery (32). Follow-up arteriography demonstrated complete aneurysmal obliteration in 77% of the cases and subtotal but >85% occlusion in 23% of cases. Permanent complications of endovascular balloon occlusion included 15 deaths (17.9%) and 10 strokes (10.7%). Ten of the 15 were due to aneurysm rupture either acutely at the time of the procedure or delayed due to subtotal aneurysm occlusion.

There are several disadvantages to direct balloon occlusion of aneurysms. The main disadvantage is that the wall of the aneurysm

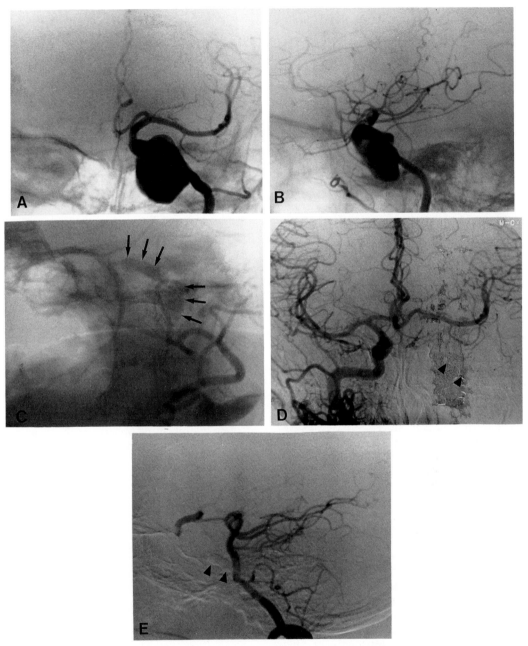

Figure 7.16. (*A* and *B*) Posterior-anterior (A) and lateral (B) left common carotid artery angiogram demonstrates a giant left cavernous carotid artery aneurysm. (*C*) Anterior oblique left common carotid artery angiogram following parent artery balloon occlusion demonstrates occlusion of left internal carotid artery. Note balloon positions (*arrows*). (*D* and *E*) Posterior-anterior right common carotid artery (D) and lateral left vertebral (E) angiograms following balloon occlusion of left internal carotid artery. There is no residual aneurysm filling. Note subtracted relief of the detached balloon (*arrowheads*).

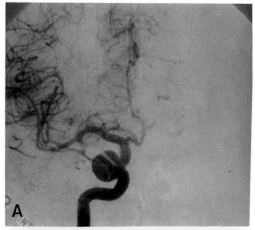

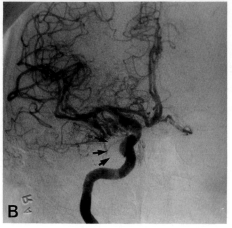

Figure 7.17. (*A*) Posterior-anterior right internal carotid artery angiogram demonstrates a right cavernous carotid artery aneurysm. (*B*) Posterior-anterior right internal carotid artery angiogram following direct aneurysm balloon occlusion (*arrows*) demonstrates no residual aneurysm filling.

may undergo stress while adapting to the shape of the balloon, thus increasing the risk of rupture during the procedure. In addition, if multiple balloons are needed it may be difficult to position them such that the entire aneurysm orifice is occluded. Also, balloon migration may occur, especially in aneurysms with thrombus at the periphery, resulting in aneurysm recanalization.

A new endovascular technique using electrothrombosis with soft detachable platinum coils (Guglielmi detachable coils) has been described recently (30). The technique involves coiling the soft platinum portion

within the aneurysm lumen. The platinum portion of the coil is bonded to a stainless steel shaft. Low-voltage current is used to detach the platinum coil from the stainless steel shaft. The positive charge induced on the coil also acts to attract negatively charged blood products, thereby promoting thrombosis.

The main advantage of the Guglielmi detachable coil technique is increased operator control of coil positioning and detachment. If an unfavorable result is obtained during coil positioning, the system can be retrieved into the catheter prior to detachment and can be repositioned. This positioning control optimizes coil placement and increases therapeutic safety.

Results of aneurysm occlusion using this method are preliminary at the time of this writing. However, trends in the results suggest that this technique is most effective in treating aneurysm of <25-mm diameter with neck widths of <4-mm diameter. Larger aneurysms with wide necks are more difficult to completely occlude using this technique. In addition, coil migration into intra-aneurysmal thrombus, with aneurysm recanalization, may occur (87).

Conclusion

The evolution of imaging techniques has allowed accurate and timely aneurysm detection and exact morphological characterization, which aid in the surgical treatment planning for aneurysm patients. Standard CT scanning as well as more advanced MRI, MRA, and CBF analysis can be used to accurately determine and follow the effects of aneurysm rupture. The advancing new frontier of endovascular therapy has increased our knowledge of aneurysm flow dynamics and allowed heretofore untreatable aneurysms to be successfully treated.

REFERENCES

1. Asari, S., Satoh, T., Sakurai, M., *et al.* Delineation of unruptured cerebral aneurysms by computerized angiotomography. J. Neurosurg. *57:*527–534, 1982.
2. Atlas, S. W., Grossman, R. I., Goldberg, H. I., *et al.* Partially thrombosed giant intracranial aneurysms: correlation of MR and pathologic findings. Radiology *162:*111–114, 1987.
3. Bannerman, R. M., Ingall, G. B., and Graf, C. J.

The familial occurrence of intracranial aneurysms. Neuroradiology 20:283–292, 1979.

4. Barkovich, A. J., and Atlas, S. W. Magnetic resonance imaging of intracranial hemorrhage. Radiol. Clin. North Am. 26:801–820, 1988.

5. Barrow, D. L., Boyer, K. L., and Joseph, G. J. Intraoperative angiography in the management of neurovascular disorders. Neurosurgery 30:153–159, 1992.

6. Belber, C. J., and Hoffman, R. B. The syndrome of intracranial aneurysms associated with fibromuscular hyperplasia of renal arteries. J. Neurosurg. 28:556–559, 1969.

7. Bert, J. W. M., Overtoom, T. M. D., Ludwig, J. W., et al. Detection of unruptured familial intracranial aneurysms by intravenous digital subtraction angiography. Neuroradiology 29:272–276, 1987.

8. Biondi, A., Scialfa, G., and Scotti, G. Intracranial aneurysms: MR imaging. Neuroradiology 30:214–218, 1988.

9. Bradley, W. G., Jr., Waluch, V., Lai, K.-S., et al. The appearance of rapidly flowing blood on magnetic resonance images. AJR 143:1167–1174, 1984.

10. Brown, M. A., Carden, J. A., Coleman, R. E., et al. Magnetic field effects on surgical ligation clips. Magn. Reson. Imaging 5:443–453, 1987.

11. Bryan, R. N., Levy, L. M., Whitlow, W. D., et al. Diagnosis of acute cerebral infarction: comparison of CT and MR imaging. AJNR 12:611–620, 1991.

12. Burt, T. B. MR of CSF flow phenomenon mimicking basilar artery aneurysm. AJNR 8:55–58, 1987.

13. Campbell, G. J., and Roach, M. R. Fenestrations in the internal elastic lamina at bifarctions of human cerebral arteries. Stroke 12:489–496, 1981.

14. Drake, C. G., Friedman, A. H., and Peerless, S. J. Failed aneurysm surgery: reoperation in 115 cases. J. Neurosurg. 61:848–856, 1984.

15. DuBoulay, G. H. Some observations on the natural history of intracranial aneurysms. Br. J. Radiol. 38:721–757, 1965.

16. Erba, S. M., Horton, J. A., Latchaw, R. E., et al. Balloon test occlusion of the internal carotid artery with stable xenon/CT cerebral blood flow imaging. AJNR 9:533–538, 1988.

17. Fisher, C. M. Clinical syndromes in cerebral thrombosis, hypertensive hemorrhage, and ruptured saccular aneurysm. Clin. Neurosurg. 22:117–147, 1982.

18. Fisher, C. M., Kistler, J. P., and Davis, J. M. Relation of cerebral vasospasm to subarachnoid hemorrhage visualized by computerized tomographic scanning. Neurosurgery 6:1–9, 1980.

19. Foster, D. M. C., Sifiner, L., Hakanson, S., and Bergvall, U. The value of repeat pan-angiography in cases of unexplained subarachnoid hemorrhage. J. Neurosurg. 48:712–716, 1978.

20. Fox, A. J., Vinuela, F., Pelz, D. M., et al. Use of detachable balloons for proximal artery occlusion in the treatment of unclippable cerebral aneurysms. J. Neurosurg. 66:40–46, 1987.

21. Fuki, M. B., Johnson, D. W., Yonas, H., et al. Xe/CT cerebral blood flow evaluation of delayed symptomatic cerebral ischemia after subarachnoid hemorrhage. AJNR 13:265–270, 1992.

22. Gean, A. D., Pile-Spellman, J., and Heros, R. C. A pneumatized anterior clinoid mimicking an aneurysm on MR imaging: report of two cases. J. Neurosurg. 71:128–132, 1989.

23. Ghoshhajra, K., Scotti, L., Marasco, J., and Baghai-Naiini, P. CT detection of intracranial aneurysms in subarachnoid hemorrhage. AJR 132:613–616, 1979.

24. Gomori, J. M., Bilaniuk, L. T., Zimmerman, R. A., et al. High field MR imaging of superficial siderosis of the central nervous system. J. Comput. Assist. Tomogr. 9:972–976, 1984.

25. Gomori, J. M., Grossman, R. I., Goldberg, H. I., et al. Intracranial hematomas: imaging by high field MR. Radiology 157:87–93, 1985.

26. Gomori, J. M., Grossman, R. I., Goldberg, H. I., et al. High field spin-echo MR imaging of superficial and subependymal siderosis secondary to neonatal intraventricular hemorrhage. Neuroradiology 29:339–343, 1987.

27. Goto, K., Halbach, V. V., Hardin, C. W., et al. Permanent inflation of detachable balloons for a low-viscosity, hydrophilic polymerizing system. Radiology 169:787–790, 1988.

28. Graeb, D. A., Robertson, W. D., Lapointe, J. S., et al. Computed tomographic diagnosis of intraventricular hemorrhage: etiology and prognosis. Radiology 143:91–96, 1982.

29. Grossman, R. I., Kemp, S. S., Yulp, C., et al. The importance of oxygenation in the appearance of subarachnoid hemorrhage on high field magnetic resonance imaging. Acta Radiol., in press.

30. Guglielmi, G., Vinuela, F., Sepetka, I., et al. Electrothrombosis of saccular aneurysms via endovascular approach. 1. Electrochemical basis, technique, and experimental results. J. Neurosurg. 75:1–7, 1991.

31. Hatfield, P. M., and Pfister, R. C. Adult polycystic disease of the kidney (Potter type 3). JAMA 222:1527–1533, 1972.

32. Higashida, R. T., Halbach, V. V., Barnwell, S. L., et al. Treatment of intracranial aneurysms with preservation of the parent vessel: results of percutaneous balloon embolization in 84 patients. AJNR 11:633–640, 1990.

33. Higashida, R. T., Halbach, V. V., Dormandy, W. L., et al. Endovascular treatment of intracranial aneurysms with a new silicone microballoon device: technical considerations and indications for therapy. Radiology 174:687–691, 1990.

34. Housepian, B. M., and Pool, J. L. A systematic analysis of intracranial aneurysms from the autopsy file of Presbyterian Hospital. J. Neuropathol. Exp. Neurol. 17:409–423, 1958.

35. Hubacek, J., Kliment, K., Dusek, J., and Hubacek, J. Tissue reaction after implantation and in situ polymerization of hydrophilic gel. J. Biomed. Mater. Res. 1:387–394, 1967.

36. Inoui, Y., Saiwai, S., Miyamato, T., et al. Post contrast computed tomography in subarachnoid hemorrhage from ruptured aneurysms. J. Com-

put. Assist. Tomogr. *5*:341–344, 1981.

37. Ishii, R., Koike, T., Ohsugi, S., *et al.* Ruptured cerebral aneurysms not diagnosed by the initial cerebral angiography: clinical and radiological study. Neurol. Med. Chir. (Tokyo) *23*:471–477, 1983.

38. Jane, J. A., Winn, and Richardson, A. E. The natural history of intracranial aneurysms: rebleeding rates during the acute and long term period and implication for surgical management. Clin. Neurosurg. *24*:176–184, 1977.

39. Jellinger, K. Pathology and aetiology of intracranial aneurysms. In: *Advances in Diagnosis and Therapy*, edited by H. W. Pia, L. Langmaid, and J. Zierski, pp. 5–19. Springer Publishing Co., New York, 1979.

40. Kassel, N. F., and Torner, J. C. Aneurysmal rebleeding: a preliminary report from the Cooperative Aneurysm Study. Neurosurgery *13*:479–481, 1983.

41. Koike, T., Kobayashi, K., Ishii, R., *et al.* Clinical analysis of cerebral vasospasm following subarachnoid hemorrhage. 2. Disturbance of cerebral circulation and cerebral infarction associated with cerebral vasospasms. Neurol. Med. Chir. (Tokyo) *20*:1015–1021, 1980.

42. Lanzieri, C. F., Tarr, R. W., Selman, W. R., *et al.* Use of the delayed mask for improved demonstration of aneurysms on intraarterial DSA. AJNR *13*:1589–1593, 1992.

43. Levey, A. S., Pauker, S. G., and Kassirer, J. P. Occult intracranial aneurysms in polycystic kidney disease: when is cerebral arteriography indicated? N. Engl. J. Med. *308(17)*:986–994, 1983.

44. Liliequist, B., Lindquist, M., and Valdimarsson, E. Computed tomography and subarachnoid hemorrhage. Neuroradiology *14*:21–26, 1977.

45. Lim, S. T., and Sage, D. J. Detection of subarachnoid blood clot and other thin flat structures by computed tomography. Radiology *123*:79–84, 1977.

46. Lin, T., Fox, A. J., and Drake, C. G. Regrowth of aneurysm sacs from residual neck following aneurysm clipping. J. Neurosurg. *70*:556–560, 1989.

47. Locksley, H. B. Report on the Cooperative Study of Intracranial Aneurysms and Subarachnoid Hemorrhage. Section V, Part I: Natural history of subarachnoid hemorrhage, intracranial aneurysms and arteriovenous malformations: based on 6368 cases in the Cooperative Study. J. Neurosurg. *25*:219–239, 1966.

48. Maurice-Williams, R. S. Ruptured intracranial aneurysms: has the incidence of early rebleeding been over-estimated? J. Neurol. Neurosurg. Psychiatry *45*:774–779, 1982.

49. McCormick, W. F. Problems and pathogenesis of intracranial arterial aneurysms. In: *Cerebrovascular Disorders*, edited by J. F. Toole, J. Moosey, and R. Janeway, Ed. 2, pp. 219–231. Grune Stratton, New York, 1971.

50. McCormick, W. F., and Costra-Rua, G. J. The size of intracranial saccular aneurysms an autopsy study. J. Neurosurg. *33*:422–427, 1970.

51. McKissock, W., Richardson, A., and Walsh, L. Middle-cerebral aneurysms: further results in the controlled trial of conservative and surgical treatment of ruptured intracranial aneurysms. Lancet *2*:417–421, 1962.

52. McKissock, W., Richardson, A., Walsh, L., *et al.* Multiple intracranial aneurysms. Lancet *1*:623–631, 1964.

53. McKusik, V. A. The cardiovascular aspects of Marfan's syndrome: a heritable disorder of connective tissue. Circulation *11*:321–328, 1955.

54. Mizukami, M., Takamae, T., Tazawa, T., *et al.* Value of computed tomography in the prediction of cerebral vasospasm after aneurysm rupture. Neurosurgery *7*:583–586, 1980.

55. Nehls, D. G., Flom, R. A., Carter, L. P., and Spetzler, R. F. Multiple intracranial aneurysms: determining the site of rupture. J. Neurosurg. *63*:342–348, 1985.

56. Neill, J. M., and Hasting, A. B. The influence of the tension of molecular oxygen upon certain oxidations of hemoglobin. J. Biol. Chem. *63*:479–484, 1925.

57. Newton, T. H., and Troost, B. T. Arteriovenous malformations and fistulae. In *Radiology of the Skull and Brain*, edited by T. H. Newton, and D. G. Potts, p. 2512. Mosby, St. Louis, 1974.

58. Nibbelink, D. W., Torner, J. C., and Henderson, W. G. Intracranial aneurysms and subarachnoid hemorrhage: report on a randomized treatment study. IV-A. Regulated bed rest. Stroke *8*:202–218, 1977.

59. Nukui, H., Imai, S., Fukamachi, A., *et al.* Bilaterally symmetrical giant aneurysms of the internal carotid artery within the cavernous sinus, associated with an aneurysm of the basilar artery. Neurol. Surg. *5*:479–484, 1977.

60. Ohta, H., and Ito, Z. Cerebral infarction due to vasospasm, revealed by computed tomography. Neurol. Med. Chir. (Tokyo) *21*:365–372, 1981.

61. Olsen, W. L., Brant-Zawadzki, M., and Hodes, J. Giant intracranial aneurysms: MR imaging. Radiology *163*:431–435, 1987.

62. Pakarinen, S. Incidence, aetiology, and prognosis of primary subarachnoid hemorrhage: a study based on 589 cases diagnosed in a defined urban population during a defined period. Acta Neurol. Scand. *43*(suppl. 29):1–128, 1967.

63. Perret, G., and Nishioka, H. Report on the Cooperative Study of Intracranial Aneurysms and Subarachnoid Hemorrhage: Arteriovenous malformations. An analysis of 545 cases of craniocerebral arteriovenous malformations and fistulae reported to the cooperative study. J. Neurosurg. *25*:467–490, 1966.

64. Pia, H. W., and Zierski, J. Giant cerebral aneurysms. Neurosurg. Rev. *5*:117–148, 1982.

65. Pinto, R. S., Cohen, W. A., Kricheff, II, *et al.* Giant intracranial aneurysms: rapid sequential computed tomography. AJNR *3*:495–499, 1982.

66. Pinto, R. S., Kricheff, I. I., Butler, A. R., *et al.* Correlation of computed tomographic angiographic and neuropathological changes in giant cerebral aneurysms. Radiology *132*:85–92, 1979.

67. Powers, W. J., Gruble, R. L., Baker, R. P., *et al.* Regional CBF and metabolism in reversible is-

chemia due to vasospasm. J. Neurosurg. *62:*539–546, 1985.

68. Ross, J. S., Masaryk, T. J., Modic, M. T., *et al.* Intracranial aneurysms: evaluation by MR angiography. AJNR *11:*449–456, 1990.

69. Sahs, A. L., Perret, G. E., Locksley, H. B., and Nishioka, H. *Intracranial Aneurysms and Subarachnoid Hemorrhage: A Cooperative Study.* J. B. Lippincott, Philadelphia, 1969.

70. Sakamoto, T., Kwak, R., Mizoi, K., *et al.* Angiographical study of ruptured aneurysm in the multiple aneurysm patients. Neurol. Surg. *6:*549–553, 1978.

71. Sano, K., and Saito, I. Timing and indication of surgery for ruptured intracranial aneurysms with regard to cerebral vasospasm. Acta Neurochir. (Wien) *41:*49–60, 1978.

72. Schievink, W. I., Limburg, M., Dreissen, J. J. R., *et al.* Screening for unruptured familial intracranial aneurysms: subarachnoid hemorrhage 2 years after angiography negative for aneurysms. Neurosurgery *29:*434–438, 1991.

73. Schmid, U., Steiger, H. J., and Huber, P. Accuracy of high resolution computed tomography in the indirect diagnosis of cerebral aneurysms. Neuroradiology *29:*152–159, 1987.

74. Sekhar, L. N., Schramm, V. L., Jones, N. F., *et al.* Operative exposure and management of the petrous and upper cervical internal carotid artery. Neurosurgery *19:*967–982, 1986.

75. Serbinenko, F. A. Catheterization and occlusion of cerebral major vessels and prospects for the development of vascular neurosurgery. Vopr. Nierokhir. *35:*17–27, 1971.

76. Serbinenko, F. A. Balloon catheterization and occlusion of major cerebral vessels. J. Neurosurg. *41:*125–145, 1974.

77. Shapiro, H. M. Anesthesia effects upon cerebral blood flow, cerebral metabolism and the electroencephalogram. In: *Anesthesia,* edited by R. D. Miller, Ed. 1, Vol. 2, pp. 795–824. Churchill Livingstone, New York, 1981.

78. Silver, A. J., Pederson, M. E., Ganti, S. R., *et al.* CT of subarachnoid hemorrhage due to ruptured aneurysm. AJNR *2:*549–552, 1981.

79. Spetzler, R. F., and Carter, L. P. Revascularization and aneurysm surgery: current status. Neurosurgery *16:*111–116, 1985.

80. Stehbens, W. E. Experimental arterial loops and arterial atrophy. Exp. Mol. Pathol. *44:*177–189, 1986.

81. Strother, C. M., Eldevik, P., Kikuchi, Y., *et al.* Thrombus formation and structure and the evolution of mass effect in intracranial aneurysms treated by balloon embolization: emphasis on MR findings. AJNR *10:*787–796, 1989.

82. Suzuki, J., Komatsu, S., Sato, T., *et al.* Correlation between CT findings and subsequent development of cerebral infarction due to vasospasm in subarachnoid hemorrhage. Acta Neurochir. (Wien) *55:*63–70, 1980.

83. Taki, W., Handa, H., Yamagata, S., *et al.* Radioopaque solidifying liquids for releasable balloon technique: a technical note. Surg. Neurol. *13:*140–142, 1980.

84. Teresi, L. M., and Davis, S. J. *Magnetic Resonance Imaging,* Vol. 1. Mosby, St. Louis, 1991.

85. Torner, J. C., Kassell, N. F., Wallace, R. B., *et al.* Preoperative prognostic factors for rebleeding and survival in aneurysm patients receiving antifibrinolytic therapy: report of the Cooperative Aneurysm Study. Neurosurgery *9:*506–511, 1981.

86. Tsuruda, J. S., Halbach, V. V., and Higashida, R. T. MR evaluation of large intracranial aneurysms using cine low flip angle gradient-refocused imaging. AJNR *9:*415–424, 1988.

87. Vinuela, F. North American experience in the embolization of intracranial aneurysms with the GDC system. In: *Proceedings of the 30th Annual Meeting of the American Society of Neuroradiology.* 1992.

88. Walton, J. N. *Subarachnoid Hemorrhage.* ES Livingstone, London, 1956.

89. Weir, B., Grace, M., Hansen, J., *et al.* Time course of vasospasm in man. J. Neurosurg. *48:*173–178, 1978.

90. Weir, B. K. A. The effect of vasospasm on morbidity and mortality after subarachnoid hemorrhage from ruptured aneurysm. In: *Cerebral Arterial Spasm,* edited by R. H. H. Wilkins, pp. 385–393. Williams & Wilkins, Baltimore, 1980.

91. Wood, E. H. Angiographic identification of the ruptured lesion in patients with multiple cerebral aneurysms. J. Neurosurg. *21:*182–198, 1964.

92. Yamamoto, Y., Asari, S., Sunami, N., *et al.* Computed angiotomography of unruptured cerebral aneurysms. J. Comput. Assist. Tomogr. *10:*21–27, 1986.

93. Yoshimoto, T., Ohi, T., and Suzuki, J. Recurrence of ruptured cerebral aneurysm during hospitalization. Acta Neurochir. (Wien) *47:*37–44, 1979.

94. Yousem, D. M., Balakrichnan, J., Debrun, J. M., and Bryan, R. N. Hyperintense thrombus of GRASS MR images: potential pitfall in flow evaluation. AJNR *11:*51–58, 1990.

95. Yuh, W. T. C., Crain, M. R., Loes, D. J., *et al.* MR imaging of cerebral ischemia: findings in the first 24 hours. AJNR *12:*621–629, 1991.

96. Zimmerman, R. D., and Deck, M. F. Intracranial hematomas: imaging by high field MR. Radiology *159:*565–569, 1986.

97. Zimmerman, R. D., Hein, L. A., Snow, R. B., *et al.* Acute intracranial hemorrhage: intensity changes on sequential MR scans at 0.5 T. AJNR *9:*47–53, 1988.

Index

Page numbers in italics denote figures; those followed by "t" denote tables.